Key Clinical Topics in

Sports and Exercise Medicine

Key Clinical Topics in

Sports and Exercise Medicine

A Ali Narvani BSc MBBS MSc(Sports Med) FRCS(Tr&Orth) MFSEM(UK)
Consultant Shoulder and Elbow Surgeon
Rowley Bristow Orthopaedic Unit
Ashford and St Peter's Hospitals NHS Foundation Trust
Surrey, UK

Panos Thomas MD CCST(Orth) MFSEM FRCS
Consultant Orthopaedic Surgeon
The Whittington Hospital
London, UK

Bruce Lynn BSc PhD
Emeritus Professor of Physiology
University College London
London, UK

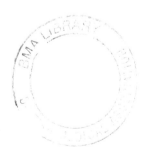

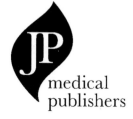

medical
publishers

London • Philadelphia • Panama City • New Delhi

© 2014 JP Medical Ltd.
Published by JP Medical Ltd,
83 Victoria Street, London, SW1H 0HW, UK
Tel: +44 (0)20 3170 8910   Fax: +44 (0)20 3008 6180
Email: info@jpmedpub.com   Web: www.jpmedpub.com

The rights of Ali Narvani, Panos Thomas and Bruce Lynn to be identified as the editors of this work have been asserted by them in accordance with the Copyright, Designs and Patents Act 1988.

All brand names and product names used in this book are trade names, service marks, trademarks or registered trademarks of their respective owners. The publisher is not associated with any product or vendor mentioned in this book.

Medical knowledge and practice change constantly. This book is designed to provide accurate, authoritative information about the subject matter in question. However readers are advised to check the most current information available on procedures included and check information from the manufacturer of each product to be administered, to verify the recommended dose, formula, method and duration of administration, adverse effects and contraindications. It is the responsibility of the practitioner to take all appropriate safety precautions. Neither the publisher nor the editors assume any liability for any injury and/or damage to persons or property arising from or related to use of material in this book.

This book is sold on the understanding that the publisher is not engaged in providing professional medical services. If such advice or services are required, the services of a competent medical professional should be sought.

Every effort has been made where necessary to contact holders of copyright to obtain permission to reproduce copyright material. If any have been inadvertently overlooked, the publisher will be pleased to make the necessary arrangements at the first opportunity.

ISBN: 978-1-907816-63-5

British Library Cataloguing in Publication Data
A catalogue record for this book is available from the British Library

Library of Congress Cataloging in Publication Data
A catalog record for this book is available from the Library of Congress

JP Medical Ltd is a subsidiary of Jaypee Brothers Medical Publishers (P) Ltd, New Delhi, India

Commissioning Editor: Steffan Clements
Editorial Assistant: Sophie Woolven
Design: Designers Collective Ltd

Indexed, typeset, printed and bound in India.

Preface

The demand for expertise in sports and exercise medicine has grown immensely in recent years. Physical activity has rightly been promoted as an effective way of preventing chronic and debilitating diseases, as well as improving quality of life. Patients with chronic conditions have been encouraged to enhance their recovery and decrease the burden of their disorder by regular exercise. One result of this is a growing number of sports injuries.

In recent years there has also been a deeper appreciation that the medical needs of elite sports competitors often require specialized care. Intense training and competition results in stress syndromes that are not often encountered in non-athletes, and there is usually huge pressure for elite athletes to return to sport as quickly as possible.

With this in mind, *Key Clinical Topics in Sports and Exercise Medicine* aims to provide sports physicians, general practitioners, physiotherapists, orthopaedic surgeons and all those involved in the medical care of athletes with a quick reference on sports and exercise medicine. The succinct style is ideal for this purpose, and we have tried to include all aspects of the subject, from abdominal injuries to urological injuries. Where possible a similar format has been used for each of the topics, which are presented in a concise manner. All sports injury topics end with a Return to Sport section, and provide an estimate of when the patient may be allowed to return to sport.

We have been influenced by our experience of teaching (and for one of us, of studying on) graduate level courses in this subject. We are particularly pleased that so many experts with national and international reputations have contributed to this book.

Sports and exercise medicine is a hugely rewarding specialty. Helping individuals to be active and healthy, helping to prevent injury and helping those injured to get back to full fitness as quickly as possible – these and other elements of sports medicine provide enormous satisfaction. We believe that this book will provide an invaluable, practical guide for all those involved in this field of medicine.

A Ali Narvani
Panos Thomas
Bruce Lynn
February 2014

Dedications

To my wife, without whose support and patience this book would not have been possible, and to whom I have promised that this is going to be my last book project.

To my mother, whose sacrifices I truly appreciate.

To Kamran and Niki, I hope this book will inspire you to seek success in whatever field makes you happy.

Thank you to my co-editors, all of the contributing authors and the publishing company JP Medical Ltd.

AN

To my parents.
To Jennie and my daughters Bethany and Jessica.

PT

To the many people - family, colleagues, friends - who have helped me in this and other endeavours.

BL

Acknowledgements

The publishers wish to thank Series Advisors Dr Tim M. Craft and Dr Paul M. Upton for their assistance during the planning of the *Key Clinical Topics* series.

Contents

Contributors

Pouya Alaghband MD
Topic 39
Ophthalmology Specialist Trainee, Bradford
Teaching Hospitals NHS Foundation Trust,
Bradford, UK

Adeeb Alam FRCR FRCS(Edin) MBChB BSc
Topics 50, 51, 52, 53, 54
Consultant Radiologist, Ashford & St Peters NHS
Foundation Trust, Surrey, UK

Ehud Atoun MD
Topics 2, 47
Head of the Shoulder and Sports Medicine
Service, Barzilai Medical Center, Ashkelon, Israel

James Calder MD FRCS(Tr&Orth) FFSEM
Topics 5, 6, 7, 49
Consultant Trauma and Orthopaedic Surgeon
Chelsea and Westminster Hospital, London, UK

Michael Carmont FRCS(Tr&Orth) FFSEM Dip
SEM GB&I
Topics 18, 69, 83
Consultant Orthopaedic Surgeon, Princess
Royal Hospital, Telford, UK

Ramsey H Chammaa MD MRCS(Eng) Dip SEM
Topics 73, 74, 94
Specialist Registrar, The Royal London Hospital
Rotation, London, UK

Rhonda Cohen PhD CPsychol AFBPsS
Topics 80, 81
Head of the London Sport Institute and Sport
and Exercise Psychologist, London Sport
Institute at Middlesex University, London, UK

Rupen Dattani BSc(Hons) MBChB MRCS MD
FRCS(Tr&Orth)
Topics 84, 90
Shoulder Fellow, The Reading Shoulder Unit,
Reading, UK

Ronen Debbi MD
Topic 2
Head of Orthopedics Department, Barzilai
Medical Center, Ashkelon, Israel

Rups Deol FRCS(Orth)
Topics 5, 6, 7, 49
Consultant in Trauma and Orthopaedic Surgery
Lister Hospital, Stevenage, UK

Simon Gilcrist B. Phty M. Phty(Sports) APAM
CSPM
Topics 78, 79, 97
Senior Sports Physiotherapist
Marylebone Physiotherapy and Sports
Medicine, London, UK

Rohit Gupta BSc(Hons) MBBS(Lond) FRCS(Eng)
FRCS(Tr&Orth)
Topics 84, 90
Consultant Orthopaedic Surgeon, Woking
Hospital, Woking, UK

Sabahat Gurdezi BPharm MBBS MRCS
Topics 44, 48
Specialist Registrar Trauma and Orthopaedics
St Peters Hospital, Chertsey UK

Stephen Harridge PhD
Topic 3
Professor of Human and Applied Physiology
King's College London, London, UK

Alison Hulme MBBS FRCS(Orth)
Topics 73, 74
Consultant Paediatric Orthopaedic Surgeon
Chelsea and Westminster Hospital NHS Trust,
London, UK

Arash Kamvari MBBS MRCGP(London)
Topic 91
General Practitioner, Kensington Park Medical
Centre, London, UK

Simon Kemp MBBS MSc(SEM) FFSEM(UK)
Topic 93
Head of Sports Medicine, Rugby Football
Union, London, UK

Tamim Khanbhai MBBS BSc(Hons) MRCGP
MFSEM
Topic 95
Club Doctor, Leyton Orient Football Club,
London, UK

Bijan Khoubehi BSc MBBS MD FRCS FRCS(Urol)
Topic 104
Consultant Urological Surgeon, Chelsea and
Westminster NHS Foundation, London, UK

Hamid Kiani DDS StR
Topic 67
Restorative Specialty Registrar, St George's
Hospital, London, UK

Sujith Konan MRCS(Tr&Orth)
Topics 58, 59, 61
Registrar Trauma and Orthopaedics, University
College London, London, UK

Ofer Levy MD MCh(Orth) FRCS
Topics 83, 84
Professor, Orthopaedic Research and Learning
Centre, Brunel University and Shoulder and
Elbow Surgeon, Reading Shoulder Unit,
Reading, UK

Bruce Lynn BSc PhD
*Topics 8, 17, 25, 26, 27, 28, 36, 37, 38, 40, 41, 42,
43, 45, 46, 68, 70, 71, 92, 98, 102, 103*
Emeritus Professor of Physiology, University
College London, London, UK

Nicola Maffulli MD MS PhD FRCP FRCS(Orth)
Topic 96
Professor of Sport and Exercise Medicine and
Consultant Orthopaedic Surgeon, Queen Mary
University of London, London, UK

Chris McLean B. Phty M. Phty(Sports) APAM
CSPM
Topics 76, 77
Senior Sports Physiotherapist
Marylebone Physiotherapy and Sports
Medicine, London, UK

Ritan Mehta MSc
Topics 20, 21, 22, 23
General Practitioner, Specialist Registrar in
Sport and Exercise Medicine and Club Doctor
for Watford Football Club, Watford, UK

Dean Michael MBBS FRCS FRCS(Tr&Orth)
Topic 100
Consultant Orthopaedic Surgeon, Ashford & St
Peter's NHS Foundation Trust, Surrey, UK

Bijan Modarai PhD FRCS
Topic 1
Consultant Vascular Surgeon, Guy's and
St Thomas' NHS Foundation Trust, London, UK

Farid Monibi BDS MClin Dent MFDS MRD RCS
Topic 67
Specialist Prosthodontist, St George's
Healthcare NHS Trust, London, UK

Reza Mobasheri BSc MBBS FRCS(Tr&Orth)
Topics 9, 10, 11, 12, 13, 14
Locum Consultant Orthopaedic Trauma and
Spine Surgeon, Imperial College Healthcare
NHS Trust, London, UK

Nazia Munir MBBCh DO-HNS FRCS (ORL-HNS)
Topic 33
Consultant ENT Surgeon, Aintree University
Hospital, Liverpool, UK

Ali Narvani BSc(Hons) MBBS(Hons) MSc(Sport
Med) FRCS(Tr&Orth) MFSEM(UK)
*Topics 4, 29, 30, 31, 32, 50, 51, 52, 53, 54, 72, 79,
85, 86, 87, 88, 99, 100, 101*
Consultant Trauma and Orthopaedic Surgeon
Ashford and St Peter's NHS Foundation Trust,
Surrey, UK

Rachel O'Connell MBBS BSc MRCS
Topic 55
General Surgical Registrar Trainee, London
Deanery, London, UK

Sam Parnia MBBS PhD MRCP
Topics 19, 34, 82
Assistant Professor, Pulmonary and Critical Care
Medicine, Stony Brook Medical Center, New
York, USA

Anant Patel MBBS MA
Topic 1
Clinical Fellow, Cambridge University Hospitals
NHS Foundation Trust, Cambridge, UK

Ioannis Polyzois MBChB MRCS CCST(Orth)
FEBOT
Topic 89
Senior Shoulder and Elbow Fellow, The Reading
Shoulder Unit, Reading, UK

Manoj Ramachandran BSc MBBS(Hons)
MRCS(Eng) FRCS(Tr&Orth)
Topic 94
Consultant Orthopaedics and Trauma Surgeon
The Royal London and St Bartholomew's
Hospitals, Barts Health NHS Trust, London, UK

Tanaya Sarkhal MBBS BSc FRCS (Tr&Orth)
Topics 44, 48
Orthopaedic Consultant, Woking Hospital,
Woking, UK

Khaled M Sarraf BSc(Hons) MBBS MRCS(Eng)
FRCS(Tr&Orth)
Topics 73, 74
Specialist Registrar (ST7) Trauma and
Orthopaedic Surgery, North West Thames
London Rotation, London Deanery, UK

Panos Thomas MD CCST(Orth) MFSEM FRCS
Topics 56, 57, 60, 62, 63, 64, 65, 66, 75
Consultant Orthopaedic Surgeon
The Whittington Hospital, London, UK

Paul Trikha MBBS(London) MRCS FRCS(Tr&Orth)
Topic 101
Consultant Orthopaedic Surgeon, Ashford & St
Peter's NHS Foundation Trust, Surrey, UK

Andrew Wallace PhD MFSEM FRACS(Orth) FRCS
Topic 89
Consultant Orthopaedic Surgeon, Hospital of
St John and St Elizabeth and King Edward VII
Hospital, London, UK

Andy Williams MBBS FRCS FRCS(Orth)
FFSEM(UK)
Topics 58, 59, 61
Specialist Knee Surgeon, Fortius Clinic and
Chelsea and Westminster Hospital, London, UK

Peter Wilmshurst BSc MBChB FRCP FISM
FFSEM
Topic 24
Honorary Consultant Cardiologist, University
Hospital of North Staffordshire, Stoke-on-Trent,
UK

Pouya Youssefi BSc(Hons) MBBS MRCS(Eng)
Topics 15, 16
Cardiothoracic Surgery Registrar,
Guy's Hospital, London, UK

Abdominal injuries in sport

Key points

- Intra-abdominal trauma in sport can be caused by blunt impacts, rapid decelerations and penetrating injuries
- Abdominal wall injuries can usually be treated conservatively but can lead to significant loss of time from training and competition
- Potentially life-threatening injuries can be masked by athletes who have substantial cardiovascular reserve

Aetiology

Around 10% of abdominal traumas are the result of sports-related activities, and this figure may be higher in children. Blunt injuries are seen more commonly in contact sports such as rugby and martial arts. The abdomen can be damaged by rapid decelerations in high-velocity sports such as skiing and equestrian events. Injuries sustained on the handlebars of bicycles are amongst the most common cause of severe abdominal trauma in children.

Penetrating injuries, frequently involving the small bowel, colon, liver and retroperitoneal organs, are associated with high-velocity sports such as motorcycling, when the injury can be sustained by impaling on a stationary object. Some sports use equipments that can directly cause penetrative injury, such as shooting and fencing.

Clinical features

Taking a careful history of the mechanism of injury and exacerbating factors should help a clinician to diagnose an abdominal wall injury. For example, a sudden pain on powerful trunk rotation, which can be reproduced upon forceful contraction of the affected muscle, suggests an acute muscle strain. Rectus sheath haematomas may be present as a painful swelling that does not cross the midline and the swelling remains palpable when the rectus sheath muscle is strained (Fothergill's sign).

Specific symptoms and signs are initially absent in as many as 20% of athletes with a serious abdominal injury; therefore, serial examinations are essential. The abdomen should be inspected for abrasions and bruising, especially to the right and left upper quadrants and flanks. Rib fractures may be present as tenderness on palpation over the rib cage or an overt chest wall deformity. A lower rib fracture will alert the clinician to the possibility of splenic or liver trauma. A splenic injury may be present with bruising on the left hypochondrium, left upper quadrant tenderness, left shoulder tip pain (Kehr's sign), tachycardia and hypotension. Liver injuries show similar symptoms, but right-sided symptoms.

Rebound tenderness, involuntary guarding and rigidity indicate peritoneal irritation by blood or visceral contents and should immediately raise the suspicion of significant intra-abdominal pathology. If abdominal pain remains unchanged or increases when the abdominal muscles are strained (positive Carnett's sign), an abdominal wall injury is more likely. Ecchymosis involving the flanks (Grey Turner sign) or the umbilicus (Cullen sign) indicates retroperitoneal haemorrhage. Penetrating wounds can be gently explored under aseptic conditions to ascertain depth of the wound and to determine whether the peritoneal cavity has been breached. Examination of the external genitalia and a digital rectal examination are mandatory.

Investigations

In the athlete with suspected intra-abdominal injury, blood tests should include a full blood count, serum amylase, group and save and a blood cross-match if the patient is haemodynamically unstable. Deranged liver function tests are associated with liver injury. A urine sample should be tested for blood and β-hCG in females.

The decision whether to perform early imaging depends on the severity and nature of the injury and also on the patient's haemodynamic status. An erect chest X-ray may show free air under the diaphragm or a ruptured hemidiaphragm. The presence of lower rib fractures should raise the suspicion of damage to the spleen or liver. On a plain abdominal X-ray, displacement of the gastric air bubble and loss of the psoas shadow are associated with splenic rupture and free intraperitoneal fluid, respectively.

An ultrasound scan (FAST, focussed assessment sonography in trauma) carried out by an experienced sonographer can detect a haemoperitoneum. Although user dependent, this noninvasive method has comparable sensitivity and specificity to diagnostic peritoneal lavage, which is now considered by some sonographers to be obsolete. A contrast-enhanced abdominal computed tomography scan is the investigation of choice in the haemodynamically stable patient and can demonstrate a pneumoperitoneum, free intraperitoneal fluid or specific signs of organ damage. This investigation is particularly useful for imaging the pancreas, duodenum and genitourinary system. The anatomical detail provided, not only provides a diagnosis but also aids treatment planning.

Management

The immediate priority in any patient with a suspected abdominal injury is to assess the airway, breathing and circulation. Two large-bore peripheral intravenous lines should be sited and used to administer 2 L of intravenous fluid. The haemodynamically unstable patient who does not respond to fluid resuscitation requires an urgent laparotomy provided that all other sources of haemorrhage have been excluded. Some of the indications for urgent laparotomy are:

- Blunt abdominal trauma with persistent hypotension despite resuscitation
- Hypotension associated with a penetrating abdominal wound
- Peritonitis
- Evisceration
- Free air seen on erect chest X-ray.

Diagnostic imaging of the haemodynamically stable patient can demonstrate injuries that are amenable to nonoperative treatment. Splenic, liver and kidney injuries are being increasingly treated conservatively.

Specific injuries

Abdominal wall injuries

Muscular strains can occur in the rectus abdominis or oblique muscles of the abdominal wall. These injuries usually result from an overloading trunk movement, such as sudden rotation or hyperextension, but can also develop insidiously in a sport that involves repetitive use of the abdominal muscles for pelvic stabilisation (e.g. track events) or for rotational movements (e.g. tennis, golf). Treatment is largely conservative, with rest and ice packs. Gentle stretching and isometric contractions, as tolerated, may aid the healing process.

Abdominal wall contusions are usually caused by direct blows in contact sports and are a common cause of pain in the athlete. A simple contusion must be distinguished from a rectus sheath haematoma, which develops after bleeding from the inferior or superior epigastric arteries. A rectus sheath haematoma can be treated conservatively if the patient is haemodynamically stable. The two treatment options for the patient requiring intervention are therapeutic angiography and embolisation, or operative evacuation of clot and ligation of the bleeding artery.

Abdominal wall hernias, commonly inguinal and femoral, can develop or worsen after heavy lifting or following a sudden increase in intra-abdominal pressure. The 'sports hernia' (athletic pubalgia, Gilmore's hernia), refers to a subtle disruption of the inguinal canal that occurs with repeated twisting and turning in sports such as ice hockey. A torn external oblique aponeurosis causing dilatation of the superficial inguinal ring, a torn conjoint tendon and a dehiscence between the torn conjoint tendon and the inguinal ligament are most often described as the causes of the sports hernia. If physiotherapy for core strengthening fails to alleviate symptoms, then the patient should be referred to a specialist for surgical repair.

Intra-abdominal trauma

Blunt injuries to the abdomen, such as a kick in martial arts or tackle in contact sports, can cause compression and crushing injuries to the solid and hollow organs of the abdomen. The organs of the upper peritoneal cavity are partly covered by the lower ribs, and therefore injury to the diaphragm, liver, spleen, transverse colon, and stomach can occur resulting in fractures of the lower ribs. Lacerations of the liver and spleen can occur in high-velocity injuries at sites of their supporting ligaments or due to blunt or penetrating trauma. Owing to their vascularity, they can cause significant intra-abdominal haemorrhage and result in hypovolaemic shock.

The small bowel, occupying most of the area of the peritoneal cavity, is at particular risk from penetrative injury and is also at risk in deceleration injuries when a tear can occur at a point of fixed attachment (e.g. the duodenojejunal flexure). Blunt abdominal injury may also cause mural haematomas of the duodenum and jejunum, whose thickening can lead to obstruction. Small bowel obstruction can result in vomiting, abdominal distension and constipation, sometimes days after the initial injury. Stable patients can be managed conservatively with nasogastric suction and intravenous fluid resuscitation.

Gastric rupture can occur with both penetrating and blunt trauma and has also been reported after swift ascent from deep scuba dives where rapid expansion of air trapped within the organ causes rupture. Presentation can be insidious with diffuse abdominal pain developing into peritonism.

Blunt tears can occur in the diaphragm (the posterolateral left hemidiaphargm is most commonly injured) and are associated with herniation of abdominal organs into the thorax, which can become strangulated. A direct blow to the abdomen can crush the pancreas against the vertebral column and cause pancreatitis. Diagnosis of this condition is notoriously difficult, and delayed recognition often worsens the prognosis.

Return to sport

Most abdominal injuries necessitating a laparotomy will require 7-10 days in hospital, and return to competitive sport may take 4 months or longer. A shorter period of 6-8 weeks is required after hernia repair. Return to sport following an abdominal muscle strain should follow a period of symptom-free muscle strengthening and can take days to weeks, depending on the severity of injury and intensity of exercise.

Further reading

Browne GJ, Noaman F, Lam LT, Soundappan SV. The nature and characteristics of abdominal injuries sustained during children's sports. Paediatr Emer Care 2010; 26:30–35.

Johnson R. Abdominal wall injuries: rectus abdominis strains, oblique strains, rectus sheath haematoma. Curr Sports Med Rep 2006; 5:99–103.

Rifat SF, Gilvydis RP. Blunt abdominal trauma in sport. Curr Sports Med Rep 2003; 2:93–97.

Related topics of interest

Achilles tendon and calf

Key points

- Calf pain causes up to 20.4% of all sports injuries
- Inflammatory cells are absent in most of tendinopathies
- Stress fractures may progress to complete fractures

Calf pain associated with exercise is a common among athletes. Some reports suggest that it is the cause of up to 21% of all sport injuries. The indiscriminant use of terminology such as 'shin splints' has resulted in ongoing confusion regarding the pathoanatomic entities associated with this pain syndrome.

Aetiology

Shin splints

One of the most common shin pathologies, also called medial tibial stress syndrome. It is an irritation of the tibia (shin bone). The exact cause is unknown. It has been attributed to inflammation of the muscles, tendons and lining of the bone ('periosteum') at this location that causes pain after repetitive activities.

Chronic exertional compartment syndrome

The leg has four osseofascial compartments: anterior, lateral, superficial posterior and deep posterior. When the volume of these compartments increases, the compartmental pressure increases, potentially affecting the movement of blood, lymph and nerve impulses through the compartment and inducing tissue ischemia. Chronic exertional compartment syndrome (CECS) is a microtraumatic condition associated with overuse and results from increased muscle volume within a compartment during exercise.

Stress fracture

An injury begins with repetitive and excessive stress on the bone. This leads to the acceleration of normal bone remodelling, the production of microfractures (caused by insufficient time for the bone to repair), the creation of a bone stress injury (i.e. stress reaction) and, eventually, a stress fracture.

Tendinopathies

It is caused by overuse in combination with intrinsic and extrinsic factors leading to a progressive interference with the healing response of the tendon. Inflammatory cells are absent in most cases; therefore, the term tendinosis is usually more appropriate than tendinitis. The most frequently involved calf tendons are the Achilles, peroneal and tibialis posterior.

Achilles rupture

Histologically, many of the torn tendons exhibit degenerative changes. This degenerative process may also be related to decreased blood supply to the tendon with increasing age. Mechanical factors such as overpronation of the foot, training errors and poor-quality of sport equipments may also play a part in increasing the stress on the tendon. There is also an association with previous history of Achilles tendon tendinopathy and corticosteroid injections.

Clinical features

Shin splints

This results in pain along the posteromedial border of the distal two thirds of the tibia, most usually localized at the intersection of the distal and middle thirds. The pain typically intensifies at the initiation of the exercise session, may subside during exercise and ends with the rest.

Chronic exertional compartment syndrome

This results in pain that begins at a predictable point after initiation of the exercise. The pain is characterized by 'cramping' or 'burning' and may or may not subside immediately after exercise.

Stress fracture

The onset of pain is usually gradual, and in early stages pain decreases with rest. Tibial stress fractures are more common than fibular ones.

Tendinopathies

The pain pattern of an athlete with tendon pain depends on the chronicity of the condition. In an early stage, the athlete may have tendon pain only after exercise. As the condition progresses, the pain may become constant with all daily activities. The pain is typically located along the course of the tendon, in some cases at the enthesis site and in other cases as the tendon passes around a bony prominence. Tendon pain is typically intensified with resisted testing of the involved muscle group.

Achilles rupture

Typically, the patient experiences sudden pain and reports that at the time of injury he thought that tendons had been struck behind the ankle. Some also report an audible snap. On examination, there is a palpable defect in the tendon; however, the bruising and the swelling might mask the gap. There may be some weakness for plantar flexion, but some active plantar flexion may be possible.

Investigations

Shin splints

A bone scan may demonstrate increased tracer uptake in the muscle or bone lining ('periosteum') of the lower leg. Magnetic resonance imaging (MRI) may similarly demonstrate some inflammation and fluid ('oedema') at this location. More importantly, however, the MRI will help to exclude a stress fracture or adjacent muscle/tendon injury in these cases.

Chronic exertional compartment syndrome

A physical examination or imaging cannot definitively diagnose the problem, but this can identify or rule out other problems. The gold standard for diagnosis of CECS is a compartment pressure test, which involves insertion of needles to the various compartments.

Stress fractures

Initially, plain radiography is usually negative but is more likely to become positive over time. Although triple-phase bone scintigraphy is highly sensitive to focal radionuclide , MRI has equal or slightly better sensitivity to higher specificity.

Tendinopathies

Imaging is usually not needed, but ultrasound and MRI may be utilized to demonstrate tendinosis in those cases that are not straightforward.

Achilles rupture

The Achilles tendon rupture is a clinical diagnosis; however, ultrasound and MRI are the studies of choice if diagnosis is in question.

Management

Shin splints

Early management often includes resting from the bruising activity, and the use of modalities such as icing and ultrasound. Other recommendations include ankle muscle strengthening, stretching, and a progressive return to sport. In recalcitrant cases, fasciotomy of the superficial and deep fascia of the posteromedial leg may be recommended.

Chronic exertional compartment syndrome

Little evidence exists to support conservative treatment for CECS. Recalcitrant cases may require compartmental fasciotomy for symptom reduction.

Stress fractures

Initial treatment should include reducing activity followed by muscle strengthening. Bone stimulation via electrical or ultrasonic impulses is an area of growing interest, but evidence is currently lacking. This may progress to complete fractures, delays in healing or nonunion that require surgical treatment.

Tendinopathies

Interventions for tendon pain are also largely based on anecdotal reports and clinical lore. Such interventions include relative rest, cross-training, stretching, strengthening, ultrasound, iontophoresis, cryotherapy, counterforce bracing, foot orthotics, nonsteroidal anti-inflammatory medications, steroid and platelet-rich plasma injections, extracorporeal shock wave therapy, and surgery.

Achilles rupture

Nonoperative treatment involves reapposing the tendon ends by immobilizing the ankle in plantar flexion and then gradually bringing the foot to neutral position over 2 months. Surgical treatment involves repairing of the Achilles tendon. There are various techniques, including open and percutaneous methods. In recent years, there has been a trend towards a more aggressive mobilization postsurgery.

Return to sport

Shin splints: It may take a week in mild cases and several weeks in severe cases.

CECS: The typical postoperative course involves nonimpact aerobic training for 2-4 weeks. Next, impact aerobic training gradually helps the patient to return to sport within 2-3 months.

Stress fractures: When the patient can perform pain-free sport-specific exercises, he can usually return within 8-12 weeks. With cortical stress, the anterior tibial midshaft recovery of fractures on average takes 6 months.

Tendinopathies: Timing of returning to sport varies from a few weeks to 6 months in the severe and postoperative cases.

Achilles tear: Returning to sport is permitted once the athlete is pain free, is able to achieve a full range of movements and has regained enough strength to perform his sport-specific activities. This may take 4 months.

Further reading

Bresler M, Mar W, Toman J. Diagnostic imaging in the evaluation of leg pain in athletes. Clin Sports Med. 2012; 31:217–245.

George CA, Hutchinson MR. Chronic exertional compartment syndrome. Clin Sports Med. 2012; 31:307–319.

Reshef N, Guelich DR. Medial tibial stress syndrome. Clin Sports Med. 2012; 31:273–290.

Related topics of interest

- Tendon overuse injuries (p. 302)
- Compartment syndromes (p. 48)

Ageing, exercise and sport

Key points

- Ageing and inactivity both cause decrements in physiological function, and it is often difficult to separate the contribution of each of these to the decline in physical performance in older people
- The decline in sporting performance is due to a number of factors that include reductions in muscle strength, muscle power, maximal rates of oxygen consumption (VO_2max) and changes in body composition
- Even very elderly people remain able to respond to the positive effects of exercise, being able to increase muscle function, VO_2max and performance

Ageing

The world is facing a demographic change such that the people, particularly in the developed countries, are living longer. In the United Kingdom, those over the age of 65 years now outnumber those under the age of 16 years. There are, as a consequence, increased numbers of frail older people who have poor health and a poor quality of life. However, at the other end of the spectrum, there are also a growing number of older people who undertake very high levels of physical activity and who still engage in competitive sport.

We actually know surprisingly little about the biology of this inherent or 'healthy' human ageing process. The Nobel Prize winning physiologist A. V. Hill once commented that a great deal of information in regard to understanding the physiology of human performance was contained in athletic records. A perusal of world records for 'master' or 'veteran' athletes reveals potentially interesting information about ageing. It seems that performance in almost all athletic events whether it is running, swimming or cycling declines in an essentially linear fashion until around the age of 70 years. There then appears to be a breakpoint, after which the rate of

decline in performance is accelerated. The decline in athletic performance in these trained people is due to the inherent ageing process, because it is now widely recognised that exercise is able to counter the negative effects of inactivity. The breakpoint itself may well represent a stage where there are more profound changes taking place in integrative physiology as a result of ageing.

The unravelling of the relationship between ageing and physical performance is hampered because (i) many studies of human ageing are of a cross-sectional design and (ii) many participants recruited into ageing studies are physically inactive. Cross-sectional study designs confound interpretation of the effects of ageing due to the inherent variability in function between individuals at any given age, whereas the incorporation of sedentary individuals into ageing studies results in an interaction between ageing and the negative and unpredictable consequences of inactivity. It has been argued that the population in whom we should be studying the effects of the inherent ageing process itself are those who are physically active, such as master athletes.

Whilst our understanding of the physiology of the human ageing process is limited and a discussion of all physiological systems beyond the remit of this short Topic, two systems are focused on here because they have particular relevance for athletic and sporting performance. These are the cardiovascular/respiratory and neuromuscular systems.

Ageing and VO_2max

The physiological gold standard of physical fitness has long been considered to be the maximal rate at which we can consume oxygen (VO_2max) during whole body exercise. Given that this involves the action and co-ordination of many systems, it is in many ways considered to be the ultimate marker of integrated physiological function and indeed has been shown to be the best predictor of all cause mortality. A comparison of VO$_2$max values of young and older (70 or more years) individuals of both sedentary and trained populations shows a clear difference in function between the two age groups. However, in the middle age ranges many subjects often show similarity of function, suggesting that the ageing process is unlikely to be linear as is generally assumed (**Figure 1**). One reason for the decline in VO$_2$max is the reduction in maximum cardiac output, which in turn is driven by an age-related decline in maximum heart rate. This occurs irrespective of activity pattern. However, this is not the only reason. It also relates to a change in body composition, particularly to a loss in the prime oxygen-consuming tissue, skeletal muscle. It is standard practice to normalise VO$_2$max to body mass (expressed as $mL \times kg^{-1} \times min^{-1}$), but ageing is generally associated with a change in body composition (e.g. increased fat and connective tissue mass) this means that the difference between young and old may be overestimated. Indeed, normalisation of VO$_2$max to estimates of muscle mass (e.g. using creatinine excretion) suggests the difference between young and old may be a lot less than when expressed relative to body mass. That said, normalisation to body mass is appropriate as regard its relevance to whole body performance (i.e. it reflects the power to weight ratio).

Loss of skeletal muscle mass and function

In addition to contributing to the decline in VO$_2$max, muscle loss with ageing is the prime reason underlying the observed declines in muscle strength and power. Master athletes who take part in explosive events such as weightlifting show that there is also an ageing effect with the amount of weight capable of being lifted in competitive performance progressively declining with age (**Figure 2**). Muscle is a tissue that is particularly sensitive to activity pattern. It atrophies when unloaded (e.g. cast immobilization, bed rest, microgravity) and hypertrophies when overloaded (e.g. resistance training). 'Sarcopenia' is the term that specifically is applied to the loss of muscle that occurs in ageing. Here, the cause appears to be an age-related loss of muscle fibres and an atrophy of the fast-contracting type II fibres. The latter is particularly important in contributing to the decline in explosive power. What are the mechanisms driving this loss of muscle mass? Again, these are difficult to dissociate from decreased activity pattern in many older people. Changes in the sensitivity to the drivers of muscle protein synthesis (feeding and exercise), decreased circulating levels of anabolic hormones (growth hormone, insulin like

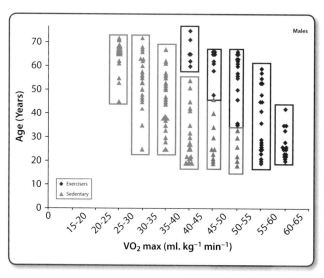

Figure 1 VO$_2$max estimates for sedentary and exercising males. The data show two salient points: (i) the superiority of function in exercisers compared to the sedentary at all ages and (ii) the nonoverlap of function between the youngest and oldest subjects, but overlap in the middle age ranges. *Lazarus NL, Harridge, SDR. Exercise, Physiological Function, and the Selection of Participants for Aging Research, J Gerontol A Biol Sci Med Sci 2010;65:851-854, by permission of Oxford University Press.*

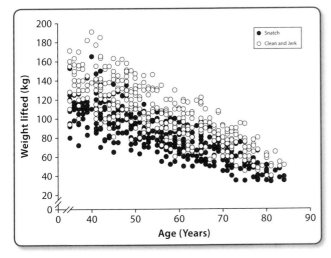

Figure 2 Performance data from the two Olympic weightlifting disciplines taken from the World Masters Weightlifting Championships 2012. The cross-sectional approach shows a decline with age, but also the remarkable functional ability of the veteran competitors.

growth factor one and testosterone), a more inflammatory circulatory environment and less efficient repair have all been implicated as contributory factors.

Adaptation to exercise training

Whilst there is clearly an ageing effect, such that older people are compromised in physiological function compared to their younger counterparts, the good news is that even very elderly people are able to adapt positively to exercise training. This is both in regard to endurance training and to more explosive strength training. Whether an older person can respond by an equal proportion to a younger individual remains difficult to answer with certainty. This is because sufficiently robust studies, which take into account the innate variability in adaptation between individuals at any age, have not been performed. However, the evidence from studies on master athletes suggests that their general physiological function is superior when compared to their age-matched counterparts, to the point where this can be expressed in terms of 'buying back' years of function. From a public health perspective, there is sufficient evidence to demonstrate that even very frail elderly people can benefit from increased exercise to improve physical function, health and quality of life.

Further reading

Klitgaard H, Mantoni, M, Schiaffino S, Ausoni S, Gorza L, et al. Function, morphology and protein expression of ageing skeletal muscle: a cross-sectional study of elderly men with different training backgrounds. Acta Physiol Scand 1990; 140:41–54.

Lazarus NL, Harridge, SDR. Exercise, physiological function and the selection of participants for ageing research. J Gerontol A Biol Sci Med Sci 2010; 65: 854–847.

Tanaka H, Seals DR. Dynamic exercise performance in masters athletes: insight into the effects of primary human aging on physiological capacity. J Appl Physiol 2003; 95:2152–2162.

Related topics of interest

Ankle – acute sprains

Key points

- Acute ankle sprains are extremely common
- Other pathologies of acute ankle injuries must be excluded
- Treatment is mainly non operative, however surgery is indicated in those patients with severe/grade III injuries, who remain symptomatic after six weeks of conservative treatment

Overview

Ankle sprains represent 15-20% of all sporting injuries, and are the most common injury sustained by athletes. Up 40% of patients with acute ankle sprains may develop some type of chronic problem such as instability, chronic pain, and recurrent swelling, particularly in those who are inadequately treated. They are more common in the younger age group as they participate more often in sports. They are also more frequent in sports that require rapid change of direction.

Pathology

Sprains of the lateral ligament complex represent 85% of all ankle sprains. The lateral ligament complex consists of the anterior talofibular ligament (ATFL), the calcaneofibular ligament (CFL), and the posterior talofibular ligament (PTFL). The ATFL has a flat band appearance and passes from the tip of the fibula anteriorly to the lateral talar neck. The CFL fans out from the tip of the lateral malleolus to the lateral side of the calcaneum. The PTFL is the strongest of the three and runs posteriorly from the fibula to the talus.

Damage to this ligament complex occurs as a result of supination and inversion of the foot with external rotation of the tibia on the fixed foot. As the foot twists medially in relation to the lower leg, the ATFL is the first ligament damaged followed by the CFL and finally the PTFL.

Traditionally these injuries are divided into 3 grades. Grade I injuries result in tearing of some fibres with minimal haemorrhage. Grade II injuries, there is an incomplete tear of the ligament and moderate haemorrhage. Grade III injuries are characterised by complete disruption of the ligament.

Clinical features

There is a history of twisting injury to the ankle. Patients may recall hearing a pop at the time of the injury. There is usually a combination of pain, swelling, weakness and instability, the degree of which is dependent on the severity and the grade of the injury:

- Grade I, mildly severe
  - Pain, but able to carry on with activity.
  - Able to weight bear
  - Mild or minimal swelling
  - Pain reproduced by stressing the ligaments but there is no laxity
  - No functional and strength loss
- Grade II, moderately severe
  - Pain severe enough to stop the patient from carrying on with activity
  - Able to weight bear
  - Moderate swelling
  - Pain on stressing the ligament with some degree of laxity, but a firm end point
  - Slight reduction in function with possible decrease in strength
- Grade III, severe
  - Pain and inability to weight bear
  - Severe swelling
  - Gross laxity without and endpoint

Investigations

Plain X-rays are important in ruling out malleolar, talus, calcaneum, base of fifth metatarsal fractures, and osteochondral injuries (however ostechondral injuries may not be apparent on the initial X-ray).

Differential diagnosis

- Fractures
  - Malleolar
  - Talus
  - Base of 5th metatarsal

- Calcaneum
- Tibial platfond
- Osteochondral injuries
- Syndesmosis injuries
- Tendon rupture
  - Tibialis posterior
  - Peroneal tendons
  - Achilles tendon
- Peroneal tendon dislocation
- Tendinopathies
- Other ligament injuries
  - Medial ligaments
  - AITFL sprain

Treatment

This can be divided into three phases irrespective of how severe the injury is, however rate of progression from one phase to another is dependent on the grade of the injury.

Phase I- *Control of pain and inflammation*. This phase starts immediately after injury and is achieved by protection, rest, ice, compression and elevation.

Phase II- *Restoration of full range of movement and of muscle strength*. There is a progression from none weight bearing to partial weight bearing to full weight bearing. Mobilization of the ankle, subtalar and the midtarsal joints commences. Muscle strengthening involves progression from active exercises to resistive exercises.

Phase III- *Restoration of proprioception function, functional exercises, restoration of general fitness and return to sport, prevention of future injuries*. Patients need to be weight bearing before this phase starts. Proprioception exercises include use of rocker boards. Functional exercises involve jumping, hopping, twisting and figure of eight running. When these exercises can be performed without pain, return to sport is permitted. Taping or bracing may offer protection and further prevention of further injury once the athlete returns to sport.

Surgery

Surgery is mainly indicated in those patients with severe/grade III injuries, who remain symptomatic after six weeks of conservative treatment. In these patients, surgical reconstruction of the lateral ligaments is recommended.

Return to sport

As with other sports injuries, return to play is permitted once the athlete is pain free, able to achieve a full range of movement and has regained enough strength to perform their sport specific activities. Exactly when this occurs, is dependent on the severity of the problem, the type of management chosen and whether this management plan has been successful or not. If the non operative regime is successful, usually athletes are able to return to play within 3 month. With surgical intervention, return to play may take 3 to 6 months following surgery.

Further reading

Kamper SJ, Grootjans SJ. Surgical versus conservative treatment for acute ankle sprains. Br J Sports Med 2012; 46(1):77-78.

Kemler E, van de Port I, Backx F et al. A systematic review on the treatment of acute ankle sprain: brace versus other functional treatment types. Sports Med 2011; 41(3):185-197.

Kerkhoffs GM, van den Bekerom M, Elders LA et al. Diagnosis, treatment and prevention of ankle sprains: an evidence-based clinical guideline. Br J Sports Med 2012; 46(12):854-860.

Related topics of interest

Ankle – persistent problems following sprains: lateral ankle instability

Key points

- Up to 20% of those sustaining an ankle sprain will go on to develop instability.
- Ligament rupture alone does not necessitate surgery unless recurrent mechanical instability results
- Early functional rehabilitation, both following acute injury and surgical reconstruction, is superior to immobilisation in restoring function

The lateral side of the ankle is stabilised primarily by the lateral ligamentous complex, composed of the anterior talofibular ligament (ATFL), calcaneofibular ligament (CFL) and posterior talofibular ligament. The lateral ligaments are often injured during supination-inversion injuries. The ATFL is the main stabiliser and also the most prone to injury, because in acts as a collateral ligament in the plantar flexed ankle, the position taken just prior to the internal rotation of foot during an inversion injury. The peroneal tendons act as secondary stabilisers of the lateral side of the joint.

Aetiology

Instability may broadly be divided into two entities:

- *Mechanical instability* is caused by loss of the lateral structural constraints that in turn allows increased talar movement in the ankle joint
- *Functional instability* occurs due to the loss of neuromuscular control over the joint that gives the athlete the subjective perception that the joint 'gives way'

Both entities may occur together, highlighting the necessity of adequate comprehensive rehabilitation.

Intrinsic factors for developing lateral instability include hindfoot varus, a previous ankle injury and loss of strength, balance and proprioception. Extrinsically, play surfaces can have an effect. In soccer, playing on artificial grass surfaces increases the risk of ankle injuries, with defenders and attackers being more prone to injury due to contact. Volleyball, netball and basketball have particularly high incidences of injuries.

Clinical features

There is invariably a history of a traumatic ankle injury, usually supination-inversion. Thereafter, the joint will recurrently give way or report the sensation that it may do so. Lateral pain, weakness and suboptimal performance will often be reported. Importantly, the ankle may give way without warning and any pain occurs after the episode and does not precede it. Patients may describe activities or manoeuvres they are apprehensive to perform that cause instability, such as walking on uneven ground. Footwear modification such as the use of high ankle boots or ankle braces may be helpful.

Examination should start with a generalised screen for laxity. Hindfoot inspection should look for varus malalignment. Diffuse swelling and tenderness will often be present over the lateral ligamentous complex. Ankle and subtalar movement should be assessed. The anterior drawer test and talar tilt test may reveal laxity causing mechanical instability, indicating ATFL and ATFL + CFL injury, respectively. The anterior drawer test is performed by placing the foot in 20° of plantar flexion, holding the tibia fixed and drawing the heel forward pulling anteriorly and medially. A positive test will elicit laxity allowing the talus to be drawn forward and medially. Comparison with the noninjured side is essential. Lateral talar tilt testing is felt to be far less reliable and useful. Peroneal tendon weakness may be present with loss of control with a resulting imbalance between inversion and eversion. This may be more apparent in functional instability. Proprioception should be formally assessed using the modified Romberg test where the patient is asked to stand with eyes closed. Loss of balance indicates loss of proprioception that may normally be compensated for by vision and vestibular function.

Investigations

Weight-bearing plain AP/lateral ankle X-rays will exclude bony fractures and malalignment at the talocrural joint. Stress radiography may show excessive talar tilt, although it can be difficult to reliably obtain from the nonanaesthetised patient. Ultrasound can be used to assess the lateral ligament complex and peroneal tendons, although it is operator dependent. Whilst arthrography is sensitive to diagnosing ligament and capsular injuries in the acute setting, it is not routinely recommended. Magnetic resonance Imaging not only provides information on acute/chronic injury to the lateral ligament complex but also the capsule, peroneal tendons, the articular surfaces and the remainder of the joint. It can help to exclude/identify concomitant pathologies, although it is not a dynamic test. Examination under anaesthesia may be necessary in certain cases and may be combined with arthroscopy to assess the joint and address other pathologies.

Management

Both functional and mechanical instability should primarily be treated nonoperatively with a patient-tailored rehabilitative programme to include strengthening, particularly of the peroneal tendons, proprioception and muscular coordination.

Following the acute injury, protection, RICE (rest, ice, compression and elevation) and the use of nonsteroidal anti-inflammatory drugs is advocated. A short period (up to 2 weeks) of rigid immobilisation in a plaster or boot can be useful. Longer periods of immobilisation are not advocated, and a functional regime should be commenced with active exercises. Nonrigid supports, lace-up braces, taping and elastic bandage supports can be useful during this stage. There is no conclusive evidence that ultrasound, laser or electrotherapy have any benefit. Surgery may be indicated in those patients who develop chronic mechanical lateral ankle instability where nonoperative measures have failed. The procedures can broadly be divided into two categories.

a. Anatomic repairs/reconstructions

When the quality of the ruptured tissue permits, anatomic repair is generally favoured.

Brostrom procedure

When there is complete rupture, ATFL ligament ends are identified and plicated. If the ligaments are intact but stretched and lax, they are incised, shortened and plicated. Suture anchors or drill holes through the distal fubula are often used to reattach ligament back on to the fibula when there has been avulsion from the bone. The Gould modification of the Brostrom procedure involves coupling the ATFL and CFL shortening with an extensor retinacular reinforcement.

Nonanatomic reconstructions

The Chrisman-Snook procedure is a reconstruction of the ATFL and CFL using half of the distal peroneus brevis tendon. The tendon remains attached distally at the 5th metatarsal base but split along its distal portion and routed through tunnels in the fibula and calcaneus. Numerous other grafts can be used to reconstruct the lateral ligaments including plantaris and gracilis hamstring autografts as well as allografts.

Traditionally, the role of acute surgery has been associated with increased stiffness and slow recovery, although much of the research in this area was based on historic literature where long periods of immobilisation were used. However, earlier mobilisation with modern functional rehabilitation, the return to sport time frames may be similar to surgical and nonsurgical groups. There is emerging opinion in the treatment of high-end elite athletes that acute primary ligamentous repair can provide a more predictable outcome and can minimise long-term problems.

Return to sport

Earlier functional mobilisation leads to an earlier return to play than immobilisation. Restoration of strength (particularly of the extensor and peroneal muscles), coordination and proprioception are the key to rapid return, with or without surgery. Return to light work can normally start at around 3 weeks even for complete ligament rupture although return to sport can be possible after approximately 8–12 weeks.

Further reading

de Vries JS, Krips R, Sierevelt IN, et al. Interventions for treating chronic ankle instability. Cochrane Database Syst Rev 2011; 10:CD004124.

Kerkhoffs GM, van den Bekerom M, Elders LAM, et al. Diagnosis, treatment and prevention of ankle sprains: an evidence based clinical guideline. Br J Sports Med 2012; 46:854--860.

Krips R, deVries J, Van Dijk, CN. Ankle instability. Foot Ankle Clin 2006; 11:311--329.

Related topics of interest

- Ankle – persistent problems following sprains: other injuries (p. 15)
- Ankle – persistent problems following sprains: overview (p. 19)

Ankle – persistent problems following sprains: other injuries

Key points

- Ankle sprains are associated with a high incidence of associated injuries
- Early diagnosis and management is key to good outcome
- Chronic multiple injuries make return to sport less predictable

Ankle sprains can damage not only the lateral ligaments but also the numerous structures around the joint. This can lead to pain, swelling and restricted performance. The causes can be divided on the basis of the location around the joint and are presented in **Table 1**. This Topic will cover common persisting conditions, such as impingement, syndesmotic injury, peroneal tendon pathology and osteochondral lesions of the talus.

Ankle impingement

This may be a bony or soft tissue phenomenon and is characterised by anterior pain, often located anteromedially or anterolaterally, with restriction of dorsiflexion.

Aetiology

In soft tissue impingement, synovitis tends to be present and fibrous soft tissue connections form either anteromedially or anterolaterally that cause impingement over the talus during ankle movement. These lesions are often meniscoid in appearance and probably develop from the torn ends of the anterior talofibular ligament. In bony impingement, synovial proliferation of the anterior tibial and talar chondral surfaces form 'kissing' osteophytes following repetitive traction and microtrauma, rather than an arthritic process (**Figure 3**). The pain is again thought to be due to the inflamed soft tissue catching on these spurs that can limit dorsiflexion. This is commonly termed 'footballers ankle' but also present in many kicking sports and dancers.

Anteromedial impingement tends to be bony, whereas soft tissue impingement tends to be anterolateral.

Clinical features

Anterior joint pain that is worse with dorsiflexion that may be restricted. Clinically, there is anterior tenderness with possible palpable bony spurs. A positive impingement sign where there is anterior pain when the athlete moves forward with the foot flat on the floor or when the ankle is pushed into

Table 1 Causes of persistent problems following ankle sprains

Anterior

Anterior impingement: bony/soft tissue

Extensor tendinopathy

Osteochondral lesions of the talus

Calcaneonavicular coalition

Lateral

Undiagnosed fibular fracture

Lateral ligament complex injury

Syndesmotic injury

Peroneal tendon disorders: tendinopathy, rupture, instability

Lateral talus fracture

Anterior calcaneal process fracture

Fifth metatarsal base fracture

Sinus tarsi syndrome

Posterior

Tendo Achilles tendinopathy

Retrocalcaneal bursitis

Posterior impingement/os trigonum syndrome

Medial

Medial malleolar stress fracture

Deltoid ligament tears

Flexor hallucis tendinopathy

Talocalcaneal coalition

Tarsal tunnel syndrome

of brevis. The tendon that ruptures will usually be tendinopathic, although as with the Achilles, there are often no preceding symptoms prior to rupture. X-rays may show an avulsion fracture or movement in position of an os peroneum. MRI scanning is the choice investigation. Treatment is with repair or tenodesis to brevis in peroneus longus ruptures and debridement and repair of peroneus brevis ruptures.

Peroneal tendon instability

Almost always traumatic, the tendons will dislocate or sublux usually following sudden forceful passive dorsiflexion of the inverted foot. An audible snap may be heard at the time of injury. The tendons can then start to recurrently dislocate, causing pain and tendinopathy. Patients can often illustrate the dislocation to the clinician. X-rays may show avulsion form the posterior aspect of the fibula, although MRI best shows the disruption of the peroneal retinaculum. A few weeks of cast immobilisation may be used following the primary injury, although this leads to a higher recurrence rate and therefore acute injury repair of the retinaculum is recommended. Recurrent instability, if pain free, can be treated conservatively. However, if symptomatic, reconstruction of the superior peroneal retinaculum will be required and if necessary deepening of the fibula peroneal groove.

Osteochondral lesions of the talar dome

Osteochondral lesions (OCLs) of the talus are a common cause of persisting pain following ankle sprains and are associated with premature ankle arthritis. Clinical features include deep pain, with locking, clicking and catching, especially in the presence of loose bodies. X-rays may not show the injury, but MRI will and is the choice investigation. An OCL may be an incidental finding on MRI and lack clinical correlation. Where the cause of pain may be unclear, the presence of bone oedema beneath the OCL may be an indicator of its activity. Where doubt exists,, single photon emission computerised tomography can give more information as to whether an OCL is the cause of pain. The size of the lesion determines treatment. Arthroscopic bone marrow stimulation with microfracture yields good results in the primary and revision setting for lesions 1.5 cm or less in size. Larger lesions will often require osteochodral autograft transplantation or mosaicplasty using osteochondral plugs taken from non-weight-bearing parts of the knee. This requires open surgery with a medial malleolar osteotomy and so longer recovery times. Newer techniques with hemicap-type osteochondral partial joint replacements and autologous chondrocyte implantation may have a role.

Return to sport

This is dependent on numerous factors. Delay in diagnosis and appropriate management will allow a less predictable return. The presence of multiple injuries can compound this problem. The importance of phased rehabilitation, as for lateral ankle instability, with restoration of strength, control and coordination is essential. Activity-specific drills must be completed without symptoms prior to return.

Further reading

Cerrato, RA, Myerson MS. Peroneal Tendon Tears, Surgical Management and Its Complications. Foot Ankle Clin 2009; 14:299–312.
Strauss JE, Frosberg JA, Lipert FG III. Chronic lateral ankle instability and associated conditions: a rationale for treatment. Foot Ankle Int 2007; 28:1041–1044.
Van Dijk CN. Anterior and posterior ankle impingement. Foot Ankle Clin 2006; 11:663–683.

Related topics of interest

Ankle – persistent problems following sprains: overview

Key points

- Persisting problems following sports-related ankle sprains are common
- Early accurate diagnosis and recognition of associated injury patterns helps to limit these problems
- Inadequate rehabilitation is a common cause of ongoing problems

Ankle sprains are very common and account for approximately one in five of all sports-related injuries. The term 'ankle sprain' comprises a large spectrum of soft tissue injury, ranging from mild ligamentous damage to a complete tear. Mechanisms of injury and forces transmitted through the joint can vary considerably. Given such a large number of structures lying in such close proximity around the ankle, surrounded by such a thin soft tissue envelope, it is no surprise that there is a high incidence of associated injuries. Multiple structures can be injured simultaneously and start to interfere with the complex coordinated movements that take place around the joint. Residual symptoms following sprains during sport can limit performance considerably and be present years after the original injury. Early, accurate diagnosis and a clear individual patient-based clear management plan from the outset is vital.

Aetiology

Incomplete diagnosis and inadequate rehabilitation are the major causes of persisting problems. Where the diagnosis is not clear, further investigation should be undertaken. Once identified, all injuries must be appropriately addressed and rehabilitation planned. The importance of phased rehabilitation cannot be overstated. Protection of the joint and 'RICE' (rest, ice, compression and elevation) is fairly consistently advised in the acute phase. The second phase of restoration of motion, strength and proprioception should not be delayed and ideally needs supervision by a physiotherapist. Prior to resumption of sport, the third phase of graduated activity specific drills must be undertaken. Failure to follow this sequence can seriously hamper the athlete's recovery.

The exact mechanism of how inadequate rehabilitation may lead to persisting pain is not clear but felt to be multifactorial. Loss of muscular strength, control and coordination renders the joint prone to instability and further injury. Synovitis can cause irritation and limit joint movement that can lead to stiffness, as can prolonged immobilisation. Scar tissue and capsular adhesions can develop further compounding the problem. Loss of proprioception or joint position sense can ensue, and the development chronic regional pain syndrome with an abnormal sympathetic response can be extremely difficult to treat.

Clinical features

At first presentation following the acute injury, swelling and pain may limit the clinical examination. Repeat physical examination 4-5 days after the traumatic injury should be undertaken as has been shown to give a better chance of arriving at the correct diagnosis.

Persisting problems symptoms fall into a number of groups that that often occur simultaneously and lead to a suboptimal performance level. Each of these should be carefully screened for in the history and examination.

1. Pain
2. Instability
3. Stiffness and decreased range of joint movement
4. Weakness
5. Loss of proprioceptive control

Injury to the superficial peroneal nerve can occur following the anterolateral severe sprain and give rise to a neuropathic pain. Examination should involve performing a

Tinels test with light percussion along its course to see if this exacerbates symptoms and assessment of any sensory loss over the dorsum of the foot.

Investigations

Plain X-rays are the first line modality to assess for bony fractures. Lateral ankle and mortise views (the leg is internally rotated 20° so the X-ray beam sits almost perpendicular to the intermalleolar line) should be obtained. Antero-posterior and lateral weight-bearing views and an oblique should be obtained to adequately assess foot injuries. The Ottawa ankle rules serve as guidelines to ascertain the likelihood of a bony injury and the necessity of X-ray evaluation and have shown to have high sensitivity and specificity. Ankle X-rays are advocated if there is distal posterior medial or lateral malleolar tenderness or inability to immediately weight bear or manage four steps in the emergency department. Foot X-rays should be obtained in there is tenderness over the 5th metatarsal base, navicular or the inability to weight bear as above.

Ultrasound has a role in assessing the soft tissues dynamically and magnetic resonance imaging gives detailed information on soft tissue, bony and chondral injuries. Computerised tomography is useful in detecting occult fractures. These will be discussed further for individual problems in the subsequent Topics.

Management

Management will be specific to the injury pattern and patient. In general terms, where possible, earlier movement and weight bearing is favourable. Once the diagnosis is clear, a comprehensive rehabilitative programme should be devised and targeted goals outlined in conjunction with the physiotherapist. Phased rehabilitation is vital.

Return to sport

Early return to sport without supervised activity specific drills can lead to an overall delay in return. Patient and injury pattern factors will also normally dictate this. This will be discussed in more detail in the following Topics.

Further reading

Kerkhoffs GM, van den Bekerom M, Elders LAM, et al. Diagnosis, treatment and prevention of ankle sprains: an evidence based clinical guideline. Br J Sports Med 2012; 46:854-860

Anandacoomarasamy A, Barnsley L. Long term outcomes of inversion ankle injuries. Br J Sports Med 2005; 39: e14.

Bassewitz HL, Shapiro MS. Persistent pain after the ankle sprain: targeting the causes. Phys Sportsmed 1997; 25: 58-68.

Related topics of interest

- Ankle – persistent problems following sprains: lateral ankle instability (p.12)
- Ankle – persistent problems following sprains: other injuries (p.15)
- Ankle – acute sprain (p.10)

Biomechanics

Key points

- Biomechanics play an important role in developing evidence-based approaches for injury prevention and treatment
- The combination of kinematics, kinetics and electromyography (EMG) can give detailed insights, for example in gait analysis
- Properties of biomaterials, such as tendon and bone, can be quantitatively assessed by stress-strain analyses

Overview

Biomechanical analysis has a long history in sports science, where sophisticated methods are increasingly used in the quest for better performance. Biomechanics is also being increasingly used in sports medicine to find ways to prevent injury and monitor rehabilitation after injury. As the technology becomes more user friendly, one can expect this trend to continue. In addition, there are major applications where bioengineering and biomechanics combine to develop aids for those disabled people who wish to take part in sports activities.

Kinematics

Kinematics is concerned with describing and analysing posture and movement. The methods include goniometry, video and specialised optoelectronic systems (e.g., Cartesian optoelectronic dynamic anthropometer, CODA). Kinematic analysis is widely used in sports medicine. A good example is the use of video analysis to sort out gait problems. A typical situation may be recurring Achilles tendon or related injuries that can be traced to excessive foot pronation during running. Video analysis allows the nature of the problem to be quantified. It can then be used to critically look at treatment options, for example looking at the effect of special orthotic running shoes on ankle alignment during running.

Kinetics

Kinetics deals with forces and moments. In other words, it is not just observing patterns of motion, but analysing in detail the ways in which those movements are brought about. The necessary equipment comprises dynamometers for measuring forces in any direction or around any joint and force plates, usually used for measuring ground reaction forces. In kinetics, life becomes seriously complicated, but the basis is still just Newton's three laws:

1. A body will remain at rest unless acted upon by a net force. Many forces may be acting but they all cancel out
2. A body (its centre of mass) accelerates at a rate proportional to the net force acting and in the direction of the force. The acceleration is inversely proportional to the mass. $F = m \times a$, where F = force in Newtons, m = mass in kg and a = acceleration in m/s^2
3. Action and reaction are equal and opposite. When we measure a force, such as the *action* exerted by a subject, an equal and opposite force, the *reaction*, acts upon the subject

EMG and anatomy

Detailed analysis of sports movements and how they may cause injury first depends on knowing the anatomy. For example, we are going to be in big trouble in trying to understand shoulder overuse problems if we have not come to terms with the complex anatomy.

However, it is the EMG analysis that often leads to the complete understanding of what has gone wrong in a repeat injury scenario. It is our muscles that drive all movements, but it is not always clear whether a particular pattern on movement reflects equal activity in all the synergists, or whether a change reflects overactivity in a particular prime mover or underactivity in a stabilising antagonist.

Gait analysis

The analysis of gait illustrates how all the methods of biomechanics can combine to give a very complete picture. The subject is monitored kinematically, either using video or optoelectronically (CODA). Usually, the side view is enough, but front, or even top views can also be analysed if necessary. Whilst being viewed kinematically, the subject steps on a force plate whose signals are synchronised with those from the kinematics. The force plate tells us about forces in three planes:

- The vertical forces associated with supporting the body and accelerating and decelerating it in the up-down direction;
- The anterior--posterior directed forces involved in forward locomotion;
- The lateral forces, which should be small and symmetrical for straight motion

Finally, information about the activity of selected muscles can be obtained, again synchronously, with all the other signals.

With all this going on, there is a potential problem with data overload. Condensing the information from just lower limb biomechanics can involve three force channels, looking at angular motion around three major joints in each leg and monitoring EMG from at least four muscles on each side. So we have 17 channels of continuous data. It is really a case of knowing what to look for, plus having a database of normal responses for comparison.

Properties of biomaterials

An important area of biomechanics is the analysis of strength and stiffness of biomaterials, particularly bone, tendons and ligaments. When a force is applied to a structure, it will deform and the extent of deformation will increase as the force increases. We normally need to know the material properties of a tissue, that is how the material responds whatever the exact shape or size of the specimen. For uniform materials (only a rough approximation for bones and tendons etc.), we can define stress as the force per unit cross-sectional area. So a thick tendon can support a greater load than a thin one, but the mechanical properties of the collagen

matrix may be the same. If this is the case, then a tendon, one-tenth the cross-sectional area of another, should stretch 10 times more under the same load. Stretch or compression also needs to be normalised to allow for differences in length of the specimen. So strain is defined as the percentage change in length. Therefore, a 5-mm long tendon will stretch only half as much as an otherwise similar tendon that is 10 mm long but the strain in each will be the same.

The ratio of stress to strain is the elastic modulus of a material. Stiffness of tendons is approximately 600 MN/m^2 (MN = mega Newtons), whereas for bone, it is 15 GN/m^2, 25 times higher. Note, however, that the strength of bone and tendon (the maximum stress that can be tolerated) is pretty much the same; it is just that tendon stretches much more before it breaks. Stress-strain relations are also important as they allow the calculation of the energy storage during, for example tendon stretch.

For acute injuries, immediate breaking strain is important. For overuse injuries, the response to repeated stresses is also important. One factor here is the viscoelastic nature of all biomaterials. They do not simply show elastic responses where it does not matter at what speed the stress is applied. Biomaterials characteristically deform further to slowly applied stresses, and show 'creep', continued slow deformation, in the face of prolonged steady stresses. With repeated brief stresses, there can be accumulation of microdamage and this can build up until failure occurs. This is, of course, not just a property of biomaterials and has been much studied by mechanical engineers in non-biological materials. Unfortunately, we still do not have a very good understanding of these phenomena in biomaterials.

Further reading

Barlett R, Bussey M. Sports biomechanics: reducing injury risk and improving sports performance, 2nd edn. London: Routledge, 2012.

Nordin M, Frankel VH (eds). Basic biomechanics of the musculoskeletal system, 4th edn. Philadelphia: Lippincott Williams and Wilkins, 2012.

Related topics of interest

Cervical spine – cervical disc injury and herniation

Key Points

- Seen in collision and contact sports
- Magnetic resonance imaging (MRI) is the investigation of choice
- Surgery is indicated if there is myelopathy, progressive neurological deficit or a failure of 3 months of non-operative measures

Overview

Cervical disc injuries pose potentially career-threatening problems for athletes. Diagnosis of disc injury and herniation is routine with MRI scanning. The athlete may potentially suffer upper limb radiculopathy, neck pain or even balance and coordination problems. Opinion regarding treatment of this condition is divided, as the long-term outcome regarding return to sports is unknown.

Contact sports such as American football can involve relatively high-speed collision, where the head and neck lead the body and can be the first point of contact with the opponent. Perhaps unsurprisingly, the incidence of cervical disc disease is higher in top American football players as compared with the general population.

Pathology

Uncontrolled lateral bending of the neck can result in acute cervical disc disruption. This may or may not lead to herniation of some nucleus pulposus through the posterior annulus. This herniated material may then in turn lead to cord- or nerve-root compression.

A second pathological process is the degeneration of the disc associated with decreased disc height and dehydration of the disc. This is a chronic process with gradual onset and slow progression of symptoms. With time, associated disc herniation and osteophyte formation may develop.

Clinical features

Symptoms and signs depend on whether or not there is any associated disc herniation. The following features are seen:
- Varying degree of neck pain
- Radiculopathy (usually with disc herniation)
- Neurologic symptoms ranging from sensory disturbance to motor weakness and coordination dysfunction usually in upper limbs in association with nerve root pathology, or lower limb involvement if spinal cord compression or injury has occurred

Investigations and differential diagnosis

- Plain radiographs (can rule out bony or unstable injuries and can indicate degenerative change).
- MRI is the investigation of choice, demonstrating the disc pathology in detail.
- Where MRI is contraindicated, computerised tomography (CT) myelography can also help rule out disc herniation.

Management

Non-operative
- Rest
- Analgesia and nonsteroidal anti-inflammatory drugs
- Immobilization
- Activity adjustment
- Epidural injections
- Exercise therapy once radicular symptoms improve

Operative
- Surgery is indicated if there is:
  1. myelopathy,
  2. progressive neurological deficit,
  3. a failure of 3 months of non-operative measures.

- Surgery is in the form of anterior cervical discectomy and fusion, although posterior cervical foraminotomy is also an option.

Return to sport

With non-operative treatment, as with muscular and ligament injuries, the athlete is permitted to return to sport once there is complete resolution of symptoms, full pain free cervical range of motion and full muscle power. They must also regain complete cervical spine sport-specific function before returning to sports.

Return to sport after surgery is dependent on the type of surgery:

- Following posterior foraminotomy and decompression on its own, the criteria for return to sports are the same as those of non-operative measures

- Athletes who have had single level anterior cervical discectomy and fusion can regain pre-injury level of conditioning within 8 weeks of surgery. A return to sport can be recommended once imaging including CT scan confirms fusion and the patient is asymptomatic and able to return to sport at a pre-injury functional level
- Athletes who have had 2 or 3 level discectomy and fusion, the prognosis for a return to sport is much more guarded and needs to be assessed on an individual basis

The incidence of adjacent level degeneration is approximately 25% at 10 years following surgery in all patients, however, it is not known if this is directly attributable to fusion surgery or is a function of a naturally degenerative process. This is unlikely to translate into deteriorating sporting ability, as most top-level athletes are unlikely to remain competitive for over a decade.

Further reading

Scherping SC. Cervical disc disease in the athlete. Clin Sports Med 2002; 21(1):37–47.

Zmurko MG, Tannoury TY, Tannoury CA, Anderson DG. Cervical sprains, disc herniation, minor fractures, and other cervical injuries in the athlete. Clin Sports Med 2003; 22:513–521.

Hsu WK. Outcomes following non-operative and operative treatment for cervical disc herniations in National Football League athletes. Spine 2011; 36:800–805.

Related topics of interest

- Cervical spine injuries (p. 38)
- Cervical spine – spinal cord injury and cervical cord neurapraxia (p. 30)
- Cervical spine fracture/dislocation (p. 33)
- Cervical spine – cervical ligament and muscle injuries (p. 25)

Cervical spine – cervical ligament and muscle injuries

Key points

- Cervical ligament and muscle injuries are common in athletes, particularly in contact sports
- Subluxations, dislocations, fractures, disc injuries and cord damage need to be excluded
- Prolonged immobilizations are generally not recommended

Overview and pathology

Strains refer to muscular stretch injuries, whereas sprains are musculotendinous unit stretch injuries. Contusion is localised muscular damage and bleeding usually caused by a direct muscular blow.

Pain is localized to the cervical spine, as is any reduction of range of motion. The neurologic examination is normal.

The lifetime incidence of neck pain and injury in athletes is as high as 50%. As such, these ligament and muscle injuries are extremely common, but are a diagnosis of exclusion, once fractures and disc injuries are ruled out.

Clinical features

- 'Jamming' the neck with resultant generalized or localized neck pain
- Limitation in range of cervical spine motion
- An absence of neurological abnormality or radicular symptoms

Investigations and differential diagnosis

Plain radiographs are normal and helpful in ruling out fractures and unstable injuries. The following radiographic features may indicate the presence of instability:

1. Vertebral subluxation
2. Vertebral compression fracture
3. Loss of normal cervical lordosis
4. Interspinous widening

Computerised tomography scanning can be helpful to exclude bony injuries not diagnosed by plain radiography, if there is clinical suspicion. MRI scanning can exclude disc, ligament and spinal cord injury.

Management

Following exclusion of unstable or bony injuries, disc herniation and nerve/cord injuries, treatment involves:

- Analgesia and nonsteroidal anti-inflammatory drugs
- Soft cervical collar for comfort in the early phase. Prolonged immobilization is not recommended as it causes atrophy and deconditioning of muscles
- Physical therapy

Return to sport

Athletes may be permitted to return to sport when they

- Are symptom free
- Have achieved full range of movement
- Have regained their neck muscle power
- Have regained their sport-specific neck function

Further reading

Zmurko MG, Tannoury TY, Tannoury CA, Anderson DG. Cervical sprains, disc herniation, minor fractures, and other cervical injuries in the athlete. Clin Sports Med 2003; 22:513–521.

Villavicencio AT, Hernández TD, Burneikiene S, Thramann J. Neck pain in multisport athletes. J Neurosurg Spine 2007; 7:408–413.

Related topics of interest

Cervical spine – nerve root and brachial plexus injuries

Key points

- Mechanism of injury includes direct blow to the head or supraclavicular region and forced compression and rotation of the extended neck towards the painful neck
- Severity of damage varies from selective demylination (neurapraxia) to disruption of axon mylin (axonotmesis) to complete disruption including surrounding connective tissue (neurotmesis)
- Athletes with three or more episodes or attacks lasting longer than 24 h may be advised to consider not returning to future play

Overview and epidemiology

Collision sports, such as American football, rugby, boxing and wrestling, are known to pose an increased risk of nerve root and plexus injuries. First described in 1965, terms commonly used to describe these injuries include stingers, burners, cervical pinch syndrome and transient brachial plexopathy and make 10% of all cervical spine injuries.

Pathology

Although the mode of injury may be similar to cervical cord neurapraxia, the mechanism of stingers can either by distraction with the head forced opposite to the side of the painful arm causing stretching of the brachial plexus, or that the hyperextended spine is rotated to the side of the painful arm and axially loaded, causing injury of cervical nerve roots tethered by fibrous tissue (**Figure 4**).

The severity of the injury correlates with the underlying pathophysiology (**Figure 4**). Neurapraxia is a selective demyelination of the nerve sheath, and it is the most benign injury. Axonotmesis is a disruption of the axon and the myelin sheath, but the epineurium is intact. The most severe injury is a neurotmesis or a compete disruption of the endoneurium. This injury is associated with the most unfavourable prognosis.

Clinical features

Commonly, the athlete can experience a sharp or searing pain radiating down one arm after collision, with loss of function in that arm. The arm weakness and burning sensation resolves. It may take up to 24 h for symptom resolution. During this time, any one of the muscle groups from the shoulder down to the wrist and hand may be weak. Symptoms can be reproduced by performing the Spurling manoeuvre, which involves extension and lateral flexion towards the injured arm with axial loading of the head. Resolution of symptoms usually occurs proximal to distal. Time to resolution is variable and may depend on type of nerve injury described above. Neurapraxia can take 3 weeks to recover, axonotmesis can take much longer and neurotmesis may take 1 year or more or may not recover at all.

Investigations and differential diagnosis

Ruling out an unstable cervical spine injury is the first role of the clinician. Generally, the patient should have a full and pain-free range of movement of the cervical spine. If this is not the case, the athlete should be withdrawn from the field and have radiological investigations to rule out an unstable injury. Any athlete with persisting symptoms should be investigated with electromyography testing approximately 3 to 4 weeks after injury.

Management

1. Initially until symptoms resolve:
   - Immediate removal of the athlete from participation
   - Sling
   - Pain management with nonsteroidal anti-inflammatory drugs and physiotherapy
2. Rehabilitation once symptoms resolve:
   - Range of movement
   - Muscle strength

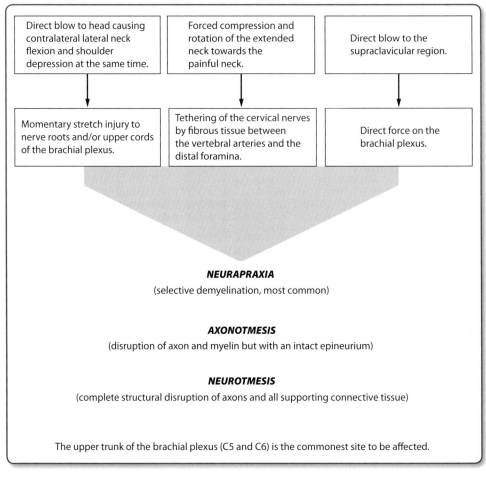

Direct blow to head causing contralateral lateral neck flexion and shoulder depression at the same time.

Forced compression and rotation of the extended neck towards the painful neck.

Direct blow to the supraclavicular region.

Momentary stretch injury to nerve roots and/or upper cords of the brachial plexus.

Tethering of the cervical nerves by fibrous tissue between the vertebral arteries and the distal foramina.

Direct force on the brachial plexus.

NEURAPRAXIA
(selective demyelination, most common)

AXONOTMESIS
(disruption of axon and myelin but with an intact epineurium)

NEUROTMESIS
(complete structural disruption of axons and all supporting connective tissue)

The upper trunk of the brachial plexus (C5 and C6) is the commonest site to be affected.

Figure 4 Pathology and features.

3. Prevention of further episodes:
   - Neck and shoulder-strengthening programme
   - Sport permitting, use of neck rolls, high-profile shoulder pads
   - Technique adjustment.
   - Some athletes may be advised not to return to their sport (see below)

Return to sport

- Following the first episode, the athlete can return to play only if:
  1. Symptoms have completely resolved within 24 h.
  2. There is full cervical spine range of movement.
  3. There is full recovery of upper limb strength.
  4. Other pathological processes have been excluded.
- The above also applies with repeat attacks if the number of episodes has been less than three
- Athletes with three or more episodes or attacks lasting longer than 24 h may be advised to consider not returning to future play

Further reading

Bailes JE, Petschauer M, Guskiewicz KM, Marano GManagement of cervical spine injuries in athletes. J Athl Train. 2007; 42(1):126–134.

Castro FP. Stingers, cervical cord neurapraxia, and stenosis. Clin Sports Med 2003; 22:483–492.

Weinburg J, Rokito S, Silber JS. Etiology, treatment, and prevention of athletic 'stingers'.Clin Sports Med 2003; 21:493–500.

Related topics of interest

Cervical spine – spinal cord injury and cervical cord neurapraxia

Key points

- This is transient neurological deficit (sensory and/or motor) of limbs as a result of transient pressure on the cervical spinal cord
- Once a prompt assessment and investigation has excluded a more significant spinal cord injury, a full recovery can normally be expected
- Risk of recurrence is particularly high in the presence of stenosis and other structural abnormalities, therefore, a recommendation may be made to cease collision sports if the athlete has had multiple neurapraxic events

Overview and epidemiology

In the USA, over 50% of spinal cord injuries occur under the age of 30, with the vast majority occurring in males. Of all spinal cord injuries, approximately half occur at the level of the cervical spine.

Cervical cord neurapraxia, also known as transient spinal cord injury (TSCI), refers to transient neurological deficits (sensory and/or motor) of limbs as a result of transient pressure on the cervical spinal cord. It is seen in sports such as American football, rugby, wrestling and boxing. Cervical spine stenosis is not uncommon in athletes and is a known radiographic finding in those with TSCI.

TSCI has become accepted to mean those instances in which sufficient forces result in temporary inhibition of spinal cord impulse transmission without causing structural damage to the vertebral column or spinal cord.

Pathology

The initial impact, with the resulting mechanical forces applied to the spinal column can cause it to fail, through the different mechanisms shown in **Figure 5**. Axial loading in a slightly flexed cervical spine or forceful extension during collision sports is a common mechanism.

Clinical features

Neurapraxia of the cervical cord was initially described by Torg in 1986. It is characterised as a transient paraesthesia and/or weakness in the arms and/or legs. Severity can be graded according to the duration of symptoms (**Figure 5**):

- Grade I: less than 15 min
- Grade II: 15 minutes to 24 h
- Grade III: over 24 h

Investigations and differential diagnosis

As previously mentioned in earlier topics, the immediate management is as per ATLS guidelines, and involves a thorough neurological examination including American Spinal Injury Association scoring. The initial plain radiographs and possible computerised tomography scans will help bony injuries, and the presence of any neurological deficit is an indication for magnetic resonance imaging scanning to assess any spinal cord, disc or ligamentous injury.

The sagittal diameter of the subaxial spinal canal typically measures 18 mm. Spinal stenosis, whether congenital or acquired, is defined as a canal size of 14 mm or less.

The Torg ratio, which is measured from plain radiograph with cervical spine in extension, is a ratio of the distance between the midpoint of the posterior aspect of the vertebral body and the nearest corresponding spinolaminar line to the anterior–posterior width of the vertebral body. A ratio of 0.8 or less is thought to indicate the presence of developmental stenosis.

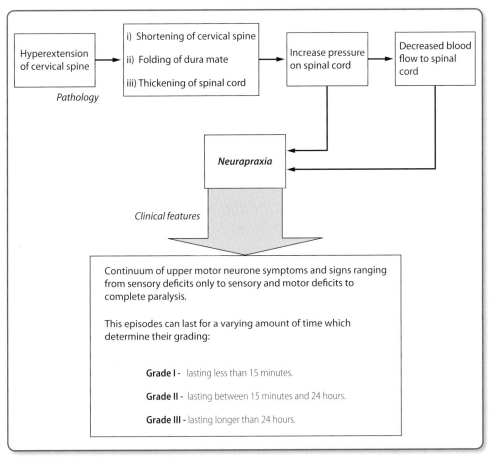

Figure 5 Pathology & clinical features.

The Torg ratio has been demonstrated to have a low positive predictive value in assessing spinal stenosis. Currently, MR imaging has become the preferred modality in assessing 'functional stenosis'.

It is important to note that neurapraxia can occur in a normal spine. However, it is also associated with acquired stenosis, ligament laxity, disc herniation and the degenerative spine.

Management

In the context of suspected neurapraxia, once a prompt assessment and investigation has excluded a more significant spinal cord injury, a full recovery can normally be expected. Unlike neurapraxia of peripheral nerves, which may take several weeks, resolution of symptoms can be relatively rapid.

Return to sport

There is an approximately 50% risk of a repeat episode if the athlete returns to sport. If radiological investigations demonstrate stenosis or structural abnormality, the risk may be higher and a recommendation may be made to cease collision sports if there have been multiple neurapraxic events.

In the case of no radiological abnormality, the athlete will make a calculated decision regarding the continuation of such sport, given the above statistics and the long-term career or financial implications it may have. An opportunity arises to educate athletes on tackling opponents more safely and avoidance of head-on collision if they decide to return to sport. As a result of work by Dr. Torg, the 'spear' tackle using the lowered head to engage the opponent has been made illegal in American football.

Further reading

Allen CR, Kang JD. Transient quadriparesis in the athlete. Clin Sports Med 2002; 1:15–27.

Castro FP. Stingers, cervical cord neurapraxia, and stenosis. Clin Sports Med 2003; 22:483–492.

Kim DH, Vaccaro AR, Berta SC. Acute sports-related spinal cord injury contemporary management principles. Clin Sports Med 2003; 22(3):501–512.

Bailes JE, Petschauer M, Guskiewicz KM, Marano, G. Management of cervical spine injuries in athletes. J Athl Train 2007; 42(1):126–134.

Related topics of interest

- Cervical spine – cervical disc injury and herniation (p. 23)
- Cervical spine – cervical ligament and muscle injuries (p. 25)
- Cervical spine – nerve root and brachial plexus injuries (p. 27)

Cervical spine fracture/ dislocation

Key points

- Principles apply in the management of any suspected cervical injury
- These injuries can be stable or unstable and may or may not be associated with neurological deficits
- Definite treatment depends on stability and is associated with neurological deficits

Overview and epidemiology

Cervical spine fractures account for 20%--30% of all spine fractures. These injuries can be stable or unstable and may or may not be associated with neurological deficits. Noncontiguous spinal fractures are seen in approximately 10% of patients.

Principles of management

The aims of managing any patient with cervical spine fracture and/or dislocation are
1. Prevention of damage to uninjured neurological tissue.
2. Realignment of the spine.
3. Obtaining stability.
4. Maximize neurologic recovery.
5. Rehabilitation.

The advanced trauma life support (ATLS) principles apply in the management of any suspected cervical injury. On a helmeted athlete, the protective helmet should not be removed until a safe controlled environment exists for cervical spine immobilization. The visor can be removed to aid airway and breathing.

A well fitting, rigid collar is applied, and lateral bolsters with tapes or straps are used to secure to a spinal backboard to prevent the movement of patient. A thorough neurological examination is performed using the American Spinal Injury Association (ASIA) standard.

Having passed the 'initial management' once, any malalignment of the cervical spine may be corrected by skeletal traction with the aid of:
- Spring-loaded Gardner Wells tongs
- Halo ring

A technical description of applying traction is beyond the scope of this topic. However, the procedure must be carried out in a fully conscious and cognitively unimpaired individual.

Further management may be non-operative or operative depending on:
1. Whether there is any compression of neural structures (as suggested by clinical exam and various imaging modalities, which include magnetic resonance imaging (MRI) and computed tomography (CT) scans).
2. Stability of the fracture. Stability is defined by White and Panjabi (see Torg, 2002) as the 'ability of the spine under physiological loads to maintain relationships in such a way that there is neither damage nor subsequent irritation to the spinal cord or nerve roots and, in addition, there is no development of incapacitating deformity and pain'. When this ability is lost, the injury is said to be 'unstable'.

Although this is a complete and comprehensive definition, clinicians need to be able to objectively assess stability. A cervical spine injury is unstable when it is associated with any one of the following:
1. Dysfunction of all the anterior elements.
2. Dysfunction of all the posterior elements.
3. More than 3.5 mm anterior–posterior displacement of one vertebral with respect to the vertebra below.
4. Angular displacement of more than 11 degrees of adjacent vertebra.

Non-operative management

Stable fractures without any compression of neural tissue may be managed with a rigid cervical collar or halo for 8 to 12 weeks. Injuries that may be treated in this way include:
- Stable compression fractures of the vertebral bodies

- Undisplaced fractures of the laminae, lateral masses and spinous process

Reduced unilateral facet joint dislocations may also be treated in a halo vest for 8 to 12 weeks.

Operative management

Surgery is indicated for unstable injuries whether or not there is a presence of any neurological deficits. Surgery is also required in patients with neurological deficits and mechanical compression of neural tissue (by definition, these are also unstable injuries). Surgery is in the form of decompression (in patients with neurologic compression) and stabilization.

Specific injuries

Cervical spine fracture and/or dislocation injuries may be divided into those that involve the occipitocervical junction and upper cervical spine (down to C2) and those that involve the lower cervical spine (C3 to C7).

Investigations and treatment

Instability is assessed once the history and physical examination is complete and imaging studies employing plain radiography (including AP/lateral and open mouth view), CT and MRI scanning, if indicated, are performed. Flexion and extension lateral radiographs may help determine instability where there is uncertainty.

Cervical spine injuries can be categorized into upper cervical and subaxial spine trauma.

Upper cervical spine injuries

Occipital condyle fracture

This is a rare injury in isolation and more commonly is associated with atlanto-occipital dislocation. Suspicion of injury may arise secondary to low cranial nerve palsy, associated head injury or basal skull fracture, or where significant neck pain is present despite normal-appearing cervical spine radiographs. This injury is usually managed with cervical collar or halo vest unless there is an evidence of ligamentous instability (see below).

Dislocation of the atlanto-occipital joint

This is a high-energy deceleration injury that causes a disruption of strong musculoligamentous attachments inherent to this region. This dislocation is usually not relevant in sports and is frequently a post-mortem diagnosis. Death occurs due to respiratory arrest. In rare survivors, cranial nerve injury VII to X can be seen. Management is surgical with closed reduction and usually posterior occiput to the C2 fusion.

Atlas (C1) fractures

This is a relatively uncommon injury. As the spinal canal is wide at this level, neurological injury is rare, but cranial nerve injury is seen. These fractures can be divided into:
- Posterior arch fractures
- Anterior arch fractures
- Burst fractures (Jefferson fracture)

Open-mouth plain radiographs or CT scan may indicate transverse ligament rupture if displacement of lateral masses of C1 relative to C2 are over 7 mm in combination. They are usually treated by rigid collar or halo vest in cases of significant displacement.

Isolated transverse ligament injuries

Usually caused by a blow to the back of the head, these injuries may involve midsubstance rupture of the ligament or avulsion with a small bone fragment of the lateral mass. Those with substance rupture require early surgery and stabilization. Those that involve bony avulsion may have a trial of non-operative management with a rigid cervical collar. Surgery is indicated in those with non-union and persistent instability after 3–4 months or those that initially have an atlanto-dens interval of 5 mm or more. Surgery is in the form of posterior atlanto-axial (C1–C2) fusion.

Odontoid fractures

These fractures can account for approximately 20% of all cervical fractures. These are classified into three types:

Type I injuries are avulsion fractures of the tip of the odontoid. These are rare, stable injuries that are not usually associated with any neurologic deficit. Most of these are treated with a rigid cervical collar.

Type II injuries refer to fractures through the neck of the odontoid process. These are associated with a high non-union rate. Optimal management remains controversial with over 400 scientific articles, but very few with level 1 or level 2 evidence. Treatment may be non-operative in the form of a cervical collar or halo vest immobilization or it can be operative. Factors increasing a risk of non-union include displacement of more than 6 mm, posterior displacement, age over 50 years and angulation on the sagittal plane of more than 10°. Non-operative care appears to be most effective for stable or minimally displaced fractures. Cervical collars are better tolerated than halo vests and have reduced complications such as pin-tract infections and loosening, but also have a lower union rate. Operative treatment is indicated if non-operative treatment has failed (continued pain and/or instability). The literature supports both anterior screw fixation and posterior fixation (several options), although each technique has its own limitations and risks.

Type III fractures extend into the cancellous bone and are associated with a much higher union rate than Type II injuries. Treatment is commonly with halo immobilization.

Hangman fractures [traumatic spondylolisthesis of C2 (axis)]

These injuries are sub classified into three types:

Type I. These are undisplaced or have an anterior translation of less than 3 mm. They are commonly treated with a rigid cervical collar.

Type II. There is anterior translation of more than 3 mm. They are initially treated with halo traction for 3 – 6 weeks followed by a halo vest for up to a further 3 months.

Type IIA. With these injuries, there is minimal translation but significant angulation.

Treatment involves reduction initially with a halo vest while applying slight compression under an image intensifier (traction is contraindicated). Once reduced, halo vest immobilization may be continued until healing occurs.

Type III. These injuries involve the posterior facets and are accompanied by unilateral or bilateral facet dislocation at C2–C3. There is significant angulation and translation. Neurological deficits are commonly present. In the vast majority of cases, treatment is in the form of attempted closed skeletal reduction followed by open stabilization. Halo vest immobilization may be required following surgery.

Lower cervical spine injuries/subaxial fractures

In the lower cervical spine, fractures are more common at C5, C6 and C7 vertebrae and dislocation/subluxations occur most frequently at C4/C5, C5/C6 and C6/C7.

Vertebral body fractures

Mechanism is commonly axial loading and compression. A wide spectrum of injuries including:

1. **Compression fractures**

   Vertbral body fractures without posterior ligamentous injury may be treated non-operatively. C3–C6 fractures can be treated in a collar, while for those at C7 or T1, a cervicothoracic brace provides better support.

   In the presence of ligamentous disruption, as indicated by MRI or significant kyphosis on CT/radiograph, surgical treatment is indicated.

2. **Burst fractures**

   These are high-energy injuries, with the presence of retropulsed fragments and, therefore, spinal cord injury is commonly seen. Imaging in the form of CT and MRI is required to assess the extent of the damage. Initially, longitudinal traction may be indicated to try to achieve some realignment. Regardless of posterior ligamentous disruption, anterior cervical surgery is performed to decompress the spinal canal and reconstruct the anterior column. If posterior ligamentous disruption is also present, then supplementary posterior instrumented fusion is carried out as a single stage or a two-stage procedure.

3. **Flexion-type teardrop fractures**

This typically occurs in young patients and involves high energy. They can be confused with burst fractures as they involve a sagittal split in the vertebral body. Patients are often presented with neurological deficit. The teardrop fragment itself is the anterior inferior vertebral body fracture. Three fracture parts may be seen with these injuries:

- Anterior–inferior teardrop fracture
- Sagittal vertebral body fracture
- Posterior neural arch disruption.

If there is no neurological deficit and the posterior ligamentous complex (PLC) is intact, there is a definite role for a rigid collar or orthosis.

Unstable fractures with or without neurological deficit are indications for surgery. An anterior vertebrectomy and decompression is performed, if indicated, followed by anterior column reconstruction. Posterior only surgery may be performed with caution, if the patient is neurologically intact with little anterior column height loss.

Facet fractures without dislocation

These injuries may be treated non-operatively in a rigid collar, provided that they occur in isolation and MRI scanning rules out a disc or ligamentous injury. Otherwise, there is an indication for surgery. Use of flexion/extension radiographs of the cervical spine can be useful in assessing stability.

Unilateral or bilateral facet dislocation

These represent a spectrum of injuries from facet capsule disruption to subluxation, and to unilateral or bilateral dislocation. The PLC is likely disrupted with bilateral injuries, whereas unilateral injuries may have spared the PLC. Non-operative treatment is reserved for unilateral injuries in those neurologically

or in those patients who are neurologically intact or those with significant co-morbidity. Persistent instability and pain are not uncommon following cervical collar or halo vest treatment.

In an athlete, early aggressive management may be preferable, though the optimal surgical treatment is still debated.

It is generally agreed that closed reduction in a neurologically intact, awake and cooperative patient is safe. Many centres will organize an MRI scan prior to reduction. Patients that have incomplete or complete spinal cord injury must have MRI to look for disc herniation.

With the reduction of dislocation, surgical planning can take place. If reduction has not occurred, there is still an indication for surgery. Debate continues over anterior versus posterior approach, or a combined anterior–posterior approach. Anterior surgical stabilization may be performed and is useful particularly if decompression of disc or bone contents from the canal is necessary, but if full reduction is not achieved, a posterior approach may be indicated at the same sitting or a staged operation to achieve circumferential fusion. Posterior approach also treats PLC injury more directly. There is little data to support combined anterior-posterior stabilization unless there is significant bony comminution or failure to achieve open anterior reduction.

The clinician should be guided by the principle of doing no harm by performing expedient reduction of these challenging injuries.

Bilateral facet dislocation

As with unilateral facet dislocations, the mechanism of injury is flexion and rotation, but neurological deficit is more common with these. They result in more than 50% anterior subluxation of one vertebra over the one below. Although close reduction is comparatively easy, redislocation rate is common with traction or a halo vest. Therefore surgery (open reduction--internal fixation) is usually indicated.

The same controversies regarding MRI scanning exist (see above).

Ankylosing spondylitis (AS) and diffuse idiopathic skeletal hyperostosis (DISH)

Although both of these conditions are less common in young athletes, they can manifest in the ageing athletes. As the spine effectively acts a solid continuous bone, any significant injury can cause a fracture with the potential for disastrous neurological consequences. The index of suspicion should be high, and injury and neck pain in those with a diagnosis of AS should be treated as an unstable fracture until proven otherwise.

Spinous process avulsion fracture

Also referred to as 'clay shoveler's' fracture, these are caused by forceful contraction of the trapezius and rhomboid muscles. It is a hyperflexion injury. These are stable injuries and are managed with a cervical collar.

Other isolated fractures

Isolated transverse process fractures can occur. The vertebral artery courses through the foramina typically C2--C6 and may be injured in transverse process fractures. MRI arteriogram can help rule out such injuries.

No specific treatment is necessary for isolated transverse process fractures.

Return to sport

Cervical spine fracture injuries can have a massive impact. Many athletes must accept that they may not be able to return to contact sport. Those who may return are generally those with (see Torg, 2002 in the Further reading list):

- Vertebral body compression fractures that meet all of the following criteria:
  - Stable
  - Healed
  - With normal neurology
  - Pain free
  - With near complete cervical spine range of movement
  - Without ligamentous laxity
  - Without posterior bony structure fractures
- Endplate fractures that meet all the above criteria mentioned for vertebral body compression fractures
- Isolated spinous process fractures that have healed

All athletes with all other cervical spine fracture injuries are generally advised against returning to contact sports.

Further reading

Banerjee R, Palumbo MA, Fadale PD. Catastrophic cervical spine injuries in the collision sport athlete, part 1, epidemiology, functional anatomy and diagnosis. Am J Sports Med 2004; 32(4):1077–1087.

Banerjee R, Palumbo MA, Fadale PD. Catastrophic cervical spine injuries in the collision sport athlete, part 2, principles of emergency care. Am J Sports Med 2004; 32(7):1760–1764.

Torg JS. Cervical spine, cervical spine injuries in adults. In: JC DeLee, D Drez, MD Miller (Eds) Orthopaedic Sports Medicine, Principles and Practice, 2nd edn. Saunders, 2002:791–828.

Related topics of interest

Cervical spine injuries

Overview

Cervical spine injuries are relatively uncommon in the general population, yet around 5%–10% of all cervical injuries are related to sports and can be potentially devastating as spinal cord function can be placed at risk.

Approximately 10%–20% of all spinal traumas are associated with spinal cord injury. Sporting activities account for more than 7% of all the spinal cord injuries and are the second most common cause of such injuries in the first three decades of life, second only to road traffic accidents.

Sporting spinal cord injuries are more common in athletes who are between 16 to 30 years of age and they predominantly occur in males. Sports such as equestrian, American football, rugby, wrestling, ice hockey, snow boarding, skiing and diving account for the majority of reported sporting injuries of the cervical spine.

The normal cervical spine is described as lordotic and allows controlled motion and force to the surrounding musculature. In a certain position, such as flexion, the lordosis is lost and thus, any direct axial load is transmitted to the vertebrae and intervertebral discs. The bones or discs can subsequently fail and risk injuring the spinal cord or neural elements.

The energy imparted to the spinal column bears a direct relationship to the injury inflicted. Second, any immediately adjacent area that is not yet damaged is susceptible to secondary pathophysiological processes that ensue. The acute processes contributing to the secondary damage include inflammatory response, free radical injury and vascular injury or ischaemia. The role of the physician is to minimize the secondary injury and create a stable environment compatible with the recovery of spinal cord function.

Management

Principles of management of cervical spine injuries are:

1. Advanced trauma life support (ATLS) management with attention to airway, breathing, circulation and disability.
2. At the same time, just as important is the prevention of further damage to spinal cord by:
   - Awareness of potential of cervical spine injury and its prompt recognition
   - Appropriate on-field management, which includes immobilization. In the field, manual immobilization of the neck is necessary until a hard collar can be applied, along with blocks on either side of the head with strapping and transfer on a rigid spinal board
   - Once off field, the detection of any neurological deficits and examination in a systematic manner
   - Detection of 'unstable' injuries. (Instability as defined by White and Panjabi is 'loss of ability of the spine under physiological loads to maintain relationships in such a way that there is neither damage nor subsequent irritation to the spinal cord or nerve roots and, in addition, there is no development of incapacitating deformity and pain'.)

A thorough assessment of the athlete, which includes history, examination and various diagnostic imaging investigations, would allow the physician to make one of the following diagnoses:

1. Cervical ligament/muscle injuries:
   - Sprains
   - Strains
   - Contusions
2. Cervical disc injuries including herniation
3. Nerve root/brachial plexus injuries
   - Stingers
4. Cervical fracture/dislocations
   - May be stable/unstable
   - May or may not be associated with neurological injury
5. Cervical cord neurapraxia
6. Spinal cord injuries (as a consequence of unstable injuries)

It is important to appreciate that a plain radiograph may not be enough to exclude unstable injuries. A computerised tomography scan is frequently used when plain radiography is insufficient to adequately visualize the cervical spine and also when a fracture has been detected to obtain further information before treatment. Magnetic resonance imaging is the investigation of choice for suspected spinal cord injury, disc herniation and posterior ligamentous disruption.

Spinal cord injury: role of steroids and early surgery

Spinal cord injury can be complete or incomplete and may result in a variety of well-known syndromes including anterior cord syndrome, central cord syndrome, Brown-Sequard syndrome and posterior cord syndrome. Further description of these syndromes is beyond the scope of this topic.

The role of high-dose corticosteroid use in acute spinal cord injury is controversial. Currently the position of the British Orthopaedic Association is to echo the British Association of Spinal Cord Injury Specialists who concluded that the use of high-dose steroid management of acute spinal cord injury could not be recommended or supported on the current evidence.

There is now evidence to demonstrate that early surgery (less than 24 h after injury) versus delayed surgery (over 24 h) after traumatic cervical spine injury results in improved clinical outcomes. The multicentre international prospective trial Surgical Timing in Acute Spinal Cord Injury Study (STASCIS) recently published an improved neurologic outcome (American Spinal Injury Association score) at 6 month follow-up after injury.

Prevention

Sporting cervical spine injuries are potentially avoidable if proper instruction and technique are provided. The advantage of coaching in certain team sports including American football and ice hockey is to train athletes to tackle and block in a safe manner to avoid potentially compromising the cervical spine. Appropriate strength training and physiotherapy are also key to prevention of injury, along with updating and modifying sports equipment to best protect the athlete in competition.

Further reading

Banerjee R, Palumbo MA, Fadale PD. Catastrophic cervical spine injuries in the collision sport athlete, part 2, principles of emergency care. Am J Sports Med 2004; 32(7):1760–1764.

The National Spinal Cord Injury Statistical Center, University of Alabama at Birmingham, NSCISC 2009 Annual Statistical Report and Facts at a Glance, 2010.

Fehlings MG, Vaccaro A, Wilson JR, et al. Early versus delayed decompression for the traumatic cervical spinal cord injury: Results of the Surgical Timing in Acute Spinal Cord Injury Study (STASCIS). PLoS One. 2012.

Related topics of interest

Chest injuries – chest wall

Key points

- Pneumothorax/ haemothorax must be excluded in patients with rib fractures
- Sternal fractures are high-energy injuries, and other associated intrathoracic injuries must be ruled out
- Thoracic outlet syndrome could arise from a number of different causes (both positional and static); therefore, accurate clinical and imaging assessment is important

Rib fracture – acute and stress

Rib fractures are one of the commonest thoracic injuries in sports with high-energy contact. Symptoms consist of pleuritic chest pain (pain on respiration) with localized tenderness and crepitus. The patient may be hesitant to breath adequately, and in extreme cases this may lead to retained secretions and chest infections. In milder cases, pain may only be present with cough/sneeze. Assessment must include examination for underlying lung injury and pleural injury (i.e. pneumothorax or haemothorax – see below). This involves chest auscultation and/or chest X-ray.

Stress fractures are related to sports with repetitive chest wall movements (i.e. rowing, tennis, golf). They are present with slowly progressive nonspecific poorly localized rib pain, which may be pleuritic and often does not get better between training sessions.

Treatment involves rest and adequate analgesia, which is important to enable the patient to breathe adequately and prevent chest infections. Sports training should be initially altered to rest the upper body, and it may take up to 6 weeks to resume normal activity.

Slipping rib syndrome

This is present with pain at the lower end of the rib cage, with associated tenderness. The cartilaginous ends of ribs 8-10 (false ribs) are hypermobile in these patients, either as a result of previous injury or a congenital defect. The ribs ride up and press on the neurovascular bundle above, thus creating symptoms. Management is rest and analgesia, although more severe cases have been treated with steroid injections or surgical resection of the anterior rib ends.

Sternal fractures

High impact/velocity blunt trauma to the thoracic cavity can cause sternal fractures. It is of vital importance to rule out other significant associated intrathoracic injuries. The patient will need to be resuscitated and managed in a hospital setting initially. Clinically, the patient will undoubtedly complain of chest pain, particularly on movement. Resuscitation according to airway, breathing and circulation needs to be instigated, and assessment made for other intrathoracic injuries. Diagnosis is made on sternal X-rays or CT. Other investigations required are ECGs, serial cardiac enzyme measurements (e.g. troponins to assess for myocardial contusion) and echo (to rule out pericardial effusion or tamponade). Commonly, all that is required is in-hospital observation for a few days, with adequate analgesia and rest. Return to sports training may take 6-12 weeks.

Costochondritis and Tietze's syndrome

Inflammation of the cartilaginous joint which connects the ribs to the sternum can present with chest pain. The key finding which differentiates this nonspecific pain from other causes is that there is marked tenderness over the costochondral joint. It is seen as an overuse injury in athletes, particularly rowers. Tietze's syndrome is similar to costochondritis; however, results from an inflammatory process and may be related to seronegative arthropathies. An additional finding in Tietze's is redness and swelling over the affected joints. The diagnosis is made clinically, and treatment in these conditions involves rest, analgesia in the form of nonsteroidal anti-inflammatories and in extreme cases corticosteroid injections.

Pectoralis major rupture

Chest wall muscle tears can occur in sports such as weightlifting, rugby, American football or ice hockey. An avulsion injury can occur at the musculotendinous junction with the humerus, as well as at the attachment to the sternum (more rare and occurs in weightlifting). Symptoms include an experienced 'snap' followed by pain, swelling, deformity and weakness. On examination, a palpable defect may be ascertained, with asymmetry of the pectoral/axillary fold. Adduction and internal rotation of the shoulder may be weakened. MRI may aid in diagnosis. Treatment involves rest and analgesia and in cases of extensive muscular tears surgical repair. Physiotherapy is very important and must include shoulder stabilizers, infraspinatus and pec minor exercises.

Thoracic outlet syndrome

The thoracic outlet is a clinical term referring to the superior opening of the thoracic cavity, the narrow passageway between the clavicle and the first rib. This small area contains the major blood vessels that exit the chest to supply the arm (the subclavian artery and vein) as well as the nerves that supply the arm from the spinal cord (brachial plexus). Thoracic outlet syndrome (TOS) refers to the clinical symptoms that arise when any part of this neurovascular bundle is compressed at the thoracic outlet.

The most common causes of TOS are trauma and repetitive exercise. A soft tissue injury or sprain, or indeed surgery, can cause excess scar formation which compresses structures later on. Clavicle fractures can also do this. First rib fractures can cause immediate brachial plexus damage, as well as delayed symptoms once the scar tissue grows around the rib and encases the vessels and nerves.

Improper weight training may also cause a muscle imbalance. Sports activities where the arms are raised above the shoulders for long periods such as swimming, weightlifting, volleyball, badminton, and rock climbing, are particularly at fault. Postural problems such as droopy shoulders are also a risk. Some people are born with an extra 'cervical rib,' which originates from C7. This protrudes into the thoracic outlet and causes fibrous changes around the brachial plexus thus inducing compression.

The main symptoms are that of pain and paraesthesia in the upper limbs and can be found from the acromioclavicular joint and biceps area down to the peripheral arm. The pain occurs on exercise as well as following exercise and at rest. Paraesthesia can be found down the arm, particularly affecting the 4th and 5th fingers. Some patients also develop motor symptoms in the form of weakness in the arms and hands. Holding the arms overhead may cause fatigue and pain.

Diagnosis is made by a combination of typical symptoms, physical examination and some routine investigations. Two physical signs which are sometimes used are Adson's sign (loss of the radial pulse in the arm by rotating head to the ipsilateral side with extended neck following deep inspiration) and the costoclavicular manoeuvure (loss of the radial pulse by drawing the patient's shoulder down and back as the patient lifts their chest in an exaggerated 'at attention posture). However, it should be noted that both these tests lack sensitivity or specificity.

Imaging takes the form of X-rays of the chest (looking for cervical rib), shoulders and cervical spine, MRI of the shoulder and cervical spine, nerve conduction studies in the arm, and arteriography/venography of the arm.

Treatment can be conservative or surgical. Conservative management involves rest, avoiding precipitating factors, anti-inflammatories and physiotherapy to strengthen muscles around the shoulder (especially deltoids and rhomboids). Surgery is indicated when the cause is due to a bony obstruction such as a cervical rib, failed medical management or in athletes who need to return to training earlier. Surgery involves decompression by removing cervical ribs and/or first ribs, dividing the scalene muscles off the first rib and division of any scar tissue.

Further reading

Gregory PL, Biswas AC, Batt ME. Musculoskeletal
problems of the chest wall. Sports Med 2002; 32:
235–250

Related topics of interest

- Cervical spine – nerve root and brachial plexus injuries (p. 27)
- Chest injuries – intrathoracic (p. 43)

Chest injuries – intrathoracic

Key points

- These could be life threatening
- Management involves adherence to ATLS and ALS protocols

Lung

Pneumothorax

Direct blunt trauma with or without rib fractures can cause a tear in the lung parenchyma leading to escape of air into the pleural cavity. The lung partially or completely collapses as the negative intrapleural pressure is lost. If the air leak is small, the lung seals itself rapidly. A tension pneumothorax is where the tear forms a one-way valve; air is allowed to enter the pleural space from the lung with inspiration, however cannot exit back into the lung with expiration (as would normally occur to some degree in a typical pneumothorax). The intrapleural pressure builds up, completely collapses the lung, and shifts the mediastinum to the contralateral side, thereby compressing the venae cavae and stopping venous return to the heart. This causes haemodynamic collapse and is life threatening if not treated immediately.

Symptoms consist of chest pain (worse with respiration), breathlessness and cough. Athletes with suspected rib fractures who continue to compete in a tournament must be closely monitored for subsequent onset of breathlessness as the pneumothorax may develop with later exertion. On examination, the classical findings are of reduced air entry on auscultation and hyper-resonant sound on percussion. There may also be surgical emphysema (air tracking in the soft tissues of the chest and neck), which will cause crepitus on palpation of the skin. In tension pneumothorax, the trachea is deviated away from the injured side and the neck veins are distended. The patient will be in extremis and cardiorespiratory arrest is imminent. The only necessary investigation is a chest X-ray; however, if tension is suspected, treatment needs to be initiated immediately without waiting for imaging.

Treatment depends on the degree of lung collapse. Airway management and oxygen therapy is necessary. In small pneumothoraces with a minor degree of lung collapse on chest X-ray, treatment is conservative and involves serial X-rays (on consecutive days) to ensure the lung collapse does not worsen. Oxygen therapy quickens the reabsorption of air from the pleural cavity. In larger pneumothoraces, or if the patient is breathless or hypoxic, management involves the insertion of a chest drain to remove the air from the pleural cavity and allow lung re-expansion. If tension is suspected, immediate treatment is insertion of a large-bore cannula in the 2nd intercostal space, midclavicular line on the affected side. This acts to remove the 'tension' component and release some of the intrapleural pressure. Subsequent chest drain insertion is mandatory.

Haemothorax

Direct blunt trauma can cause bleeding into the pleural space, particularly with fractured ribs. Typically, bleeding comes from the sheared intercostal muscles, or more seriously from intercostal vessels. Bleeding from other intrathoracic structures can be life threatening. As blood accumulates, it exerts pressure on the adjacent lung which will start to collapse. This may happen in conjunction with a pneumothorax and is called a haemopneumothorax.

The patient can complain of chest pain and shortness of breath. If bleeding is substantial, there will be haemodynamic compromise with tachycardia and hypotension. Chest auscultation will reveal reduced breath sounds, and percussion will be dull. A chest X-ray will give the diagnosis, and computerised tomography (CT) can isolate the source.

Treatment involves resuscitation according to airway, breathing and circulation. This encompasses oxygen therapy, fluid resuscitation (and possible blood transfusion) and chest drain insertion. If bleeding is substantial or the patient is haemodynamically unstable, surgery in the form of exploratory thoracotomy may be necessary.

Lung contusion

Blunt trauma to the chest can cause lung parenchymal damage. This often occurs in conjunction with rib fractures and other intrathoracic injuries such as pneumo/haemothorax; however, it can occur even in the absence of these other injuries. The trauma causes lung parenchymal bleeding and oedema, with associated localized lung collapse and mucous retention. Symptoms include breathlessness and hypoxia, and possibly haemoptysis. These typically exhibit some hours after the injury. Imaging is important to rule out other injuries. Typically there will be collapse consolidation of parts of the lung on X-ray and CT, but these changes may again take many hours to show up. Treatment involves oxygen therapy with ample pain relief and physiotherapy to ensure adequate breathing and clearing of secretions. There should be a low threshold for use of antibiotics for chest infection. These patients need close monitoring as they can rapidly deteriorate and may even require ventilation.

Heart
Commotio cordis

Commotio cordis, or cardiac concussion, is sudden cardiac arrest directly following a blow to the chest. It is a condition which occurs mostly in young teenagers because of their compliant chest wall. Despite being rare, it is still one of the most common causes of sudden death in sport in young athletes. In contrast to other causes, this occurs in structurally normal hearts. The mechanism is a precordial impact on a compliant chest wall which occurs at a point in the cardiac cycle corresponding to just before the T-wave (ventricular repolarisation phase). This initiates ventricular fibrillation (VF) instantly which causes a loss of cardiac output and arrest.

Most reported cases have occurred in young athletes playing baseball, as well as other sports such as football, ice hockey and martial arts. The patient typically collapses and loses consciousness immediately after a precordial injury. If the patient is connected to a defibrillator monitor, it will most likely show VF. Treatment is with immediate basic life support and resuscitation, a precordial thump if trained personnel are available, and prompt defibrillation.

Cardiac contusion

Blunt precordial trauma, such as with contact sports like rugby and American football, as well as high-velocity ball sports like baseball, can cause myocardial damage. This may cause the same symptoms as myocardial infarction, with chest pain, tachycardia and dyspnoea. There may be electrocardiographic changes (such as ST segment changes) and arrhythmias, and myocardial enzymes such as troponins may be elevated. Treatment is supportive. The patient needs to be monitored in hospital with serial electrocardiograms and troponin measurements and echocardiograms to assess for ventricular dysfunction and acute valve dysfunction.

Cardiac tamponade

Significant blunt chest trauma can rarely cause bleeding within the pericardial sac containing the heart (usually from right ventricular tears or epicardial vessel tears). This is a life-threatening condition as build-up of blood within the noncompliant pericardial sac compresses the venae cavae and the right-sided chambers causing reduced venous return. This can cause reduction and eventual loss of cardiac output.

Clinically, the patient may be dyspnoeic and possibly may have altered consciousness, tachycardia, hypotension, distended neck veins and quiet heart sounds. Diagnosis is made with echocardiogram. Cardiac tamponade is potentially fatal. The patient must be oxygenated and fluid resuscitated for shock and treated as per resuscitation guidelines. Definitive treatment is emergency exploration through a thoracotomy or sternotomy.

Further reading

Maron BJ, Link MS, Wang PJ, Estes NA III. Clinical profile of commotio cordis: an under appreciated cause of sudden death in the young during sports and other activities. J Cardiovasc Electrophysiol 1999; 10: 114–120.

Related topics of interest

• Chest injuries – chest wall (p. 40)

Cold – hypothermia

Key points

- Take special care if air temperature is less than –20°C
- In dealing with hypothermia, take the rectal temperature, handle patient avoiding bumps or knocks, rewarm slowly
- No one is dead until warm and dead
- Sport and exercise in the cold are safe and enjoyable as along as clothing and training are suitable for the conditions

Exercise in the cold

Exercise in the cold is perfectly safe and enjoyable as long as clothing, equipment and training are suitable – witness the many people who enjoy skiing holidays every year. Basic clothing advice is to wear plenty of it, in multiple layers. If in doubt, people should wear extra layers — it is usually possible to remove or loosen clothing if too hot. A waterproof outer layer is important if it starts raining or snowing. Participants should be taught that if they are venturing away from immediate support, then there is a need to learn basic survival skills and carry emergency rations and kit (e.g. survival bags).

Decisions about playing

Consider cancelling and certainly instigate increased safety surveillance at –20°C (American College of Sports Medicine (ACSM) guidance). At this temperature, there is a real risk of frostbite within 30 minutes on any exposed areas. If there is wind, calculate wind chill temperature and increase surveillance at a wind chill temperature of –27°C. To estimate wind chill, for a light–moderate wind (16 km/h) subtract 8°C from the air temperature; for a stronger wind, 32 km/h, subtract 13°C. Note that these are speeds well within the range of running and cycling.

During activity in the cold the high metabolic rate is a great protection against hypothermia. Postactivity, or when exhausted, participants should take immediate steps to keep warm.

Treating hypothermia

Incidents of hypothermia regularly occur related to sports, notably with water sports and mountain sports. It is essential, therefore, to understand some of the basics related to hypothermia. Remember that when dealing with likely hypothermia, this will sometimes have occurred because of an accident and that other injuries may be present.

When faced with a hypothermic subject:

- As far as possible protect from getting any colder
- Try to get rectal or aural temperature
- Exercise care with moving the subject: jerky movements or knocks may trigger ventricular fibrillation if hypothermia is moderate to severe (see **Table 2** for classification)

Rewarming

The general rule is to go slowly, not using strong surface heating due to the risk of burn injury and the problem of peripheral vasodilatation while the heart is still slow.

Table 2 Classification and features of hypothermia		
Core temperature (°C)	Designation	Comments
33–35	Mild	Shivering, may become confused
31–33	Moderate	Semiconscious, no longer able to help themselves
28-31	Severe	Loss of consciousness, stop shivering, areflexic, heart very slow
<28		Onset of ventricular fibrillation, death

From mild hypothermia

Wrap the subject up. Give a hot drink. Space blankets are not practical (too fragile and only help with radiant heat, which is not the main route of loss). You can immerse the patient in a hot bath, but it is advisable to keep his/her legs and arms elevated to maximise venous return.

From moderate/severe hypothermia

Passive rewarming is usually best, leaving the subjects to slowly warm up from their own metabolic heat. If in a hospital intensive care unit, then internal rewarming from an extracorporeal blood shunt or other method can be attempted. For very severe hypothermia, this may be necessary as the metabolism is too low. Remember, however, this practice needs a lot of care. Breathing warmed air is thought to help. The total heat gain is small, but some heat may reach vital structures in nearby brainstem. Portable equipment for warmed oxygen is available for use by sea/mountain rescue teams. Once a subject is at 34°C, it is possible to use more active methods. Note that due to immersion diuresis there may be a need to give intravenous fluids.

The general rule is that no one is dead until warm and dead.

Cold can cause problems even if core is OK

Accidents

Cold in the threshold range leads to an increase in accidents in factories, so it probably does in sports activities too. For example, with cold the hands become numb, cannot hold on or do precise manual tasks.

Frostbite

If the extremities are frozen, warm them up. Warm up. Only debride after delay to allow area of necrosis to become clearly defined.

Immersion

Hypothermia is a particular danger in water sports. Water has 23 times the thermal conductivity of air and a much higher thermal capacity. Remember the *Titanic*. Almost all who ended up in the water died; almost all who ended up in lifeboats survived.

During removal of a subject from the water, if possible keep him or her horizontal. Subject can die on the winch to helicopter if upright. The reason is circulatory collapse. Immersion diuresis reduces blood volume, vessels are dilated due to the cold, plus loss of water pressure causes venous pooling in the lower half of the body, venous returns then falls catastrophically and the heart fails.

Acute immersion death

Regularly people drown in cold water well before they become hypothermic. The diving reflex on cold immersion can stop the heart. A more common sequence is tachycardia, vasoconstriction, hypertension and increased cardiac work – a sequence that is a particular risk for anyone with threshold cardiac disease. Another problem is cold-induced hyperventilation, leading to hypocapnia, reduced brain blood flow, disorientation and clouding of consciousness – disastrous in water.

Further reading

Brukner P, Khan K. Clinical sports medicine, 4th edn. New York: McGraw-Hill. 2012; 1146-1157.
Castellani JW, Young AJ, Ducharme MB, Giesbrecht GG, Glickman E, et al. American College of Sports Medicine position stand: prevention of cold injuries during exercise. Med Sci Sports Exerc (2006); 38:2012–2029.

Related topics of interest

- Thermoregulation and fluid balance in hot conditions (p. 310)

Further reading

Murdoch M. Compartment syndrome: a review of the literature. Clin Pod Med Surg 2012; 29(2):301–310

Roberts A, Franklyn-Miller A. The validity of the diagnostic criteria used in chronic exertional compartment syndrome: a systematic review. Scand J Med Sci Sports 2012; 22:585–595.

Shuker FD. Physicians ability to manually detect isolated elevations in leg intra-compartment pressure. J Bone Joint Surg Am 2010; 92:361–367.

Related topics of interest

- Nerve entrapment syndromes – lower limb (p. 199)

Diabetes and exercise

Key points

- Exercise is a keystone to good diabetic care
- Patients should be evaluated for the existence of diabetic complications before an intense exercise regimen
- Exercise may require alterations in the medications being used for diabetic care

Background

Although exercise – along with diet and medication – has been considered one of the major cornerstones of diabetes management, patients should be evaluated before an exercise program is commenced.

Evaluation of the diabetic patient before recommending an exercise programme

Patients should, in particular, be assessed for conditions that might contraindicate certain types of exercise or predispose to injury (e.g. severe autonomic neuropathy, severe peripheral neuropathy or preproliferative or proliferative retinopathy).

Pre-exercise assessment: exercise stress testing with and without electrocardiogram monitoring

Previous guidelines have suggested that before beginning a vigorous or moderate exercise program, an exercise electrocardiogram (ECG) stress test should be carried out for all diabetic individuals aged >25 years in the presence of even one additional cardiovascular risk factor (**Table 3**).

However, this recommendation should be balanced against the fact that the lower the absolute CAD (coronary artery disease) risk, the higher the likelihood of a false-positive test. Therefore, some now propose that this test should be particularly directed at those people with diabetes with a 10-year CAD

Table 3 Risk factors for the development of cardiovascular disease in the presence of diabetes
Diabetes duration >10 years for type 2 diabetes
Diabetes >15 years for type 1 diabetes
Hypertension
Dyslipidemia
Smoking
Proliferative retinopathy
Nephropathy including microalbuminuria
Peripheral vascular disease
Autonomic neuropathy

risk of at least 10% (1% per year) and so in the absence of contraindications, maximal exercise testing could be considered in all diabetic individuals in order to assess maximal heart rate, set exercise intensity targets, and assess functional capacity and prognosis. A graded exercise test with ECG monitoring should be seriously considered before undertaking aerobic physical activity with an intensity exceeding the demands of everyday living (more intense than brisk walking) in previously sedentary diabetic individuals whose 10-year risk of a coronary event is >10%.

Frequency of exercise

The amount and intensity recommended for aerobic exercise vary according to goals.

- To improve glycaemic control, assist with weight maintenance, and reduce risk of cardiovascular disease (CVD), it is recommended to perform at least 150 minutes per week of moderate intensity aerobic physical activity (40-60% of VO_2max or 50-70% of maximum heart rate) and/or at least 90 minutes per week of vigorous aerobic exercise (>60% of VO_2max or >70% of maximum heart rate). The physical activity should be distributed over at least 3 days per week

- Performing >4 hours per week of moderate to vigorous aerobic and/or resistance exercise is associated with greater CVD risk reduction compared with lower volumes of activity
- For long-term maintenance of major weight loss (>13.6 kg [30 lb]), larger volumes of exercise (7 hours per week of moderate or vigorous aerobic physical activity per week) may be helpful

Resistance exercise

Because of the increased evidence for health benefits from resistance training during the past 10-15 years, the American College of Sports Medicine now recommends resistance training for healthy young and middle-aged adults, older adults, and adults with type 2 diabetes.

Exercise and nonoptimal glucose control

Hyperglycemia

When type 1 diabetics are deprived of insulin for 12-48 h and ketotic, exercise can worsen the hyperglycaemia and ketosis. It has been suggested that physical activity be avoided if fasting glucose levels are higher than double the upper limit of normal and ketosis is present and caution be exercised in the cases where glucose levels are >300 mg/dL even if no ketosis is present. In the absence of very severe insulin deficiency, light- or moderate-intensity exercise would tend to decrease plasma glucose. Therefore, provided the patient feels well and urine and/or blood ketones are negative, it may not be necessary to postpone exercise based simply on hyperglycaemia.

Hypoglycaemia

In individuals taking insulin and/or insulin secretagogues, physical activity can cause hypoglycaemia. Guidelines suggest that added carbohydrate should be ingested if pre-exercise glucose levels are <100 mg/dL. This applies for individuals on insulin and/or an insulin secretagogue. However, supplementary carbohydrate may generally

not be necessary for individuals treated without insulin or a secretagogue. These patients should check capillary blood glucose before, after and several hours following physical activity. Those who show a tendency toward hypoglycaemia during or after exercise, doses of insulin or secretagogues can be reduced before physical activity, and extra carbohydrate can be consumed before or during physical activity, or both.

Retinopathy

Resistance or aerobic exercise are not known to have adverse effects on the progression of nonproliferative diabetic retinopathy or macular oedema. However, in the presence of proliferative or severe nonproliferative diabetic retinopathy, vigorous aerobic or resistance exercise may be contraindicated because of the risk of triggering vitreous haemorrhage or retinal detachment. Advice should be sought regarding the optimal time to commence exercise following photocoagulation therapy.

Peripheral neuropathy

In the presence of severe peripheral neuropathy, it may be best to encourage non-weight-bearing activities such as swimming, bicycling or arm exercises in order to avoid skin breakdown and joint damage.

Autonomic neuropathy

Autonomic neuropathy can increase the risk of exercise-induced injury by decreasing cardiac responsiveness to exercise, postural hypotension, impaired thermoregulation due to impaired skin blood flow and sweating, impaired night vision due to impaired papillary reaction, impaired thirst increasing risk of dehydration and gastroparesis with unpredictable food delivery. Autonomic neuropathy is also strongly associated with CVD in people with diabetes. People with diabetic autonomic neuropathy should definitely undergo cardiac investigation before beginning physical activity more intense than that to which they are accustomed.

Microalbuminemia and nephropathy

Physical activity can increase urinary protein excretion in proportion to the acute increase in blood pressure. This has led some to recommend that people with diabetic kidney disease perform only light or moderate exercise, such that their blood pressure during exercise would not rise above 200 mmHg. Some data however suggest that improved diabetes control may improve protein excretion. Therefore, there may be no need for any specific exercise restrictions for people with diabetic kidney disease.

Summary

Lifestyle changes and a structured exercise program may prevent the progression of diabetes, but exercise programmes should be individualized.

Further reading

Colberg SR, Sigal RJ, Fernhall B, Regensteiner JG, Blissmer BJ, et al. Exercise and Type 2 Diabetes – The American College of Sports Medicine and the American Diabetes Association: joint position statement. Diabetes Care 2010; 33:e147–e167.

Sigal R, Kenny GP, Wasserman DH, Castaneda-Sceppa C, White RD. Physical activity/exercise and type 2 diabetes – a consensus statement from the American Diabetes Association. Diabetes Care 2006; 29: 1433–1438.

Zisser H, Gong P, Kelley M, Seidman JS, Riddell MC.. Exercise and diabetes. Int J Clin Pract 2011; 65(Suppl. 170):71–75

Related topics of interest

Disability and sport – classification

Key points

- Classification is essential in Paralympic sport to ensure fair competition among all athletes
- The International Paralympic Committee defines which impairments are eligible to take part in Paralympic sport, comprising 10 physical, visual and intellectual impairments
- The classification system used in each sport is determined by the individual sports federations

Introduction

In all sports, it is important that athletes are competing on a level playing field. Classification of disabled athletes is required to minimize the impact of the disability on sport performance, ensuring fair competition among all athletes. Success is therefore not determined by degree of impairment but by the same factors that determine success in sport for able-bodied athletes, such as skill, coordination, power, fitness and mental strength.

The paralympic movement - eligible impairments

The Paralympic Movement, which is governed by the International Paralympic Committee, offers sport opportunities for athletes that have at least one of the following 10 physical, visual or intellectual impairments:

Physical impairments
- Impaired muscle power, e.g. due to spinal cord injury
- Impaired passive range of movement (this does not include acute conditions)
- Loss of limb or limb deficiency
- Leg length difference - significant difference due to congenital deficiency or trauma
- Short stature, e.g. dwarfism
- Hypertonia, e.g. cerebral palsy

- Ataxia, e.g. cerebral palsy
- Athetosis, e.g. choreathetosis, cerebral palsy

Visual impairment
- Damage to one or more components of the vision system, including eye, optic nerve and visual cortex

Intellectual impairment
- Significantly limited intellectual functioning and adaptive behaviour, originating before the age of 18 years

Classification systems

there are a number of classification systems that are used. These are broadly based on type of disability, degree of disability, functional performance or more commonly a combination of these factors. The classifications vary by sport as each sport has different requirements in terms of ability. The international federations for each sport determine the classification system used by their sport. In individual sports, athletes will compete against other athletes within their specific class. In team sports, such as wheelchair basketball, athletes with varying degrees of disability can play together. The athletes are allocated points that indicate their degree of disability with a lower point indicating a greater degree of disability. A team is only allowed to field at any one time a team with a maximum sum of points to ensure fair competition.

Classification process

athletes are classified by a panel of trained certified experts with either a medical background or technical expertise in the sport. The process usually involves:
- Verification of the presence of an eligible impairment (as above)
- Physical and technical assessment
- Allocation of a sport class
- Observation in competition

The class allocated to the athlete may change over time as a result of improvements in the impairment through training or through deterioration in ability due to the progressive nature of some conditions.

Classification is not an easy process with some medical assessments open to subjective interpretation and occasionally abuse. The Spanish Intellectual disability basketball team in the 2000 Paralympic Games won gold medal, but were later stripped of their medal as no members of the team were found to have an intellectual disability.

The accuracy and reliability of the classification is vital as even small changes in classification can have disastrous affects in an athlete's chance of competing at the highest level.

Further reading

Tweedy S, Vanlandewijck Y. International Paralympic Committee position stand – background and scientific principles of classification in Paralympic sport. Br J Sports Med 2011; 45: 259–269.

Related topics of interest

- Disability and sport – overview (p. 63)
- Disability and sport – medical problems (p. 59)
- Disability and sport – equipment (p. 56)

Disability and sport – equipment

Key points

- The technological advancements in equipment for athletes with disabilities has revolutionised Paralympic sport
- There are four main types of wheelchairs used in sport – general sport, racing, throwing and motorised wheelchairs
- Lower limb prosthetics have improved so much in recent times that some Paralympic athletes are now able to actively compete against their able-bodied counterparts

Background

The advancements in specialised equipment for individuals with disabilities have dramatically enhanced their quality of life and provided opportunities for them to take part in many sports. The improvements have been most striking in amputee runners, who have been able to compete against able-bodied athletes at an elite level, by using prosthetic limbs. Although this is a controversial area, it shows how far the advancements have come and the impact they can have. Unfortunately, the availability of such equipment is not easily accessible in all parts of the world. Further investment is necessary to help drive forward Paralympic sport on a global scale.

The equipment used by athletes with disabilities can be divided into three main categories:

- Wheelchairs
- Prosthetics
- Other sport-specific specialised equipment

Wheelchairs

Wheelchair sports have greatly increased over the years. There are universal properties that all wheelchairs require which include stability, efficiency and manoeuvrability. However, the degree to which these factors are required differ for each sport, hence the need for specialised adaptations. In general, there are four major types of wheelchairs:

- General sports wheelchairs
- Racing wheelchairs
- Throwing wheelchairs
- Motorised wheelchairs

General sports wheelchairs

These are not too dissimilar to everyday wheelchairs, and often the athlete will use these for their everyday use. Specific features include:

- The hand rims are moderately large to improve efficiency and enable the athlete to start, stop, accelerate and change direction with minimal effort
- They usually have a negative camber angle of 12-15°, meaning the top of the wheels are closer together than the bottom. This increases stability, manoeuvrability and reduces risk of finger injuries from collisions
- They occasionally have small rear wheels to prevent tipping over

Racing wheelchairs

In these wheelchairs, stability and manoeuvrability are sacrificed to a degree for increased velocity. The technology and design of these wheelchairs have been derived from the advancements in cycle technology. Specific features include:

- Three wheels instead of four wheels
- Two large rear wheels and smaller wheel at the front
- Commonly have a lower body position
- The body position is forward leaning although the position will vary depending on whether the athlete is seated or kneeling
- Increased negative camber angle.

Throwing wheelchairs/chairs

These chairs are usually used for events such as javelin, shot-put and discus. The most important factor with these chairs is stability. Specific features include:

- Most wheelchairs/chairs do not have wheels. If wheels are present they are only for transporting the chair
- The seats may be hard and rigid to ensure maximum transfer of energy to the thrown object
- The body position is as high as is possible permitted under the International Paralympic Committee regulations

Motorised wheelchairs

These are designed for athletes who are unable to use general sport wheelchairs due to the degree and severity of their disability. They are used for sports such as wheelchair football and hockey. Specific features include:

- These chairs weigh a great deal due to the motor and battery, making them stable but not very mobile
- They are not practical for transport, and hence the majority of recreational athletes will use their own everyday wheelchair for the sport

Prosthetics

Prosthetics have revolutionised sports for athletes with limb deficiency or amputation. Lower limb prosthetics are the most common but the number of sports involving the use of upper limb prosthetics is increasing. A major limitation of prosthetics is the significant cost of them, which affects their accessibility and availability worldwide.

Lower limb prostheses

- many of these are based on the design developed by Van Phillips and Dale Abildskov, which involves a carbon fibre material cut into an L-shaped foot attached to a prosthetic socket above and a sole below
- The theory behind the design is the simulation of the spring action of a normal foot, with absorption of energy on foot strike and release of energy on push off.
- Depending on the deficiency of the limb, the prosthetic limb may or may not have an axial joint for articulation

- In athletes with an above knee amputation, advances in microprocessor technology have enabled computer-controlled activation of the swing phase of the prosthetic knee, automatically adjusting to activity levels
- Many sports require their own specific adaptations, for example
  - Swimmers can choose prostheses with a fin rather than a foot design
  - Cyclists may require a pedal-binding system
  - Skiers need prostheses that can be directly linked to the ski binding
  - Climbers benefit from prosthesis with a high friction sole to enhance grip

Upper limb prostheses

- Advances in technology have resulted in the design of specialised upper limb prostheses for a wide range of sports including basketball, cycling, hockey, volleyball, golf, swimming and tennis. Broadly, upper limb prostheses can be divided into three main categories (however, special adaptations have to be made for each specific sport):
  - Passive function prosthesis - most frequent type used by athletes
  - Mechanical prosthesis - consists of pulleys and cables
  - Myoelectric prosthesis - prosthesis receives the translated electromyography signals of the residual limb

Other sport-specific specialised equipment

It is beyond the scope of this topic to cover all the adapted equipment utilised by the disabled athlete. These specialised equipments allow the disabled to compete as other athletes, improve their performance and reduce the risk of injury.

Further reading

Burkett B. Technology in Paralympic sport: performance enhancement or essential for performance? Br J Sports Med 2010; 44:215–220.

Burkett B. Paralympic sports medicine – current evidence in winter sport: considerations in the development of equipment standards for Paralympic athletes. Clin J Sports Med 2012, 22: 46–50.

Related topics of interest

- Biomechanics (p. 21)
- Disability and sport – classification (p. 54)
- Disability and sport – medical problems (p. 59)

Disability and sport – medical problems

Key points

- Healthcare professionals involved in looking after athletes with disabilities must be aware of the wide variety of specific medical problems that occur in these athletes
- Athletes with spinal cord related disability are at high risk of developing medical emergencies such as hyperthermia, hypothermia and autonomic dysreflexia.
- Athletes using wheelchairs commonly develop upper limb injuries affecting the shoulder and hands

Introduction

There are specific medical problems encountered by athletes with disabilities due to their altered anatomy, physiology and biomechanics as well as the special equipment used by some. It is of vital importance that all members of the medical team are aware of and understand these differences.

Athletes with spinal cord related disability

Spinal cord related disabilities are usually secondary to an acquired lesion, such as trauma or due to congenital abnormalities such as spina bifida, with the level of the lesion affecting the associated motor, sensory and autonomic nervous system changes. Common problems encountered by athletes with spinal cord related disabilities include the following:

Impaired thermoregulation
- These athletes are vulnerable to heat-related illness and hypothermia.
- The problem is worse with high spinal cord level injuries with impaired autonomic nervous system dysfunction.
- There may be sensory deficits resulting in absent afferent input for the thermoregulation centre.

- The efferent arm of the system can also be affected with reduced or inadequate vasomotor, sweating and shivering responses
- Heat-related illness can occur following exercise in hot climates. Attempts to reduce the risks include:
  - Decreasing exposure to extreme temperature and sunlight
  - Appropriate clothing
  - Adequate hydration
  - Acclimatisation and preparation
  - Cooling strategies, such as cold wet towels, ice jackets and sprays
- Hypothermia can be an issue when undertaking exercise in cold, wet and windy environments. Preventative measures include:
  - Adequate clothing
  - Keeping dry
  - Blankets

Pressure sores
- These occur due to prolonged pressure over an insensitive area of skin below the level of the spinal cord lesion, leading to local ischaemia and skin breakdown
- Common areas include sacrum, ischial tuberosity, hip and posterior aspect of knee, foot and scapula
- Preventative measures to reduce these occurring are essential as the development of these sores can lead to unnecessary prolonged absence from the sport. The measures used include:
  - Regular skin checks
  - Appropriate padding of surfaces in contact with common pressure sore areas
  - Keeping the skin dry
  - Regular 'weight shifts' (changing position)

Bladder and bowel problems
- Autonomic nervous system dysfunction can lead to a neuropathic bladder resulting in urinary retention, recurrent urinary infections, renal calculi and incontinence

- Measures taken to reduce the risk of urinary tract infections include:
  - Intermittent self catheterisation
  - Adequate hydration
  - Particular attention to hygiene
  - Availability of accessible bathroom and catheterisation facilities
- Bowel incontinence and constipation occur in athletes with disability and can be a cause of low mood, reduced self-esteem and occasionally result in a fear of competing due to risks of accidents. A regular bowel regime is essential for the optimal health of the athlete

Autonomic dysreflexia (boosting)
- This is a medical emergency occurring as a result of an exaggerated sympathetic response to a painful stimulus below the level of the spinal cord lesion
- The trigger is usually due to trauma, infection, bladder distension from a blocked catheter, constipation or renal calculi
- It occurs in individuals with high spinal cord lesions above the level of T6
- The increased sympathetic discharge can lead to:
  - Profound hypertension
  - Sweating
  - Peripheral vasoconstriction and skin blotching
  - Severe headache
  - If untreated it can progress to cerebral haemorrhage, seizures, myocardial infarction, arrhythmias and eventually death
- Management involves removal of the trigger if possible, maintaining an elevated head and trunk position and medication to lower the blood pressure such as nifedipine
- Unfortunately, some athletes have actively sought to induce this state of autonomic dysreflexia as they have found it can reduce their perceived exertion for a given exercise, allowing them to push themselves further and improve performance. This is commonly known as 'boosting.'
- The methods used by some athletes included electric shocks to the lower limbs, clamping of a catheter, application of tight straps and sitting on a sharp object
- This was originally banned by the International Paralympic Committee in 1994 under the doping regulations but later removed as it could occur without intent and was a medical safety issue rather than doping
- Current measures put in place to reduce the risk of boosting involve precompetition measurements of blood pressure. If athletes are found to have a systolic blood pressure above 180 mmHg, they are removed from competition on medical safety grounds but do not face any further penalties

Impaired cardiovascular response to exercise
- In high spinal cord lesions, the heart can become sympathectomised, which results in a decrease in maximal heart rate response to 110-130 beats per minute
- This can affect maximal cardiac output, exercise capacity and also the ability to target training to a percentage of maximum heart rate

Compromised ventilator capacity
- The respiratory response to exercise may be reduced due to absent innervation of intercostals muscles resulting in their dysfunction

Reduced bone mineral density
- In athletes with spinal cord lesions and paralysis, it is important for medical professionals to be aware of the risk of progressive loss of bone mineral density resulting in osteopenia and osteoporosis
- The athlete is therefore at higher risk of stress and fragility fractures

Athletes with limb deficiency or amputation

The cause of limb deficiency or amputation in these athletes can vary. The commonest acquired cause is due to road traffic accidents. However, there is an increasing contribution from the military and war-related trauma. The athletes can either compete with a prosthesis, without a prosthesis, or in a wheelchair. Common medical issues arising in these individuals include:

Stump and prosthesis-related problems
- It is of vital importance that the prosthesis fits well, as an ill-fitting prosthetic limb can result in skin blisters, abrasions, ulceration and infection
- Careful management of the stump with regular skin checks, keeping it dry and appropriate padding is essential
- As the prosthetic limb is often shorter to enable it to swing through whilst running, the altered biomechanics can lead to lower back and hip pain. There is also thought to be an increased risk of premature degeneration of joints due to the altered loading patterns

Impaired thermoregulation
- Due to the reduced surface area available for heat loss, these athletes are at increased risk of heat-related illness
- Overheating and excess sweating can also lead to loosening of the prosthesis causing it to slip

Visually impaired athletes

Acute injuries in visually impaired athletes frequently occur due to collisions and falls. The visual impairment can also lead to alterations in balance and gait patterns predisposing to biomechanical-related overuse injuries.

In athletes with glaucoma, it is important to avoid sports such as weight lifting and diving where rises in intraocular pressure can occur.

Athletes with cerebral palsy

Cerebral palsy is a group of conditions in which impairment to the immature brain affects body movement and muscle coordination. The specific problems faced by athletes with cerebral palsy are determined by the type of movement disorder (spastic, choreoathetoid, mixed), its severity and the number of limbs affected.
- Spasticity is the most prevalent problem affecting athletes with cerebral palsy, causing pain and impairment in joint and muscle range of motion. However, overenthusiastic therapy to reduce the spasticity can lead to deterioration in performance due to reliance on the increased tone for joint and trunk stabilisation
- Individuals with cerebral palsy often have associated medical problems such as epilepsy, intellectual impairment, deafness, reduced visual acuity and speech and feeding difficulties
- Approximately half of all athletes with cerebral palsy will compete using a wheelchair

Athletes using a wheelchair

Athletes with spinal cord lesions, limb deficiency or amputation or cerebral palsy take part in sport using wheelchairs. Due to the inherent nature of using wheelchairs, upper limb injuries are not uncommon. They frequently affect the shoulder and hands.

Shoulder injuries
- Common shoulder injuries include acromio-clavicular joint (ACJ) pathology, impingement syndrome, rotator cuff tears and tendinopathy (see p. 000)
- These occur secondary to overuse and poor muscular movement patterning

Elbow injuries
- Throwing-related elbow injuries such as lateral epicondylitis occur in wheelchair sports that involve throwing such as club, discus, javelin and shot-put (see p. 000)

Hand and wrist injuries
- Blisters, callosities and cuts are frequently encountered by wheelchair athletes. Measures to prevent these occurring include wearing of gloves, taping and padding of rims
- Sprains of fingers and wrist joints are common

Nerve entrapments
- Median nerve entrapment (carpal tunnel syndrome) is thought to occur in up to 70% of wheelchair users
- Ulnar nerve entrapment is seen following compression in Guyon's canal and occasionally around the elbow in throwing athletes

Further reading

Patel D, Greydanus D. Physically challenged athletes, Paediatric Practice Sports Medicine. New York; New York; McGraw-Hill, 2009; 435–445.

Webborn N. The disabled athlete. In: Brukner P and Khan K (eds), Clinical sports medicine, 3rd edn.

New York; McGraw-Hill, 2006:778–786.

Webborn, N, Van de Vilet. Paralympic medicine. Lancet 2012; 379: 65–71.

Related topics of interest

- Biomechanics (p. 21)
- Shoulder – impingement syndrome/rotator cuff disease (p. 259)
- Thermoregulation and fluid balance in hot conditions (p. 310)

Disability and sport – overview

Key points

- There are increasing numbers of individuals with disability taking part in sport and physical activity with significant physical, psychological and social benefits
- There are a number of barriers that make it harder for individuals with disabilities to take part in sport that need to be overcome
- It is essential that individual with disabilities are given appropriate advice and guidance in choosing the right sport that meets their needs and abilities

Background

Physical activity participation in people with disabilities has greatly increased over the past 60 years as a result of the vision and contribution of Sir Ludwig Guttmann. He was in charge of the Spinal Injuries Unit at Stoke Mandeville Hospital and used sport as part of the rehabilitation process for patients with spinal cord injuries. On the opening day of the Olympic Games in London in 1948, he arranged an archery tournament at the hospital. Following its success, the contest developed into the International Stoke Mandeville Games and since the formation of the International Paralympic Committee in 1989, the Games are now known as the Paralympic Games. In 2012, London hosted the largest ever Paralympic Games with 4237 athletes participating from 164 National Paralympic Committees.

The benefits of physical activity are well known, and these are likely to be even greater in individuals with disabilities. Physical benefits include improvements in muscle strength, balance and flexibility, in addition to a reduction in osteoporosis, cardiovascular disease, obesity and diabetes. There are also significant psychological and social benefits of increased self-esteem and social integration.

Barriers

Participation in sport and physical activity is a right that should be afforded to all individuals. Unfortunately, several barriers exist that make it much harder for those with disabilities. It is important for all healthcare professionals and those that work with disabled individuals to appreciate these barriers and help in overcoming them. The barriers include but are not limited to the following:

- Facilities
  - Accessibility/transport
  - Adaptation of changing rooms and bathrooms
  - Availability of specialist equipment
  - Availability of coaches who understand disability sport
- Acceptance and understanding of disability sport by:
  - Coaches, managers, administrators
  - Medical personnel
  - Other athletes and team mates
- Financial
  - Cost of specialised equipment is usually more than for able-bodied participants
  - Cost of adapting facilities to cater for individuals with a disability
- Disabled individual
  - Self-esteem, picturing themselves as an athlete
  - Motivation to overcome barriers
- Lack of opportunity during childhood
- Parental and medical overprotection
- Cultural perceptions

Choosing the right sport

To ensure active and long-term participation in sport by an individual with a disability, it is important that they are given advice on choosing the sport that best suits their needs and abilities. There are several factors that should be considered:

- Individual preference – This is the most important factor as it is likely to help overcome any barriers that arise.
- The particular disability and its effect on:
  - Physical limitations
  - Cognitive ability
  - Social skills
  - Associated medical conditions (see p. 000)

- Characteristics of the sport
  - Physiological and physical demands
  - Risk of collision
  - Co-ordination skills required
- Facilities and equipment
  - Availability of adapted facilities in the local region
  - Availability of coaching staff
  - Cost and availability of specialist equipment

Travel

The increasing numbers of athletes with disabilities taking part in sport worldwide has been inspiring for all. However with this international expanse, arise certain challenges, particularly with regard to travel. From a logistical perspective, there may be difficulties in transporting specialised equipment such as wheelchairs and prostheses, in addition to the accessibility and adaptability of airplanes to carrying large numbers of athletes with various disabilities. Healthcare professionals travelling with athletes with disabilities will need to be aware of the usual risks of travel such as deep vein thrombosis and dehydration but also the possibility of aggravating medical problems that commonly occur in these athletes such as epilepsy, pressure sores and autonomic dysreflexia.

Further reading

Disability. In: MacAuley, D (ed), Oxford handbook of sport and exercise medicine. Oxford: Oxford University Press, 2007:657–674.

Webborn N. The disabled athlete. In: Brukner P and Khan K (eds), Clinical Sports Medicine, 3rd ed. McGraw-Hill, Australia, 2006:778–786.

Related topics of interest

- Disability and sport – medical problems (p. 59)
- Disability and sport – equipment (p. 56)
- Exercise and health (p. 106)

Diving – breath-hold and scuba

Key points

- Changes in pressure when diving cause barotrauma, nitrogen narcosis, acute oxygen toxicity and decompression illness
- Immersion and cold also cause problems
- Governing bodies set medical standards for divers

Introduction

Underwater swimming, when breath holding or using self-contained underwater breathing apparatus (scuba), is performed for both recreation and competitive sports, such as underwater hockey (breath-hold) and underwater orienteering (scuba).

Divers are exposed to conditions of high ambient pressure, cooling and circulatory changes that result in diseases unique to divers. Because an incapacitated diver usually drowns and because certain medical conditions predispose to diving-related illnesses, governing bodies set medical standards for participants.

Pressure at depth

At sea level, we breathe air (approximately 78% nitrogen, 21% oxygen and 1% other gases) at 1 bar pressure. (In fact, a standard atmosphere = 101 kPa = 1.013 bar.) For every 10 m that a diver descends, the pressure increases by 1 bar (100 kPa). Thus at 30 m, the ambient pressure on the diver is 4 bar and the partial pressures of constituent gases are increased fourfold. High partial pressures of gases are responsible for gas toxicity, including nitrogen narcosis and acute oxygen toxicity, and for decompression illness.

Breath-hold diving

During a breath-hold dive, the gas–containing spaces in the diver (lungs, middle ears, sinuses) are compressed in proportion to the pressure. One might imagine that a breath-hold diver could not descend to greater depths than will compress lungs fully inflated on the surface to residual volume at depth. In fact the record is deeper than 200 m or 21 bars. At that depth, the airspaces are compressed to about 300 mL and much of that gas is in rigid airspaces, for example the trachea. This can only be achieved because abdominal viscera and blood are displaced into the chest. The changes in gas volume can cause barotrauma of descent, such as a perforated eardrum.

The real risks are on ascent, usually triggered by the desire to breathe. At depth reduced lung volume causes reduced buoyancy. If the lungs are compressed by 5 L, the buoyancy loss is equivalent to carrying a 5-kg weight. So ascent to the surface requires strength and uses oxygen. During ascent, ambient pressure decreases, the lungs expand and the alveolar partial pressure of oxygen falls in proportion to the reduction in pressure. So does arterial partial pressure of oxygen. The reduction in brain oxygen tension may cause unconsciousness. As a result, a negatively buoyant diver will sink and drown. The risk of such 'shallow water blackouts' is increased by hyperventilation before a breath-hold dive. By blowing off carbon dioxide, hyperventilation increases the dive duration by delaying the stimulus to breathe until hypoxic drive is stimulated and a further reduction in partial pressure of oxygen on ascent causes unconsciousness.

Scuba diving

A scuba diver's breathing gas is delivered at his mouth at ambient pressure by his regulator or demand valve. At 30 m, the gas is delivered at 4 bars. If the breathing gas is air, the nitrogen contributes 78% of the total pressure, 3.12 bar, and oxygen 21%, 0.84 bar. Nitrogen dissolves in tissues and at depth the increased partial pressure results in more nitrogen dissolving in the diver's tissues. The raised partial pressures of nitrogen cause nitrogen narcosis. This causes progressive impairment of cognition as depth increases and is generally considered unacceptably dangerous when diving deeper than 50 m breathing air.

Drugs in sport – anabolic steroids

Key points

- Testosterone and related compounds have anabolic as well as androgenic actions
- They are abused by those aiming to increase muscle bulk – so the problem is in power events (sprints, shot-put, etc.)
- Widespread abuse in past – much more and effective testing now
- Major health risks and side effects
- Effects such as cardiac myopathy do not reverse on stopping taking the steroids

Testosterone and other steroids

Steroid hormones fall into four groups:
- Glucocorticoids (e.g. cortisone)
- Mineralocorticoids (e.g. aldosterone)
- Female sex steroid hormones (oestrogens, progesterone)
- Male sex steroid hormones (testosterone)

In sport, it is testosterone and related natural and synthetic steroids, the anabolic androgenic steroids (AASs), that are taken for their muscle-building action. However, the main actions of testosterone are on the male reproductive system:
- Development of male secondary sexual characteristics
- Control of spermatogenesis
- Feedback to hypothalamus to regulate follicle stimulating hormone (FSH), luteinizing hormone (LH)

Testosterone has the standard four-ring steroid structure with two additional methyl groups, making it a 19-carbon steroid. In the body, it is synthesised in the testes, ovaries and adrenal cortex. An isomer, epitestosterone, is always synthesised at the same time in a fixed ratio of testosterone: epitestosterone. Some testosterone is converted into oestradiol in the body by a process called aromatisation. This only becomes of interest when excess amounts of testosterone are present. Under these conditions, enough oestradiol can be produced to cause feminising effects in males (see below).

Plasma levels of testosterones average 0.6 mg/dL in males and 0.03 mg/dL in females, indicating immediately the likelihood that testosterone will improve performance in females more than in males. In the blood it is mostly bound to sex hormone-binding globulin. Nevertheless, enough of the compound is filtered into the urine to make urine testing straightforward. Testing using gas-liquid chromatography and mass spectroscopy is now technically very sophisticated. It is possible to look not just at single compounds but at the pattern of precursors and metabolites. This is important in testing for some steroids that occur naturally in small quantities (e.g. nandrolone) and for assessing the testosterone:epitestosterone ratio (1:1 is normal; anything above 4:1 is investigated further). It is also possible to examine carbon -12 to carbon -13 isotope ratios, and in this way reveal a synthetic origin for naturally occurring compounds.

Actions and effects

Testosterone acts on intracellular, cytoplasmic receptors. The receptor-hormone complex then translocates to the nucleus where it acts on DNA transcription. Steroid hormones thus have a direct action on patterns of protein synthesis in cells. A well-controlled study using large doses, closer to those used by steroid abusers, showed significant increases in muscle bulk and strength. It also found that these effects are additive to the effects seen with strength training. A 10-week programme of testosterone at supraphysiologic doses gave a 16% increase in strength on a squat test. The same treatment combined with intense strength training produced a 38% rise in strength.

What is the extent of abuse?

First some history, **Figure 7** shows the winning distances in the women's shot-put in Olympic Games from 1952 to 2012. For

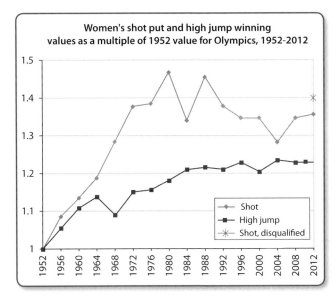

Figure 7 Women's shot-put and high jump winning value as a multiple of 1952 value for Olympics 1952–2012.

comparison, the winning heights for the high jump are plotted, with both expressed as a percentage of the 1952 level. In the 1950s and early 1960s, both events show a steady increase, probably reflecting the growth in athletics participation amongst women. From the early 1960s, the shot-put winning distance starts to increase rapidly until, by 1972, it is a remarkable 40% above the 1952 value. At this point the trend levels off. After 1988, the winning distance does something remarkable — it falls in every subsequent Olympics until 2004 when it was back to close to the high jump trend.

What does this graph represent? Two events were probably crucial. In 1976, the International Olympic Committee introduced testing for steroids. But most important of all, in 1989 the Berlin Wall came down and East and West Germany merged. From papers discovered after the fall of the wall, a major nationally sponsored programme of steroid administration in East Germany was revealed. All the shot-put winners in the years 1968-1988 were from Eastern Europe, with one exception. Notice the dip in 1984? This was the Los Angeles Olympics that were boycotted by the Russians and East Germans. Finally note the extra point in 2012. The winner on the day (from Belarus) put the shot 3% further, but tested positive for metenolone,

a synthetic anabolic steroid. So the gold medal went to the New Zealand athlete who had been second at the end of competition. Steroid use in power events may have fallen since the 1980s, but it has not gone away entirely.

What is the extent of steroid abuse now? With effective testing, both in and out of competition, the level of abuse has certainly fallen in recent years. If the shot-put trends are typical it may even be that top-level Olympic sports now have a relatively low level of abuse. But positives still occur. And the discovery in 2003 of THG (tetrahydrogestrinone, a previously unknown steroid) in urine samples from several top sprinters, American footballers and baseball players, shows how difficult it can be to be certain that steroids are not being used. Several cyclists giving evidence to the United States Anti-Doping Agency in the Lance Armstrong enquiry also admitted regular use of testosterone in a manner that mostly avoided detection.

Steroid abuse is not only a problem in sport. Abuse is widespread in bodybuilding with magazines openly on sale that advertise anabolics with no realistic discussion of the health risks. And anabolics are widely available over the internet. Surveys in the early 1990s in the United Kingdom show about 10% of gym users admitted using steroids. In surveys in the United States, including among high school children, higher figures have been reported. This is predominantly a problem in young men. There is little evidence of anabolic steroid use by women outside competitive power sports. The situation is complicated by the finding that many anabolic users also take other hormones (growth hormone, insulin, human chorionic gonadotropin) and are also often users of other illicit drugs such as heroin and cocaine.

The health risks and side effects

- Cardiac myopathy
- Liver toxicity and liver cancer
- Male sterility, gynaecomastia
- Masculinisation in females
- In children, stunting of growth
- Other side effects: acne, baldness, aggression

NB: Despite what the adverts say, all anabolic steroids are androgenic.

The cardiac and liver problems represent major health risks. A recent examination using echocardiography in power lifters and weight lifters indicated an unhealthy thickening of the left ventricular wall in those using steroids. And importantly, very little recovery in those who had stopped using

steroids for at least 1 year (and on average 2 years). This lays to rest another myth amongst abusers that any bad effects will rapidly reverse on stopping use.

Is there excess mortality among anabolic steroid users? The answer, at least, in Finnish power lifters, appears to be yes. At a 12-year follow-up, out of 62 champion power lifters from the period 1977-1982, eight were dead (13%). This was five times the mortality in a matched control group. There is also concern that long-term problems associated with the increase in use in young males in the 1980s have yet to surface.

Other banned substances related to AAS abuse

The beta-2 agonist clenbuterol has been abused for its supposed anabolic action and is on the prohibited list. Antioestrogen compounds are banned as they are used to control feminising side effects of taking large amounts of testosterone. It is one of the paradoxes of AAS abuse aimed at developing a muscular body that sterility results, plus breast growth in males. The latter is due to conversion of excess testosterone to oestradiol in the body, with the inevitable consequences. Antioestrogens can inhibit this effect. The only male competitors likely to be taking them are AAS users, hence they are banned and urine samples are checked for them.

Further reading

American College of Obstetricians and Gynecoligists (ACOG). ACOG Committee Opinion No. 484: Performance enhancing anabolic steroid abuse in women. Obstet Gynecol 2011; 117:1016–1018.

Baggish AL, Weiner RB, Kanayama G, Hudson JI, Picard MH, et al. Long-term anabolic-androgenic steroid use is associated with left ventricular dysfunction. Circ Heart Fail 2010; 3:472–476.

Cooper C. Run, swim, throw, cheat. The science behind drugs in sport. Chapt 6, pp131-158. Oxford, Oxford University Press, 2012.

Kanayama G, Hudson JI, Pope HG Jr. Long-term psychiatric and medical consequences of anabolic-androgenic steroid abuse: a looming public health concern? Drug Alcohol Depend 2008; 98:1–12.

Ungerleider, S. Faust's gold. Inside the East German doping machine. 2nd Edn. CreateSpace Independent Publishing Platform, 2013.

Related topics of interest

Drugs in sport – blood doping, erythropoietin and altitude training

Key points

- Performance in endurance events can be improved by increasing the oxygen-carrying capacity of the blood
- This can be achieved by blood transfusions or by injecting erythropoietin (EPO) or related drugs
- It is important that endurance sports move to regular blood sampling to detect suspicious changes in haematological measures
- Altitude training provides a legal way to elevate blood haemoglobin although endurance performance gains may be small

Haemoglobin and performance

The basic idea is to raise the oxygen-carrying capacity of the blood and improve performance in events involving aerobic exercise, that is any events lasting more than 1-2 min. This can be done by increasing the haemoglobin (Hb) content in the blood either by legal means (altitude training) or illegal means (blood doping or 'boosting' or use of the hormone EPO).

We have 3×10^{13} red blood cells, containing a total of 900 g of haemoglobin. Red cells last on average 120 days, so we need to replace 1/120 every day, that is 2.5×10^{11} cells, or 3 million every second. This massive production of red cells takes place in the bone marrow.

Table 5 shows the normal ranges of haemoglobin and haematocrit.

Blood doping

This is the direct method. Blood, or more usually concentrated red cells, is transfused via an intravenous catheter. If blood cells from a donor are used, this is heterologous

Table 5 Normal ranges of Hb and haematocrit		
	Men	**Women**
Hb, g/dl	14-16	12.5-15
Haematocrit	42-50%	38-47%

Hb: Amount of this oxygen-carrying protein within red blood cells. Units g/decilitre blood (1 decilitre = 100 dL).

Haematocrit: Proportion of red blood cells to the total blood volume (= packed cell volume).

transfusion. Alternatively, the athlete's own blood can be collected, stored, then transfused back – this is autologous transfusion. Either way, careful storage of red cells is necessary. Blood boosting definitely works, although estimates vary of the extent of improvements in performance. Laboratory studies show that endurance performance is typically improved by 2-3% and maximal oxygen uptake (VO_2max) up by 13%.

Although blood doping clearly works and so demonstrates the usefulness of boosting blood oxygen-carrying capacity for endurance events, there are a number of difficulties. If heterologous transfusion is used, then great care needs to be taken over tissue matching. In addition, there is always the risk of getting a blood-borne infection such as AIDS or hepatitis. Autologous transfusion means long periods out of competition as it takes 4-6 weeks to recover from a blood donor session. In addition, the effects of the donation begin to wane within 3-4 weeks.

Blood doping was extensive in professional cycling in the late 1990s and throughout the 2000s. First, there was the finding by Spanish police as part of Operation Puerta of blood transfusion equipment and stored blood. The stored blood could be traced to a number of top cyclists and the start of the 2006 Tour de France was affected in a major way with the last-minute withdrawal of several top riders.

More recently, the evidence garnered by the United States Anti-Doping Agency as part of its Lance Armstrong enquiry has filled in much of the detail. With the introduction of Athlete Biological Passports it will be much more difficult in future, but there are questions about just how sensitive this programme will be. It has been suggested that relatively small transfusions (1 unit) will still not be detected. Blood doping has also been detected in endurance track athletes, with several top runners barred from the 2012 Olympics on the basis of anomalies in their haematological data.

Erythropoietin

EPO is a hormone that is released from the kidney in response to tissue hypoxia and travels to the bone marrow. It is a large peptide (or small protein) comprising 165 amino acids with a large number of attached carbohydrate residues (it is 30% glycosylated). In the bone marrow, it stimulates production of pronormoblasts (immediate red blood cell (erythrocyte) precursors) from committed unipotential colony-forming unit - erythroid cells. Pronormoblasts, in turn, develop into normoblasts. The normoblasts start to lose their nucleus and become reticulocytes. The reticulocytes enter the blood system and finally develop into red blood cells with no nuclear material visible at all.

Recombinant human EPO is used to treat anaemia associated with kidney failure, for example for those on dialysis, and so is widely available. EPO-induced increases in blood Hb, like blood doping, increase performance in endurance exercise tests in the laboratory.

It is important not to get Hb too high. The effect of blood viscosity on haemodynamics means the heart works harder, and so there is an increased risk of heart problems. Pathologically elevated red cell counts also lead to a higher risk of clots. But many people who live at altitude have elevated Hb without any circulatory or cardiac problems – but maybe have made compensating adaptations. A spate of unexplained sudden deaths in cyclists in late 1980s was attributed to the arrival of EPO on the scene. There have also been problems with side effects in some long-term dialysis patients.

Some sports (e.g. cycling) set upper limits on haematocrit (50% for male competitors) and ban on health grounds (i.e. risks due to increased blood viscosity). But 1% of the normal population (and 20% of native highlanders) have haematocrits at or above this level. Cyclists apparently get by the haematocrit test by having saline infusions shortly before being tested at the start of events. The short-term boost to blood volume may also aid performance. Others use high molecular weight expanders. But these are easily detected over a long period, as almost the entire Finnish cross-country skiing team found to their cost at the world championships in 2001 when hydroxy-ethyl starch was detected.

Detecting EPO use

It is possible to distinguish recombinant EPO from endogenous EPO, and this can even be done in urine samples. Unfortunately, EPO has a short life in the body and is only detectable for 1–2 days. As blood cells last 120 days, single tests at the time of competition are useless. Interestingly, a longer lasting version of EPO is now available for clinical use – darbepoetin or Aranesp. This is effective for longer, so patients (or athletes) need fewer injections, and this is more convenient and cheaper. It does make it easier to detect, however, and this version of EPO was in fact successfully detected in competitors in the 2002 Winter Olympics. Continuous erythropoietin receptor activator (CERA) is also now available, and injections are only needed every 3–4 weeks. But this agent can be detected in urine. After testing became available in late 2008, several medal winners from the 2008 Beijing Summer Olympics were disqualified following retrospective testing for CERA.

Another approach to EPO detection is to count the number of immature red cells (reticulocytes) in the blood. This rises in a characteristic way with EPO supplementation and the effect is detectable for several weeks. Counts of reticulocytes form part of the Athlete Biological Passport.

It seems likely that EPO use is on the wane thanks to more extensive testing, particularly in those sports that are taking blood samples and implementing the biological passport. A relevant observation here is that average speeds in the major cycling road races peaked in 2003 and have fallen slightly since then.

Altitude acclimatisation

Living at altitudes above about 2000 m leads to enough tissue anoxia to stimulate EPO release and red cell production. For example, a group who spent 30 days at the top of Pikes Peak in Colorado had average increases in Hb from 13.7 on arrival to 16.2 at departure, with parallel increases in haematocrit (from 43 to 48%). These are similar to the increases seen with blood doping or EPO use. However, on return to sea level, little if any increase in endurance performance is found. The reasons are complex. Firstly, it is not possible to train at maximum intensity at altitude just because the atmospheric oxygen levels are lower. Secondly, the adjustments of the circulation to altitude involve more than just an increased Hb. Hyperventilation, a normal response to the lowered oxygen level, leads to increased carbon dioxide excretion and eventually to a reduction in the buffering power of the blood. This may reduce performance levels as lactic acid produced during high-intensity exercise will not be so well neutralised. There may also be reductions in blood volume and shifts in the Hb dissociation curve, changes that may impair performance. Note, however, that for competitions held at altitude, suitable acclimatisation is essential.

To get round some of these problems, coaches have developed the 'live high, train low' approach. You live and sleep up the mountain, but travel down to sea level to train. This option is now available to those of us who do not live conveniently close to a suitable mountain – the nitrogen tent or house. Athletes live in nitrogen tents with the oxygen level reduced to 15-16% (equivalent to being at 2500 m altitude). They can therefore train in the normal way, but should get a useful boost in blood Hb due to the time spent at simulated altitude. There will still be problems with other, disadvantageous, circulatory adaptations. Most experimental studies have shown useful gains in Hb and performance, but the only double blind study in well-trained athletes found no significant increases. The possibility of placebo effects cannot be ruled out.

Altitude (real or simulated) acclimatisation is not the same as blood boosting as the overall changes to blood and circulation are more complex, and deliver smaller, if any, advantages in terms of sea-level performance.

Further reading

Armstrong DJ. In: Mottram DR (Ed). Drugs in Sport, 5th edn. Abingdon: Routledge,, 2010, chapts. 9 and 24.

Lombardi G, Banfi G, Lippi G, Sanchis-Gomar F. Ex vivo erythrocyte generation and blood doping. Blood Transfus 2013; 11:161-163.
Perneger TV. Speed trends of major cycling races: does slower mean cleaner? Int J Sports Med 2010; 31:261-264.

Siebenmann C, Robach P, Jacobs RA, Rasmussen P, Nordsborg N, et al. 'Live high-train low' using normobaric hypoxia: a double-blinded, placebo-controlled study. J Appl Physiol 2012; 112:106-17.
United States Anti-Doping Agency. Reasoned decision of the United States Anti-Doping Agency on disqualification and ineligibility, claimant v. Lance Armstrong, Respondent. 2012. http://d3epuodzu3wuis.cloudfront.net/ReasonedDecision.pdf. Accessed 13 Nov 2013.

Related topics of interest

- Drugs in sport – overview (p. 74)
- Drugs in sport – anabolic steroids (p. 68)
- Drugs in sport – the administrative framework: doping control procedures (p. 78)
- Gene doping (p. 135)

Drugs in sport – overview

Key points

- Education is the key to minimise drug use in sport
- Anti-doping policy is organised on an international level, the key organisation being the World Anti-Doping Agency (WADA)
- The major classes of doping agents are anabolic steroids, erythropoietin and stimulants

Introduction

Several topics will be devoted to aspects of drug abuse in sport. However, right from the outset, it is important to stress education. The best way to ensure that those involved in sport do not resort to performance-enhancing drugs or procedures is by creating the correct climate. The fundamental issue is to ask what the sport is about? If it is not about fair competition, then really it has lost its value. This is certainly true for the individual. If you know you won only because you cheated, what is the point? Hence, education programmes run by anti-doping agencies, such as the '100% Me' in the UK and 'I compete clean' in the USA, are important in the fight against drug cheating. A key role for sports doctors and other health professionals is in education about health risks - which for many drugs are only too real (see Anabolic steroids and Blood doping).

Winning by cheating may be viewed by some as simply about obtaining a lot of money (and peer popularity). So highly paid professional sports are likely to need to be policed particularly closely. Here education is still important, but this time, educating the audience. While people are still happy to pay money to watch drug cheats, then there is clearly a major job of public education waiting to be done.

Anti-doping policy and WADA

Anti-drugs policies operate within an administrative and legal framework that is now well established. The formation of the World Anti-Doping Agency (WADA) in 1999 has provided the machinery for moving the policy forward and we now have internationally agreed systems for penalties and for the regular review of the list of banned drugs and methods. We have a Court of Arbitration in Sport. We have a major research programme concerned with improving the information about performance-enhancing drugs and how best to detect them. Pretty much everyone is signed up - all the Olympic sports, plus most of the professional ones (e.g. FIFA for association football).

Testing continues to improve and to become more fair and rigorous. However, one point worth stressing here is the need for effective out-of-competition testing. Many of the most abused drugs have effects that last significantly longer than the time for which they can be detected. So sports that really want to deal with drugs, such as anabolic steroids or erythropoietin, need to test potential winners before the competition, either with home or training ground visits. And these visits must be unannounced. Many sports now have a very thorough 'Whereabouts' programme to enable effective out-of-competition testing. More on this and other administrative issues is given in Drugs in sport – the administrative framework.

The main classes of drugs that are abused are stimulants, anabolic steroids, erythropoietin (plus illegal blood doping), hormones affecting growth and opiate painkillers. The classes as listed by WADA are given in **Table 6**. Other substances that are banned for specific sports are alcohol and beta blockers. Very detailed information on banned substances is held on the web-based Global Drug Reference Online (Global DRO) run by a partnership between UK Anti-Doping, the Canadian Centre for Ethics in Sport and the United States Anti-Doping Agency. Usefully, this database lists by proprietary names as well as generic ones and is updated every year. The current version is available at http://www.globaldro.com/.

Steroids get their own topic in this book, as do blood doping and erythropoietin. Other

Table 6 WADA 2013 prohibited list – summary of classes of substance and methods banned to different extents		
Prohibited substances		**Prohibited methods**
1. Substances and methods prohibited at all times (in- and out-of-competition)	S0. Non-approved substances Any pharmacological substance which is not addressed by any of the subsequent sections of the list and with no current approval by any governmental regulatory health authority for human therapeutic use (e.g drugs under pre-clinical or clinical development or discontinued, designer drugs, substances approved only for veterinary use) is prohibited at all times. S1. Anabolic agents S2. Peptide hormones, growth factors and related substances S3. Beta-2 agonists S4. Hormone and metabolic modulators S5. Diuretics and other masking agents	M1. manipulation of blood and blood components M2. chemical and physical manipulation M3. gene doping
2. Substances and methods prohibited in-competition In addition to the categories s0 to s5 and m1 to m3 defined above	S6. Stimulants S7. Narcotics S8. Cannabinoids S9. Glucocorticosteroids	–
3. Substances prohibited in competition in particular sports	P1. Alcohol Alcohol (ethanol) is prohibited in the following sports Aeronautic, archery, automobile, karate, motorcycling, powerboating P2. Beta-blockers Prohibited in the following sports. Archery (also prohibited out-of-competition), automobile, billiards (all disciplines), darts, golf, shooting (also prohibited out-of-competition), skiing/snowboarding in ski jumping, freestyle aerials/halfpipe and snowboard halfpipe/big air	–

banned substances will be briefly discussed now.

Stimulants

These are the traditional performance enhancers and all are nearly based either on adrenaline (epinephrine) or amphetamine. They need to be taken at the time of the event and so can be detected readily by testing during competitions. A problem has been cough and cold remedies that include significant amounts of adrenaline-related compounds. Fortunately, pseudephedrine has now been removed from the banned list. Many others, however, remain. A rather different stimulant is caffeine. There used to be a threshold for this, but it has now been removed altogether from the list (but keep an eye on the Global DRO – drugs can be reinstated). Another stimulant, modafinil, has also been the cause of positive drug tests. It is an essential role of the sports doctors to advise clearly on what is allowed and what is not. A useful resource for this is the Global DRO mentioned above.

Hormones

Various hormones that affect growth have been abused and are on the prohibited list, including growth hormone, human chorionic gonadotrophin (hCG) and insulin. Growth hormone has been used to increase muscle growth and reduce body fat. The evidence that it is performance enhancing is quite weak. However, it is thought that the main abusers may use it in combination with anabolic steroids and possibly insulin. No controlled trials of these combination treatments have been carried out. However, there are no legitimate reasons for a sports person to be taking growth hormone and there are health risks (e.g. cardiac effects). Testing was introduced in 2010 using a test based on the ratio of different isoforms. The recombinant rHGH is a single isoform whereas in the body, several are secreted. A new test based on abnormal levels of endogenous compounds that are directly affected by growth hormone (insulin-like growth factor-I and the amino terminal pro-peptide of type III collagen (P-III-NP) was introduced for the 2012 Olympics and Paralympics. This resulted in two positives for powerlifters in the 2012 Paralympics. Both tests require a blood sample.

hCG is used by males to boost testosterone production from the testes. It appears to be mainly used as an adjunct to androgenic steroid administration (see Anabolic steroid abuse in sport). Exogenous administration of testosterone or analogues leads to reduced gonadotropin release via the normal physiological feedback to the hypothalamus and pituitary. Thus, while exogenous steroids raise the hormone levels, endogenous secretion shuts down. hCG can counter this effect and maintain testicular function. Abuse of hCG is thought to be widespread. It can be detected in urine so standard testing procedures can pick up hCG abuse and several positives have been reported, including cases in major league baseball and American football.

Opiate painkillers

Morphine and related narcotics are banned. Only codeine is allowed. Again, these are likely to be in the body at the time of competition so detecting them with testing at events is straightforward.

Diuretics

These are banned principally as they can cause a urine sample to become very dilute, thus making illegal compounds harder to detect.

Other banned compounds

Beta blockers are banned in competition in sports like shooting as they reduce tremor. Steroids of the glucocorticoid family are generally allowed out of competition, but are banned in competition. However, preparations for skin use are not banned. And steroid inhalers are permitted as long as a Therapeutic Use Exemption (TUE) has been obtained. A TUE requires application in advance using a standard form, with appropriate medical support and information. This is an important system that ensures that where a banned drug is essential for medical purposes, it is still possible for an individual to compete. More information on TUEs will be given in the next topic.

Is drug testing worth the effort?

The complexities of anti-doping regulations and the cost of effective testing programmes can lead to an attitude that says, well maybe we should just let people do what they want to improve performance. After all, the sport would still be entertaining. But a moment's reflection shows that the fight against drug cheats is worth it. Why are we entertained by sport? Why do we encourage our children to play sports? It is to improve our and their lives, to broaden our humanity. Cheating, often with health-damaging drugs, is the antithesis of these things. If we want sport to continue as a vehicle for improving ourselves and our society, then we must educate people so that drug cheating becomes marginalised further. And we must be vigilant — and pay the price in money terms and in inconvenience — to ensure that no one, for monetary or other motives, undermines one of the greatest human endeavours.

The ultimate horror that awaits any laissez-faire attitude is gene doping. This is the use of gene therapy methods to artificially alter an individual's physiology to improve performance. This route could lead to sport as a gene-fuelled freak show. Some of the issues involved in gene doping are discussed in a separate topic. But let us hope that this problem can be defeated by a combination of education and scientific methods for detecting the practice.

Further reading

Cooper, C. Run, swim, throw, cheat. The science behind drugs in sport. Oxford: Oxford University Press, 2012.

Mottram DR (ed.) Drugs in sport, 5th edn. Abingdon: Routledge, 2010.

Related topics of interest

- Drugs in sport – anabolic steroids (p. 68)
- Drugs in sport – blood doping, erythropoietin and altitude training (p. 71)
- Drugs in sport – the administrative framework: doping-control procedures (p. 78)
- Gene doping (p. 135)

Drugs in sport – the administrative framework: doping-control procedures

Key points

- The formation of the World Anti-Doping Agency (WADA) has established an almost universally accepted set of rules for dealing with doping violations, the WADA code
- Key features of the code are:
  - it is only necessary to provide evidence 'to the comfortable satisfaction of the hearing body'
  - a standard 2–year ban is imposed for a first violation, a lifetime ban for a second
- Therapeutic use exemptions (TUEs) allow athletes to compete when receiving a substance on the banned list for medical purposes
- Doping control procedures involve the supervised collection of urine sample, plus sometimes a blood sample, and their analysis by a WADA-accredited laboratory using the latest analytical methods

WADA and antidoping organisations (ADOs)

The legal and administrative framework for antidoping programmes has much improved in recent years due to international cooperative action. The key event was the setting up of an independent body, the WADA, in 1999. This body is jointly funded by the Olympic movement and national governments. It has moved rapidly to bring uniformity into policy and practice across all sports and all countries. A detailed WADA code covering antidoping policy has been adopted by all major sports organisations. This code now forms the basis of a UNESCO convention and has so far been ratified by 171 of 195 UNESCO member states.

Within each sport, international governing bodies supervise the antidoping policy. These bodies have all signed up to the WADA code. Within many countries, there are national antidoping agencies, often set up as independent bodies (e.g. the US Anti-Doping Agency (USADA) and UK Anti-Doping (UKAD)). Much practical antidoping activity for individual sports is provided by national antidoping bodies. The best thing about this practice is, it is best practice that the national antidoping agency is independent of both national sports bodies and international sports federations. This is because there is an obvious conflict of interest for sports organisations when a star athlete tests positive. It is likely that such an individual would have become very useful to senior administrators as the public face of their sport, so they would have no interest in seeing them banned.

Key points from the WADA code

The WADA code runs to 135 pages, but much of this is commentary explaining the individual articles. After some initial definitions, there are four main sections. The largest section deals with doping control (see the next paragraph). Three shorter sections deal with education and research, with the responsibilities of signatories such as national governing bodies and international associations, and with acceptance, compliance, modification and interpretation.

Doping control in the WADA code

Article 2 covers rule violations and article 2.1.1 restates what was already the accepted principle, i.e. 'It is each athlete's personal duty to ensure that no Prohibited Substance enters his or her body.' Rule violations related to trafficking, failure to provide whereabouts information and tampering with doping control are also covered. Article 3 covers the important issue of burden of proof. Crucially, it is not necessary to establish doping 'beyond reasonable doubt'. A lesser criterion is given: 'to the comfortable satisfaction of the hearing body'. This is more than just a 'balance of probabilities', but less than 'beyond reasonable doubt'. WADA's role in taking over publication of the Prohibited List is covered in article 4 of the code. This section also covers standardisation of procedures for TUEs. Articles 5 and 6 cover aspects of testing and analysis. The accreditation of laboratories becomes the responsibility of WADA. Article 7 covers the tricky area of results management. Who tells whom, what and when? When the A sample has given an adverse result, the athlete is informed by the ADO involved and can request that the B sample be checked. Provisional suspension from competition can be imposed before the B sample results are available. Various safeguards are set out in detail. Exactly who is responsible for publishing details of the violation is not set out in the code. Article 10 covers sanctions against the athlete and here the simple rule is: a 2-year suspension for first violation and lifetime ban for the second one. This was one of the most contentious compromises in the code. But in the end, there was an agreement that it was best to have a single 'across the board' rule that would be simple to administer and difficult to appeal. In practice, many cases of shorter bans have occurred. Article 13 deals with appeals and sets up a Court of Arbitration for Sport (CAS) to which international-level competitors can appeal. Interestingly, it is also possible for the International Olympic Committee or WADA to appeal a result.

Therapeutic use exemptions

An important role for sports doctors is to ensure that any necessary medication involving a prohibited agent is notified to the relevant authority by requesting a TUE. A TUE application must be made and approved before competition and lasts for a specified period (whose duration depends on the condition being treated). For international-level competitions, and for international-level athletes in any competition, the form must be submitted to the international governing body. For national-level competitors, the form goes to the relevant national federation or to the national ADO. The form requires the notifying medical practitioner to justify not using a different medication that is not on the banned list (e.g. a nonsteroidal anti-inflammatory rather than a steroid). Appropriate documentation is required (including test results, images, etc.) along with dosage information. If a TUE is denied, the athlete can appeal, if necessary all the way to the CAS.

Procedures vary a little between sports, and with the level of competition, so it is necessary to be familiar with any special rules that may apply. Until recently, a lot of TUEs were for beta-2 inhalers. However, since 2010-12, inhaled salmeterol, salbutimol (up to 1600 µg/day) and formoterol (up to 36 µg/day) are no longer prohibited. However, terbutaline is still on the banned list and so still needs a TUE.

Doping control procedures

This section deals with some of the important 'nuts and bolts' aspects of drug testing in sport, including sample collection rules and laboratory methods. For athletes, governing bodies and other ADOs, WADA has developed a web-based database management system, the anti-doping administration and management system (ADAMS). This simplifies the daily activities for everyone involved in the antidoping system and, at the same time, allows central bodies to monitor the pattern of antidoping activities and to gather statistics.

Samples may be collected at events 'in competition' or during training 'out of competition'. At major events, a team from the relevant antidoping agency will set up a doping-control station and generally test all winners plus a random sample of non-winners. Subjects for out-of-competition testing generally include only elite level performers likely to figure in national championships or international events. WADA, in its out-of-competition testing, also looks out for athletes showing unexpected increases in form.

At doping control, the subject urinates into a suitable container under observation from a member of the doping control team. This is necessary, as attempts have been made in the past to substitute someone else's urine. The sample is divided between two containers, A and B. The samples are taken to an accredited laboratory, of which there are now 33 worldwide. There the B sample is stored and the A sample is analysed. Key analytical methods are gas chromatography, high-pressure liquid chromatography, mass spectroscopy (combined with gas chromatography) and immunoassay. Similar steps are used for taking blood samples. Blood sampling will become more and more common as certain agents can only be detected from blood samples (e.g. growth hormone) and haematological data is important for building the athlete's biological passport (see below). However, blood sampling is more expensive so most doping control still depends on urine samples. At he London Olympics in 2012, for example, 4,686 antidoping tests were carried out, of which 3,729 were on urine samples and 957 on blood.

Whereabouts

For out-of-competition testing, essential for detecting steroid and erythropoietin use, the ADOs need to know where athletes are. So all athletes are now required to provide 'whereabouts' information. They must provide a time and place for 1 h every day. If they fail to do this, or are not at the designated location, on three occasions within 18 months, they receive a ban for 1 to 2 years. Procedures have been simplified since the start of the system to try to avoid unintentional mistakes. Athletes can enter the information using ADAMS via the web. They can also update information by phone or e-mail. The importance of enforcement is demonstrated by the evidence collected by the USADA in the Lance Armstrong enquiry. Here, top cyclists confessed to 'hiding' from the doping control officers, who at this time were not rigorously following up what was at the time (late 1990s, early 2000s), a less formalised system.

Biological passports

As mentioned above, in several sports (cycling, athletics, swimming, triathlon and modern pentathlon), the longitudinal pattern of test results is being studied to see if doping is occurring. At present, this is only for haematological parameters (blood count, percentage reticulocytes etc). However the intentions are to extend this to steroid levels. There is a lot of variation in hormone levels and blood measures between individuals. However, in a given individual, the measures will be pretty stable. It should therefore be easier to detect new use of endogenous compounds such as testosterone, and also blood doping, by comparing new test values with those collected in the past. A number of doping bans have already resulted from abnormal patterns seen in the biological passport.

Further reading

Cooper, C. Run, swim, throw, cheat. The science behind drugs in sport. Oxford: Oxford University of Press, 2012:223-242.

Green GA. Doping control for the team physician: a review of drug testing procedures in sport. Am J Sports Med 2006; 34(10):1690--1698.

WADA Code: Published on the Internet. Available at http://www.wada-ama.org/en/World-Anti-Doping-Program/Sports-and-Anti-Doping-Organizations/The-Code/. Accessed 13 Nov 2013.

Very useful and clear information is on the USADA site: http://www.usada.org/program/. Accessed 13 Nov 2013.

Related topics of interest

Elbow – instability

Key points

- The commonest mechanism for elbow dislocation is falling on an outstretched hand leading to axial compression in combination with supination and valgus force on the elbow
- This combination of forces leads to a 'circle' of soft tissue and/or bone damage that starts from the lateral side and progresses medially through stages
- Once reduced, most acute elbow dislocations that are not associated with fractures could be treated nonoperatively whereas chronic posterolateral instability commonly requires surgery

Overview

The primary function of the elbow joint is to place the hand in a variety of positions around the body and space. To achieve this, it requires absolute mobility and stability.

The elbow joint complex consists of three distinct joints: the humero-ulnar joint, the humero-radial joint and the proximal radio-ulnar joint. The stability of this complex is dependent on both static and dynamic factors. The primary static stabilisers include humero-ulnar articulation, the medial collateral ligament (MCL) and the lateral collateral ligament (LCL) (**Figure 8**). Secondary static stabilizers include the capsule, radial head and flexor/extensor origins. Dynamic stability is provided by all the muscles around the elbow complex. These structures may be damaged by a number of mechanisms in athletes causing significant functional deficit and resulting in a variety of conditions that can manifest as elbow instability.

Pathology

There are a number of different mechanism by which elbow ligaments may be damaged.

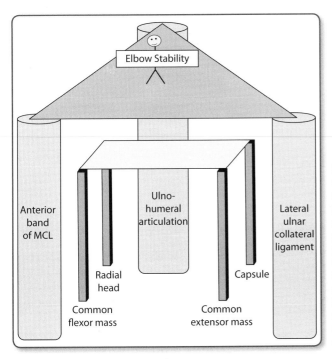

Figure 8 The primary stabilisers of the elbow are anterior band of MCL, ulnar component of LCL and the bony constrains of ulno-humeral articulation (as presented by the large pale grey pillars). With dysfunction of any one of these primary stabilisers, then stability is dependent on the secondary stabilizers (as presented by the smaller dark grey pillars), which include common flexor and extensor mass, radial head and the capsule.

Posterolateral rotatory subluxation or dislocation of the elbow (acute)

This is the most common mode of elbow dislocation (more common than varus posteromedial injuries (PMRI)) (see below). Falls on extended elbow and outstretched hand leads to external rotation moment of the forearm and internal rotation moment of the humerus on the elbow joint. In addition, there is also a valgus force resulting in a combination torque of external rotation, valgus and axial compression on the elbow. This combination of forces lead to a 'circle' of soft tissue and/or bone damage that starts from the lateral side and progresses medially through stages (**Table 7**). Whether the disruption progresses to the next stage or not is dependent on the energy of the injury.

Clinical features of each stage are different as presented in **Table 7**. Treatment is dependent on the stage of injury, as demonstrated in the algorithm in **Figure 9**.

Acute varus injury damaging LCL

Acute LCL injuries usually occur as part of the posterolatral rotatory subluxation/dislocation spectrum (see above), so management would be as that presented by the algorithm for the treatment of acute posterolateral rotatory subluxation/dislocation.

These injuries are also often associated with radial head or coronoid process fractures. When these fractures are treated by operative fixation, LCL must also be repaired.

Acute isolated LCL injuries are usually treated nonoperatively.

Chronic posterolateral rotator instability (PLRI)

These are secondary to insufficiency of the lateral ulnar collateral ligament. This sufficiency may be secondary to:
- Posterolateral rotatory subluxation or dislocation of the elbow (i.e. previous acute elbow dislocation, see above)
- Latrogenic damage to LCL, i.e. in tennis elbow surgery

Table 7 Posterolateral rotatory subluxation or dislocation of the elbow: soft tissue damage progresses in a circle from lateral to medial resulting in a spectrum of damage (the Hori circle of soft tissue injury)				
Stage 1 (PLRI)	Stage 2 (perched)	Stage 3 (dislocated) (3 parts)		
		Stage 3a	Stage 3b	Stage 3c
– Ulnar band of LCL is distrupted – Postero-lateral rotator subluxation which reduces spontaneously – Elbow stable throughout ROM, but positive lateral pivot shift test	– Other lateral structure as well as anterior and posterior capsule are damaged – Concave medial edge of ulna rest on the trochlea – Can be reduced by minimal force or self manipulation – Ulno-humeral gapping in extension but elbow is stable	– Disruption extends to MCL including posterior band, but anterior band of MCL is preserved – Reduction usually easily achievable with gentle manipulation – Elbow unstable in extension, but becomes stable with pronation (pronation locks the lateral side) – Radial head and coronoid fractures may be seen in this stage	– Disruption includes the entire MCL complex including anterior band – Elbow unstable in extension even with pronation – Elbow may become stable in flexion	– Disruption of the entire soft tissue from the humerus – >90°C of flexion is required to maintain the reduction

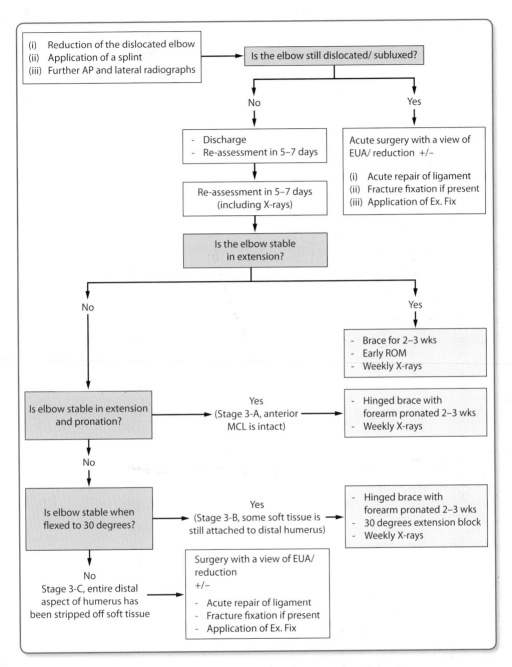

(i)   Reduction of the dislocated elbow
(ii) Application of a splint
(iii) Further AP and lateral radiographs

Is the elbow still dislocated/ subluxed?

No

Yes

- Discharge
- Re-assessment in 5–7 days

Acute surgery with a view of
EUA/ reduction +/–

(i)   Acute repair of ligament
(ii) Fracture fixation if present
(iii) Application of Ex. Fix

Re-assessment in 5–7 days
(including X-rays)

Is the elbow stable
in extension?

No

Yes

- Brace for 2–3 wks
- Early ROM
- Weekly X-rays

Is elbow stable in extension
and pronation?

Yes
(Stage 3-A, anterior
MCL is intact)

- Hinged brace with
  forearm pronated 2–3 wks
- Weekly X-rays

No

Is elbow stable when
flexed to 30 degrees?

Yes
(Stage 3-B, some soft tissue is
still attached to distal humerus)

- Hinged brace with
  forearm pronated 2–3 wks
- 30 degrees extension block
- Weekly X-rays

No
Stage 3-C, entire distal
aspect of humerus has
been stripped off soft tissue

Surgery with a view of EUA/
reduction
+/–

- Acute repair of ligament
- Fracture fixation if present
- Application of Ex. Fix

Figure 9 Algorithm for the management of acute posterolateral rotatory elbow dislocation.

- Previous acute varus injury damaging LCL,
- LCL chronic attenuation as a result of:
  - Long standing cubitas varus deformity
    (traumatic/ atrumatic)
  - Long-term crutch users, and
  - Inflammatory elbow conditions

Clinical features

Symptoms may include:
- Previous injury/ dislocation, surgery or
  history of inflammatory elbow conditions
- Lateral elbow pain

Particular motions that aggravate the lateral elbow pain include:

- Pushing up from a chair to stand up (see below)
- Lifting weights with a supinated forearm
- Mechanical symptoms such as locking or clicking
- Elbow not feeling quite stable

Examination findings may include:

- Elbow deformity (i.e. cubital varus)
- Scars from previous surgery (i.e. lateral epicondylitis surgery)
- Forced external rotation in of the semiflexed elbow joint produces pain and discomfort
- Positive 'pivot shift' test

Elbow is extended while applying valgus and external rotation to the forearm. In presence of PLRI, as the elbow is extended, radial head subluxes posteriorly from the humerus. With flexion, it relocates back into the joint. This manoeuvre may also lead to apprehension without any radial head subluxation. This may need to be performed under anaesthesia.

- Positive 'push up' test
- Pushing body weight up from an armchair leads to pain or apprehension

Investigations

- Plain radiograph (X-ray)
- Deformity/previous fractures/subluxation of radial head
- Examination under fluoroscopy provides additional information,
- Magnetic resonance imaging (MRI) Accuracy may be improved with MRI arthrogram

Treatment

Management of chronic PLRI is mainly operative with reconstruction or 'refixation' of the lateralm ligament complex. In presence of significant deformity, osteotomy must also be considered.

Return to sport

Generally speaking, following the reconstruction, athletes should not return to contact sport for about 6 months after surgery.

Posteromedial complex instability

Varus PMRI are certainly less frequent than the posterolateral elbow instability. The mechanism of the injury involves a fall onto the extended elbow with the forearm in pronation. With this forearm pronation on the humerus, distraction forces on the lateral joint line result in failure of the LCL. In addition, humeral trochlea impacts on the anteromedial coronoid facet resulting in fracture of this facet. There is subluxation of the joint although this, in some cases, may only be appreciated with stress views. MCL injuries and complete dislocation may fallow with continued force.

These are usually unstable injuries with potential persistent elbow incongruity and surgery is generally indicated. Surgical steps include:

Examination Under Anaesthesia (EUA).

Coronoid fracture must be addressed. The exact surgical option is dependent on the size of the fragment.

LCL must be repaired.

Acute injury after trauma in valgus direction

See topic on Elbow-throwing injuries.

Valgus extension overload syndrome

See topic on Elbow – throwing injuries.

Further reading

O'Driscoll SW, Morrey BF, Korinek S, An KN. Elbow subluxation and dislocation: a spectrum of instability. Clin Orthop Relat Res 1992; 280:186–197.

O'Driscoll SW. Classification and evaluation of recurrent instability of the elbow. Clin Orthop Relat Res 2000; (370):34–43.

Sanderhof-Olsen BS. Lateral collateral ligament complex injury. In: Eygendaal D (ed.), The elbow. Nieuwegein: Arko Sports Media, 2009:187–194.

Eygendaal D. The assessment and management of posterolateral instability. In: Stanley D, Trail I (eds.), Operative elbow surgery. Elsevier: Churchill Livingstone, 2012:385–397.

Cohen MS. The assessment & management of posteromedial instability. In: Stanley D, Trail I (eds.), Operative elbow surgery. Elsevier: Churchill Livingstone, 2012:399–406.

Related topics of interest

- Elbow – throwing injuries (p. 92)

Elbow – lateral epicondylitis (tennis elbow)

Key points

- Common cause of elbow pain
- Diagnosis is clinical
- Most patients respond to nonoperative management

Overview

This condition was first described in 1873. It is often referred to as 'tennis elbow' although tennis contributes to less than 10% of the cases. It is common in manual workers, but also seen in swimmers and climbers.

Epidemiology

Lateral epicondylitis is the most common cause of lateral elbow pain in adults and some reports estimate it to affect between 7% and 10% of the adult population at any point of time. It is more common in patients who are 30 to 60 years old and perform some type of repetitive motion with their upper arm, but it can affect athletes of any age. Its incidence is equal among males and females.

Pathology

Lateral epicondylitis is thought to represent a repetitive overuse injury to common wrist extensors at the lateral epicondyle. The pathology appears to be at the origin of the tendinous origin of the extensor carpi radialis brevis, however tendinous origins of the extensor carpi radialis longus and the extensor digitorum communis may also be involved. In some cases, there is partial or complete tear of the extensor tendon with disruption of the normal collagen architecture and ingrowth of fibroblastic and granulation tissue. Acute and chronic inflammatory cells are often absent. This appearance has been referred to as microtearing followed by incomplete healing.

Predisposing factors

Long duration and increased intensity of arm use predisposes to the described tendinopathy. Therefore, this condition occurs more commonly in patients whose profession places a high demand on their upper extremity. Other factors that may be important include inadequate or compromised musculoskeletal conditions, incorrect techniques and genetic predisposition.

Clinical features

There is pain over the lateral epicondyle, which may extend proximally or over the forearm. Initially this pain may be elicited by activities of daily living and made worse by lifting, gripping or repetitive wrist activity. This may be followed by rest pain once the pathological changes become more extensive.

On examination, typically there is localised tenderness over the extensor mass just distal to the lateral epicondyle. This is made worse by resisted wrist extension or passive wrist flexion.

Investigations

Plain X-rays are normal in majority of the patients with lateral epicondylitis, but some patients may have calcification in soft tissue adjacent to the epicondyle. They do, however, help to exclude other pathologies. The use of ultrasound in diagnosis of lateral epicondylitis is not widespread yet (it can demonstrate a degree of tendon damage and increased blood flow over the extensor mass). Magentic resonance imaging will confirm the diagnosis and exclude other pathologies.

Differential diagnosis

Other causes of lateral elbow pain include posterior interosseous nerve entrapment, synovitis, loose bodies, oesteochondral defects, posterolateral impingement and cervical radiculopathy.

Treatment

The steps in the management of lateral epicondylitis as other tendinopathies involve:

- Control of pain and inflammation
- Promotion of healing process
- Restoration of flexibility and strength
- Restoration of general fitness
- Control of force loads and correction of predisposing factors
- Platelet-rich plasma (PRP) injection
- Surgery if all steps listed above fail

Control of pain and inflammation

This includes protection, rest, ice, compression, elevation, medication (nonsteroidal anti-inflammatory drugs) and other modalities. Corticosteroid injections have therapeutic and diagnostic values but recurrence of symptoms is not uncommon. Modalities used include ultrasound, heat/ cold modalities, shock wave therapy, laser, iontophoresis, acupuncture and massage therapy.

Promotion of healing process

This may be achieved by rehabilitative exercises, massage therapy, high-voltage electrical stimulation, extracorporeal shockwave therapy and absence from abuse. Long-term studies are, however, lacking with many of these techniques.

Restoration of flexibility and strength

Physical therapy involves stretching the extensors followed by light progressive, pain-free active and isometric strengthening.

Control of force loads and correction of predisposing factors

Counterforce bracing may have a role in some patients. It is thought to offload the wrist extensor origin during repetitive activity. It should be applied approximately 5-cm distal to the epicondyle. Correction of predisposing factors involves assessment of technique and equipment (i.e. grip size).

Platelet-rich plasma

Platelet-rich plasma has been gaining popularity in recent years for management of tendinopathies. PRP contains high concentrations of platelets (which release growth factors by degranulation) as well as cytokines, thrombin and other factors that are involved in tissue healing. PRP is prepared by centrifugation of patients owning peripheral blood to obtain a preparation with high concentration of platelets and cytokines. This preparation is then injected around the pathological tissue. Although there have been some reports of very encouraging outcomes following PRP in tendinopathies, further well-designed randomised control studies are required to clarify the PRP role. Part of the problem is that there are a number of different commercially available PRP systems with varying preparation protocols. As a result, the absolute number of platelets, concentration of white blood cells and the mode of platelet activation differs in each system. This makes comparison of different studies extremely difficult.

Surgery

Surgical intervention is recommended to those who do not respond to conservative management. Techniques include:

- Open
- Percutaneous
- Arthroscopic

Return to sports

If it is a first-time injury, proper care and sufficient healing time before resuming activity should prevent permanent disability. Healing time can be between 3 to 8 weeks depending on the severity of the injury.

Further reading

Bisset L, Paungmali A, Vicenzio B, Beller E. A systematic review and meta-analysis of clinical trials on physical interventions for lateral epicondylalgia. Br J Sports Med 2005; 39(7):411–422.

Krogh TP, Fredberg U, Stengaard-Pedersen K, et al. Treatment of lateral epicondylitis with platelet-rich plasma, glucocorticoid, or saline: a randomized, double-blind, placebo-controlled trial. Am J Sports Med 2013; 41(3):625-35.

Lopez-Vidriero E, Goulding KA, Simon DA, Sanchez M, Johnson DH. The use of platelet-rich plasma in arthroscopy and sports medicine: optimizing the healing environment. Arthroscopy 2010; 26(2):269–278.

Related topics of interest

- Elbow – medial epicondylitis (golfer's elbow) (p. 89)
- Tendon overuse injuries (p. 302)

Elbow – medial epicondylitis (golfer's elbow)

Key points

- Less common than lateral epicondylitis.
- Pathology is at the origin of the flexor-pronator musculotendenous region of the medial epicondyle
- Treatment is mainly nonoperative with surgery reserved only for those that do not respond

Overview

Although less common than lateral epicondylitis (tennis elbow), this condition can be seen in those athletes who are involved in golf, tennis, squash, baseball, cricket, javelin throwing, American football, weight lifting and all other throwing and racquet sports.

Epidemiology

It is more common in second to fifth decades of life, but can occur in other age groups as well. With majority of athletes, this condition involves the dominant arm.

Pathology

Like lateral epicondylitis, medial epicondylitis is thought to represent a repetitive overuse injury. The pathology is at the origin of the flexor-pronator musculotendenous region of the medial epicondyle with pronator teres and flexor carpi radialis being affected more often than palmirus longus , flexor digitorum superficialis and flexor carpi ulnaris. In most cases, there is partial or complete tearing of the flexor tendon with disruption of the normal collagen architecture and ingrowth of fibroblastic and granulation tissue. Acute and chronic inflammatory cells can be absent. This appearance has been referred to as microtearing followed by incomplete healing and degeneration that may be referred to as tendinopathy.

Predisposing factors

As with other sports injuries these can be classified as:

Sports related:
- Participation in sports that require high demand on the upper extremity, i.e. racquet and throwing sports

Athlete related:
- Previous injury
- Inadequate management and recovery from previous injury
- Inadequate or compromised musculoskeletal condition (muscle weakness, poor flexibility, lack of fitness)
- Genetic predisposition

Technique related:
- Poor technique (excessive grip tension, poor forehand and serve in tennis, incorrect golf swing)

Training related:
- Recent history of increase in intensity and duration of training, and lack of warm up

Equipment related:
- Wrong grip size
- Old tennis balls
- Too tight strings

Clinical features

Pain over the medial epicondylitis.
- Made worse by gripping, repetitive wrist activity and lifting
- Varying severity

Localised tenderness over flexor mass, just distal to the medial epicondyle.
- Made worse by:
  - passive wrist extension
  - resisted wrist flexion and forearm pronation

There may be a reduced range of movement of the elbow joint.

There may be features of ulnar nerve dysfunction (in up to 20% of the athletes).

Ulnar collateral ligament injury must be excluded, as it could coexist, particularly in throwing athletes.

Investigations

Plain radiograph

- Normal in majority of athletes
- May show calcification
- Will aid to exclude other pathologies (see topic on throwing injuries)

Ultrasound and MRI

As well as helping to exclude other pathologies, these investigations may demonstrate features of tendinopathy.

Differential diagnosis

These include:
Elbow related:
- Elbow ulnar collateral ligament injury
- Posterior olecranon impingement
- Stress fractures
- Osteoarthritis
- Loose bodies
- Osteochondral defects
- Medial epicondyle apophysitis

Nerve related:
- Cervical radiculopathy
- Ulnar nerve neuropathy

Treatment

The steps in the management of medial epicondylitis as other tendinopathies involve:
- Control of pain and inflammation
- Promotion of healing process
- Restoration of flexibility and strength
- Restoration of general fitness
- Control of force loads and correction of predisposing factors
- Platelet-rich plasma
- Surgery if above fail

Control of pain and inflammation

This includes protection, rest, ice, compression, elevation, medication (nonsteroidal anti-inflammatory drugs) and other modalities. Corticosteroid injections have therapeutic and diagnostic values, but recurrence of symptoms is not uncommon (must be extremely careful not to inject the ular nerve). Modalities used include ultrasound, heat/cold modalities, shock wave therapy, laser, iontophoresis, acupuncture and massage therapy.

Promotion of healing process

This may be achieved by rehabilitative exercises, massage therapy, high-voltage electrical stimulation, extracorporeal shockwave therapy and absence from abuse. Long-term studies are, however, lacking with many of these techniques.

Restoration of flexibility and strength

Physical therapy involves stretching the flexors followed by light progressive, pain-free active and isometric strengthening.

Control of force loads and correction of predisposing factors

As with lateral epicondylitis, counterforce bracing may have a role in some athletes. It is thought to offload the wrist flexor origin during repetitive activity. It should be applied approximately 5-cm distal to the epicondyle. Correction of predisposing factors involves assessment of technique and equipment (see above).

Platelet-rich plasma (PRP)

See the topic elbow – lateral epicondylitis.

Surgery

Surgery may be offered to those athletes who are still symptomatic despite 3 to 6 months of adequate nonoperative program when all other cause of elbow pain have been excluded. There are a number of techniques but most of them involve identification and excision of torn and scar tissues which may be followed by some form of repair of the healthy tendon. As well as identifying and protecting the ulnar nerve, it may be necessary to perform ulnar nerve decompression or transposition.

Return to sport

As with other sports injuries, return to sport is permitted once the athlete is pain free, able to achieve a full range of movement and has regained enough strength to perform their sport specific activities. With nonoperative management, return to play usually takes 6 to 12 weeks. Return to play following operative management may take 3 to 6 months.

Further Reading

Ciccotti MC, Schwartz MA, Ciccotti MG. Diagnosis and treatment of the medial epicondylitis of the elbow. Clin Sports Med 2004; 23:693–705.

Van Hofwegen C, Baker CL 3rd, Baker CL Jr.Epicondylitis in the athlete's elbow. Clin Sports Med 2010; 29(4):577–597.

Related topics of interest

- Elbow – lateral epicondylitis (tennis elbow) (p. 86)
- Elbow – throwing injuries (p. 92)
- Nerve entrapment syndrome – upper limb (p. 203)
- Tendon overuse injuries (p. 302)

Elbow – throwing injuries

Key points

- Elbow injuries are common in throwing sports
- In the late cocking and the early acceleration phases of throwing motion, the elbow is placed under tremendous valgus forces, which can result in damages to medial, lateral and posterior compartments of the elbow
- Most conditions are overuse and chronic injuries, and include medial collateral ligament damage, posterior olecranon impingement, olecranon stress fracture, medial epicondyle apophysitis and osteochondritis dissecans, medial epicondylitis and ulnar nerve dysfunction

Overview

With throwing sports, excessively large forces are generated at the elbow joint. Therefore, elbow injuries are not uncommon in athletes who participate in sports that involve throwing, such as cricket, baseball, some track and field sports and American football, in particular those with poor technique. As the frequency of participation in many of these sports is increasing, sports clinicians' appreciation and understanding of 'throwing elbow injuries' is of vital importance.

Pathology. Throwing may be divided into five phases, which include:

- Wind up
- Early cocking phase
- Late cocking
- Acceleration
- Deceleration

In the late cocking and the early acceleration phases, the elbow is placed under tremendous valgus forces, which also result in large compressive forces on the lateral radiocapitellar articulation (as much as 500 N). Such forces can cause damage to medial, lateral and posterior compartments of the elbow.

Figure 10 illustrates the different conditions encountered by the throwing athlete. Medial collateral ligament injury of the elbow, posterior olecranon impingement, olecranon stress fracture, medial epicondyle apophysitis and osteochondritis dissecans are described in this Topic, while medial epicondylitis and ulnar nerve dysfunction are described elsewhere.

Medial collateral ligament injuries

Medial collateral ligament (MCL) consists of an anterior bundle, a posterior bundle and a transverse bundle. The anterior bundle plays a vital role in providing medial stability to valgus force in the range of 30°–120° of flexion. It is therefore subjected to extremely high forces during the late cocking and the acceleration phases of the throwing motion. As a result, medial collateral ligament injuries occur in sports that involve a throwing motion.

Pathology

Common causes of MCL injury include:

- Acute
  - Elbow dislocation
  - Acute valgus injury
- Chronic
  - MCL attenuation in throwing/racquet athletes

Clinical features

Presentation may be chronic, acute or acute on chronic.

- Athletes may recall an acute injury that started the symptoms. This acute injury may have caused elbow dislocation
- Medial pain during throwing (in most athletes in the acceleration phase)
- In most athletes, pain usually improves with rest
- May complain of popping in elbow while throwing
- Medial elbow tenderness
- Valgus stress to the elbow flexed 20°–30° reproduces the pain and causes medial joint opening (up to 1 mm medial joint opening is normal)

Investigations

Plain radiograph

- In acute setting will exclude elbow dislocation and/or fractures

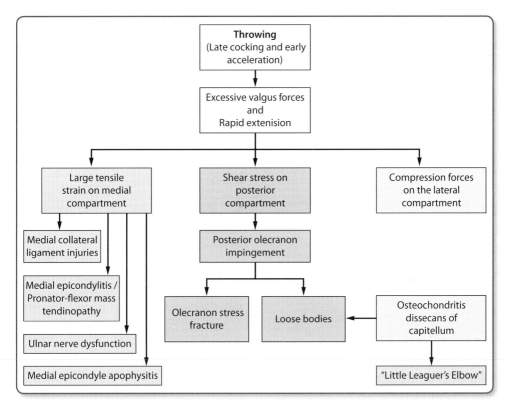

Figure 10 Elbow-throwing injuries.

- May demonstrate an avulsion fragment
- Will aid to exclude other causes of elbow pain
- Stress radiographs, with valgus stress, will demonstrate increased medial opening

Ultrasound
- Dynamic ultrasonography may have a role in evaluating injuries to medial collateral ligament but it is operator dependent

Magnetic resonance imaging
- With contrast, this is the investigation of choice and will demonstrate any presence of damage to the medial collateral ligament and whether or not this damage is partial or full thickness tear
- Magnetic resonance imaging (MRI) will also aid to exclude other injuries

Computed tomography
- As well as helping to exclude some of the other injuries, computed tomography

(CT) arthrogram can also be useful in illustrating the medial collateral ligament injuries

Differential diagnosis
These include:
1. Medial epicondylitis
2. Cubital tunnel syndrome
3. Elbow chondropathy
4. Synovial plica
5. Snapping triceps

Treatment
Nonoperative
- Short-term elbow rest (usually 3–6 weeks but avoiding valgus load for 3–6 months)
- NSAIDs
- Once pain is controlled:
  - Range of movement exercises
  - Supervised and progressive return to throwing

Operative

- Surgery is indicated:
  - In throwing athletes with complete tear (in order for the athlete to return to their throwing sports)
  - In those throwing athletes with incomplete tears in whom adequate nonoperative management has failed
  - In non-throwing athletes who remain symptomatic despite adequate nonoperative measures
- In most athletes, surgery involves reconstruction of the medial collateral ligament using tendon autograft

Return to sport

With nonoperative treatment, return to play is permitted once athletes have completed their rehabilitation programme pain free. This may take anything from 6 weeks to 6 months.

With operative treatment, the athlete is usually allowed to return to play 4–6 months following surgery.

Posterior olecranon impingement

This is not an uncommon condition among throwing athletes and occurs as the valgus extension force to the elbow during throwing leads to impingement of the posteromedial olecranon tip against the olecranon fossa. This repeated impingements will, in time, cause soft tissue hypertrophy and osteophyte formation, which will further worsen the impingement. As the condition progresses, these osteophytes may fracture and form loose bodies.

Clinical features

- Postero-medial elbow pain in acceleration phase of throwing
- Athlete may not be able to fully extend the elbow
- Tenderness in the posterior medial tip of the olecranon
- Repeated forced hyperextension and valgus force to the elbow provokes postero-medial pain (Valgus Extension Overload test)

Investigations

- Plain radiograph may show the presence of osteophytes, loose bodies or fractures
- Bone scan, CT or MRI will help to exclude stress fractures

Treatment

Nonoperative

- Short-term elbow rest
- NSAIDs
- Once pain is controlled:
  - Range of movement exercises
  - Supervised and progressive return to throwing

Operative

- Surgery is indicated in those athletes who do not respond to nonoperative treatment. The option in these athletes is arthroscopic or open excision impinging soft tissue and osteophytes ± removal of the loose bodies

Return to sport

Throwing athletes are allowed to return to play once they are pain free and have achieved full range of movement and strength. Following surgery, this may take 6 weeks to 3 months.

Olecranon stress fractures

Repeated impingement of the olecranon in throwing athletes (see above) can lead to stress fractures.

Clinical features

- Posterior elbow pain in the acceleration phase of throwing. Pain can persist after throwing
- Localised tenderness over the fracture site

Investigations

- Although plain radiograph may show the fractures in some athletes, it may be normal as in other athletes with stress fractures
- Bone scan, CT or MRI are the investigations of choice if stress fractures are suspected clinically

Treatment

Nonoperative
- Rest from throwing
- Once pain is controlled:
  - Range of movement exercises
  - Muscle strengthening exercises
  - Supervised and progressive return to throwing

Operative
- Surgery is indicated in those athletes who do not respond to nonoperative treatment. Surgical option in these athletes includes:
  - Open internal fixation
  - Arthroscopic internal fixation
  - Excision of olecranon tip

Medial epicondyle apophytis

In skeletally immature throwers, the medial epicondyle appears to be weaker than the ulnar collateral ligament; therefore, repetitive valgus force encountered during throwing results in its apophyseal fragmentation or avulsion rather than rupture of the medial collateral ligament. These injuries are thought to be most common in 9–12-year-old athletes, especially in young baseball pitchers but are also seen in sports such as tennis (serving) and javelin throwing. Together with osteochondritis dissecans of the capitellum (see below), these injuries form a group of conditions that are sometimes referred to as 'little leaguer's elbow'.

Clinical features
- Medial elbow pain
  - Usually in the dominant arm
  - Commonly insidious onset
- Impaired throwing and performance (reduced throwing effectiveness and distance)
- Swelling
- Localised tenderness
- Decreased range of movement of the elbow joint

Investigations

Plain radiograph
Anteroposterior, lateral, right and left oblique views may need to compare with films of the uninjured side

- May reveal:
  - Enlargement of the elbow
  - Apophyseal irregularities
  - Apophyseal fragmentation
  - Apophyseal separation
  - Epicondyle beaking
- Will aid to exclude other causes of medial elbow pain

Bone scan, CT and MRI
- Can be helpful in those with very subtle plain film features as well as in excluding other causes of elbow pain

Treatment
This may be both nonoperative or operative.

Nonoperative
- Rest from throwing (4–6 weeks)
- Ice
- NSAIDs
- Splint immobilisation for undisplaced or minimally displaced medial epicondyle avulsion fractures
- Once pain is controlled:
  - Range of movement exercises
  - Supervised and progressive return to throwing
- Activity modification and correction of any predisposing factors that could have contributed to the condition (i.e. poor technique, rules concerning intensity of throwing and training in young athletes, education of coach and athlete)

Operative
- Open reduction internal fixation is indicated in those who are young with significantly displaced medial epicondyle avulsion fractures

Return to sport
Young athletes are allowed to return to throwing once they are pain free and have achieved full range of movement and strength. This return must be cautious and gradual in order to prevent recurrent injury. Time taken for return to play is dependent on the exact pathology and can range from few weeks to a whole season.

Osteochondritis dissecans of capitellum

This condition, seen in adolescent throwing athletes, also belongs to the group of conditions sometimes referred to as 'little leaguer's elbow'. It occurs as a consequence of the compressive forces between the radial head and the capitellum during throwing, which in turn are thought to disturb the subchondral blood supply. The end result is osteochondral injury, which may be associated with loose body formation.

Clinical features

- Elbow pain
  - Commonly insidious onset
- Impaired throwing and performance (reduced throwing effectiveness and distance)
- Localised tenderness
- Flexion contracture and decreased range of movement of the elbow joint

Investigations

Plain radiograph

- May reveal:
  - Rarefaction
  - Irregular ossification
  - Subchondral rarefied crater in the capitellum
  - Enlarged radial head
  - Loose bodies

Contrast tomograms, MRI and arthroscopy

- Can be helpful in evaluating the lesions of the articular surface and subchondral bone in detail

Treatment

This may be both nonoperative or operative.

Nonoperative

- Rest from throwing
- Ice
- NSAIDs
- Splint immobilisation
- Once pain is controlled:
  - Range of movement exercises
  - Supervised and progressive return to throwing
- Activity modification and correction of any predisposing factors

Operative

- Indications for surgery are:
  - Presence of loose bodies
  - Presence of mechanical symptoms
  - Persistent symptoms despite adequate nonoperative management
- Surgical options include:
  - Arthroscopic:
    - Removal of loose bodies
    - Abrasion chondroplasty
    - Capitellum drilling
  - Open
    - Removal of loose bodies
    - Abrasion chondroplasty
    - Capitellum drilling
    - Humeral osteotomy

Further reading

Caine EL, Dugas JR, Wolf RS, Andrews JR. Elbow injuries in throwing athletes: a current concept review. Am J Sports Med 2003; 31:621–634.

Rahman RK, Levine WN, Ahmad CS. Elbow medial collateral ligaments injuries. Curr Rev Musculoskelet Med 2008; 1:197–204.

Related topics of interest

ENT conditions in sport medicine

Sports-related ear, nose and throat (ENT) conditions are common. This Topic aims to provide a succinct overview of the commonest conditions rather than an exhaustive text on the subject.

Head and neck injuries should initially be managed as closed head injuries with appropriate evaluation of airway with cervical spine control, breathing and circulation. Bleeding is often a feature and should not distract from prompt and systematic evaluation of the patient.

Nasal injuries

Key points

- Soft tissue injury in combination with nasal bone fracture often seen
- Septal trauma is common – septal haematoma is uncommon but must be excluded
- Cerebrospinal fluid leak is a rare occurrence

Overview

Nasal injury may result in a combination of soft tissue injury, nasal bone fracture, septal dislocation/fracture, septal haematoma or cerebrospinal fluid (CSF) leak.

Epidemiology

Nasal fractures are the most common facial fracture, and occur twice as often in males than females.

Pathology

The nose is particularly susceptible to injury due to its prominent location and low strength of its skeletal support.

Clinical features

Symptoms of nasal injury include epistaxis, cosmetic deformity, nasal airway compromise, periorbital and subconjunctival ecchymosis.

Investigations

Radiological investigations are not required, but have a role to play if additional facial fractures are suspected.

Differential diagnosis

Nasal trauma often occurs in conjunction with other maxillofacial injuries and these need to be fully evaluated.

Treatment

Soft tissue injuries

Wounds should be cleaned thoroughly. Abrasions are best left open to heal. Steri-strips may be used to close small lacerations; larger lacerations should be sutured. Tetanus status should be assessed and cover provided.

Epistaxis

The majority settles with direct pressure. Persisting epistaxis in the presence of a nasal fracture may settle following fracture reduction. In cases where epistaxis fails to resolve by these measures, nasal packing may be required.

Nasal bone fracture

Uncomplicated fractures without a cosmetic or functional deficit do not require treatment. In simple displaced fractures, closed reduction under local or general anaesthetic can be carried out, either immediately after the injury or 5–7 days after the injury once any swelling subsides. Fracture reduction should not be delayed for longer than 2 weeks after the injury, due to the bone healing and callus formation – manipulation can be difficult or impossible. More extensive injuries may require open reduction. Cases of functional or cosmetic deformity may require a septorhinoplasty at a later date.

Septal haematoma

Haematoma may be unilateral or bilateral. Cartilage necrosis occurs if the haematoma is left untreated for more than 48 h. The usual presentation of a septal haematoma is progressive nasal obstruction after trauma. On examination, a soft swelling may be noted in the nasal airway. The definitive treatment is drainage. In early cases, needle aspiration may suffice; however, once organised clot has formed, an incision and drainage is required.

If left untreated, a septal abscess and cartilage necrosis follows, resulting in cosmetic and functional deficit.

CSF leak

CSF leak should be suspected in the presence of clear rhinorrhoea following nasal injury. Diagnosis can be confirmed by testing for b-2 transferrin in the fluid. Most leaks heal spontaneously. Persistent leaks require surgical repair. The patient is at risk of developing meningitis until the leak stops and they should be made aware of this.

Return to sport

Following nasal fracture requiring manipulation, 6 weeks should be given prior to return to sport.

Ear injuries

Key points

- The anatomical location of the pinna makes it prone to sporting injuries
- Most tympanic membrane perforations heal spontaneously
- Otitis externa/swimmer's ear is a commonly encountered condition

Overview

The pinna is an unprotected appendage readily accessible to trauma. Injury to the ear can result in pinna haematoma and tympanic membrane perforation. Otitis externa/swimmer's ear is commonly seen in those involved in water sports.

Epidemiology

Traumatic injury to the pinna is common especially in contact sports, and otitis externa affects around 10% of the population at some point.

Pathology

Auricular haematoma

Blunt injuries produce shearing forces, disrupting the adherence of auricular perichondrium to the underlying cartilage. The subperichondrial space becomes filled with blood, depriving the cartilage of nutrition.

Tympanic membrane perforation

Sports-related blunt trauma or barotrauma from swimming/diving can result in perforations.

Otitis externa

Swimmer's ear is a term used to describe an acute inflammatory condition affecting the external auditory canal (otitis externa). Subsequent bacterial infection can exacerbate the changes to the external ear skin. The main pathogens are pseudomonas and *Staphylococcus aureus*.

Clinical features

Auricular haematoma

Presents with pain, fluctuant swelling/distortion and bruising over the pinna.

Tympanic membrane perforation

Patients can be asymptomatic, or complain of hearing loss, vertigo, otorrhoea or ear discomfort. Perforation is seen on otoscopy.

Otitis externa

Discomfort or itching of the external auditory canal progresses to tenderness and pain. There may also be a sensation of fullness and reduced hearing. On examination, the canal appears erythematous and oedematous.

Investigations

Head injuries can occur concurrently and should be investigated. Inspection of the external ear and otoscopy are often the only examinations required.

Differential diagnosis

Soft tissue swelling and bruising to the pinna may be mistaken for an auricular haematoma.

Treatment

Auricular haematoma

If left untreated, infection and cartilage necrosis and remodelling occur, causing 'cauliflower ear'. Treatment involves incision and drainage and application of a pressure dressing to prevent re-collection.

Tympanic membrane perforation

Most perforations heal spontaneously. The ear should be kept dry until this happens. If the perforation fails to heal, surgical intervention can be considered to repair the defect.

Otitis externa

Patients should be advised to keep their ears dry and avoid instrumentation. Treatment is with topical medication containing antibiotics and steroid. In severe cases, aural toilet and insertion of an aural wick may be necessitated to augment the topical therapy.

Return to sport

Patients with auricular haematomas should avoid contact sports until the condition has fully resolved. Those suffering with otitis externa should avoid water sports until the inflammation has settled. Water precaution advice should be given.

Throat injuries

Key points

- Laryngeal injury is extremely rare but can be life-threatening, therefore a high index of suspicion should be maintained to avoid fatal misdiagnosis

Overview

Injuries to the larynx may result following trauma to the neck and can lead to airway compromise if not recognised and managed promptly.

Epidemiology

Sports-related laryngeal injuries are rare, and account for less than 1% of all blunt traumas.

Pathology

The larynx is formed by a complex arrangement of cartilage, nerves and muscles covered by a mucous membrane. Laryngeal cartilage can be fractured or dislocated resulting in life-threatening airway compromise.

Clinical features

Severe injuries are usually evident. Less severe injuries may present with hoarseness/change in voice, dysphagia, odynophagia and anterior neck pain. Clinical findings include dyspnoea, stridor, surgical emphysema, haemoptysis and soft tissue swelling/ecchymosis.

Investigations

Expert endoscopic visualisation of the larynx is vital. X-rays of the cervical spine and chest are also used in initial assessment and to rule out underlying spinal injury. A computed tomography (CT) scan provides more detail of the underlying injury.

Differential diagnosis

Trauma to the neck may lead to soft tissue injury without any underlying damage to the larynx.

Treatment

Management of the patient should be as per ATLS guidelines with airway protection and maintenance being the most immediate concern. Cervical spine injury must be excluded.

Return to sport

This is dependent upon the severity of the injury and should be discussed with the consulting ENT team.

Further reading

Flint PW, Haughey BH, Lund VJ et al. Cummings otolaryngology: head and neck surgery, 5th edn. Philadelphia; Mosby, 2010.

Roland NJ, McRae RDR, McCombe AW. Key topics in otolaryngology, 2nd edn. Oxford; BIOS Scientific Publishers Ltd, 2001.

Related topics of interest

Epilepsy and exercise

Key points

- Choices about whether participation in particular sports need to be individualised
- Most exercise activity is safe in epilepsy
- Regular monitoring for changes in the patient's epilepsy control is needed

Aetiology

Although concerns regarding participation in sports and epilepsy exist, the latest evidence suggests the need for a reasoned approach. This Topic reviews clinically relevant aspects of the relationship between epilepsy and exercise.

Clinical features

Seizures, epilepsy and the risk of injury during seizures

Seizures are classified as either generalised or partial seizures and assessing each seizure type provides the basis for understanding how harm may occur during a seizure.

Generalised seizures

Generalised tonic–clonic seizures result in unprotected falling followed by rhythmic clonic jerks. Atonic seizures consist of sudden loss of muscle tone with unprotected falling, both of which can result in serious injury. Absence seizures consist of brief (typically 3–10 s), motionless, nondistractible staring, but balance is usually maintained. Therefore, absence seizures do not usually cause falling injuries.

Partial seizures

Simple partial seizures begin in such a small part of the brain that consciousness is not altered. These are thus unlikely to cause unanticipated injury to sports participants. Complex partial seizures are defined by alteration (but not loss) of consciousness, usually of 1–2 min duration, followed by a few minutes of confusion, thus rendering the participant unable to participate for a few minutes. Seizures that begin as partial seizures may generalise, with the same implications as primary generalised seizures noted above.

Potential of athletics to exacerbate seizures

Athletic participation can be associated with factors that could alter seizure threshold, including repeated head injury during contact sports, excessive aerobic exercise, hyperventilation and changes in drug metabolism.

Repeated head injury

Despite concerns that repeated head injury during contact sports could trigger seizures, there is little evidence to support this. One reason may be the fact that most patients are dissuaded or prohibited from participating in contact sports and thus there is little experience on which to base this judgement.

Aerobic exercise

Aerobic exercise occasionally causes seizure exacerbations, but on average, it improves seizure frequency. Overall, aerobic exercise has great benefit to general health. Therefore, it is recommended for most patients, although it must be recognised that it may trigger seizures in some.

Hyperventilation

Hyperventilation performed at rest can trigger an absence seizure, but there is little evidence to indicate that exercise-induced hyperventilation can also do the same.

Drug metabolism

Physical training induces hepatic microsomal enzymes, and this may be important for patients on antiepileptic drugs, such as phenytoin. Therefore, altered pharmacokinetics may lead to alterations in the dose of medication required to control their seizures.

Sports as a cause of seizures and epilepsy

Seizure-like episodes can immediately follow a severe head injury, yet these typical concussive convulsions are not actually seizures. There is epidemiological evidence that severe head injuries may cause epilepsy. In the severe cases of penetrating-missile head injury, epilepsy may occur in up to 50%.

However, there is no consistent association of the development of epilepsy from typical mild head injury during typical sporting activities. The paucity of reports of epilepsy following participation in contact sports such as boxing also suggests that this is uncommon.

Investigations

Routine investigations include a head computed tomography (CT) and electroencephalography (EEG) as well as bloods tests to exclude an infection or imbalanced metabolic state. Other testing is dependent on the specific case.

Management

Patients should be managed in consultation with a neurologist. While, there is little evidence of increased risk of exercise, and clear evidence of benefit there are some risks for certain patients. Decision-making should thus be individualised.

Return to sport

Water sports (swimming, rowing, boating, canoeing, rafting, sailing, fishing, scuba diving)

Water sports present a particular problem due to the risk of drowning. Yet, it is generally recommended that water sports be permitted with appropriate precautions. The risk of drowning during a seizure is extremely low with close supervision in the shallow, clear water of a swimming pool. Patients should generally be allowed to swim with direct visual supervision. Rowing, boating of any type and fishing pose a risk from falling into open water and patients should always wear floatation devices. These activities should be avoided if seizures are frequent.

Scuba diving is prohibited for patients with active epilepsy and is not recommended even if seizures are controlled by medication. According to the medical committee of the British Sub-Aqua Club (BSAC), people taking anti-epileptic medication are more likely to experience 'nitrogen narcosis'. They suggest that people should be seizure free and off

medication for 5 years (3 years if seizures only occur during sleep) before they consider scuba diving.

Competitive underwater swimming and diving pose problems similar to scuba diving and should be avoided.

Sports at heights (sky diving, hang gliding, flying, climbing, bungi jumping, gymnastics, horseback riding)

Sky diving, hang gliding and free climbing would place a patient at considerable risk if a seizure was to occur, and should be discouraged. Epilepsy presents no specific additional risk as regards bungi jumping. Gymnastics may pose a risk for activities that involve swinging from parallel bars or other acrobatic activities, but other activities are not discouraged. There is significant risk of injury due to falls during equestrian sports, so horseback riding should generally be avoided for patients with active epilepsy.

Contact sports (boxing, football, American football, hockey, rugby)

There are no strict prohibitions on contact sports, due to a lack of evidence that repeated mild blows to the head exacerbate seizures. However, it seems prudent to advise against them when seizures are newly diagnosed and their course for a given patient has not been defined.

Aerobic sports (running, track and field, ice skating, skiing)

There are no prohibitions to aerobic exercise and there is evidence that it reduces seizure frequency. Appropriate head gear and safe practices should be followed during ice skating and skiing. A consideration for skiers is whether a seizure might occur on a ski lift and whether the patient would fall out of a lift chair.

Wheeled sports (cycling, rollerblading, skateboarding)

There are no specific prohibitions for wheeled sports. It is prudent to restrict these activities, however, if seizures are frequent or of as-yet-undetermined frequency.

importance. This may be handwritten or using medical software

Training

- Working as a doctor in an event is likely to be outside your normal practice. Therefore, it is imperative to undertake recognised regular training, so that the skills you require are up to date
- The requirements for an event may vary but a recognised prehospital care course is a minimum
- If working regularly as an event doctor, then more advanced training should be undertaken, e.g. BASICS (British Association for Immediate Care) with the aim to undertake a Diploma in Immediate Medical Care (or equivalent)

Medical event organiser

- Organising a medical event can be a serious undertaking. You need to coordinate everything from basic first aid to major incident planning
- Whether organising an event or working as the crowd doctor, ensure a risk assessment has been carried out to evaluate the level of medical support required for the event. There need to be first aiders, crowd doctors (at least one doctor is required if more than 2000 spectators) and ambulance provision (at least one ambulance with a paramedic if over 5000 spectators but this will vary as numbers increase). You will need to ensure they have the necessary qualifications for their roles
- You need to arrange for all medical equipment and supplies. Depending on the number of officials and spectators, this will determine how much emergency equipments, such as defibrillators, airways, splints, bandages, medications and so on you will require
- Knowing the layout of the event arena is essential especially for transporting unwell persons.
- Know the number and sizes of first aid/ medical rooms – ensure they are large enough for couches and secure for equipment (minimum is 15 m^2)

- Where the command and control systems will be
- Ambulance access points and egress routes
- Coordinate the structure of the team, with all individuals being aware of their roles and responsibilities throughout the event
- Decide if staff training prior to the event is required
- Information on local emergency department hospitals
- Other issues such as weather, monitoring equipment levels and daily briefings need to be considered
- Have a medical plan easily accessible for all healthcare professionals, which relate the above information
- If organising endurance events, then a number of first aid/medical rooms will be required along the course, usually one every 3–5 km with regular drink stations. Multiple different healthcare professionals will be required from doctors (anaesthetists, emergency medicine doctors, sports medicine physicians), to physiotherapists, sports therapists and podiatrists. Medical tents towards the end of the courses will require equipment to deal with severe illnesses like hyponatraemia and hyperthermia. There needs to be access to diagnostic equipment for electrolyte analysis, stretchers, blankets, ice water baths, advanced medical equipment and medications, intravenous (iv) fluids and drugs and full resuscitation facilities

Major incident planning

- Examples of major incidents are stand collapses, fires, bombs or anything that puts a strain on medical resources above and beyond normal incidents
- During a major incident, there is a clear hierarchical structure in place with gold, silver and bronze commanders. Each team should know their roles and responsibilities
  - Gold commander is usually the chief police or fire officer and is in overall control. They will have a team that liaise with the hospitals and any other

national services that are required for the incident
- Silver commander is the strategic commander, not normally at the scene but coordinates bronze team leaders
- Bronze commander is at the incident and controls the situation at ground level
- Depending on your level of expertise, you may be at either bronze or silver if you are the medical event organiser

- A doctor can be at an operational level or assisting paramedics and so on with the triage and treatment of individuals
- The plan must describe the locations for triaging and treating individuals in addition to clear routes for emergency services into and out of the event
- Make sure that all emergency services (police, fire and ambulance services) are aware and have agreed the plan – keep a copy in the medical room

Further reading

Department for culture, media and sport. Guide to safety at sports grounds. 5th edn. London; TSO publishing, 2008.

Noakes T. Medical coverage of endurance events. In: Brukner P, Khan K (eds), Clinical sports medicine, 3rd edn. Australia: McGraw-Hill, 2006:969–975.

Related topics of interest

- Drugs in sport – overview (p. 74)
- Team physician (p. 298)
- Thermoregulation and fluid balance in hot conditions (p. 310)

Exercise and health

Key points

- The evidence linking a sedentary lifestyle to poor health and an early death is unassailable
- Diseases that have a higher incidence in people with a sedentary lifestyle include coronary heart disease, many cancers, stroke, diabetes, osteoporosis and depression
- The relative risk in sedentary individuals of getting many of these diseases is roughly twice the risk for a person with a physically active lifestyle
- Quality of life is also reduced in sedentary individuals, for example poorer mental health

London bus drivers and conductors

Knowledge about the devastating effects of a sedentary lifestyle has emerged steadily since the pioneering epidemiological studies of Prof Jerry Morris and colleagues in the early 1950s. The evidence base is now massive and this Topic will review some of the highlights.

Data on the incidence of heart attacks (acute myocardial infarction or MI) and on the immediate morbidity of MIs were obtained for thousands of drivers and conductors on London's double-decker buses during 1949 and 1950. It showed that drivers were roughly twice as likely as conductors to suffer an acute MI. What is more, increased mortality within the first 3 days was even more elevated. Consideration of all the possible differences between drivers and conductors led Prof Jerry Morris and colleagues to propose the following hypothesis: 'Men in physically active jobs have a lower incidence of coronary artery disease in middle age than have men in physically inactive jobs'.

This hypothesis has been examined by many subsequent studies and fully supported, and significant extensions have been made. The importance of all physical activity, not just physical activity at work, has been established. Thus, it is the overall level of physical activity, including work, leisure time and travelling, that is important. And a wide range of other diseases have been shown to be increased in incidence in sedentary individuals. These include stroke, colon cancer, breast cancer, diabetes, osteoporosis and depression (see **Table 8**).

Longitudinal studies

A number of large studies have followed groups of individuals for several years. These have shown, importantly, that within the subpopulation who switch from a sedentary to an active lifestyle, there is a substantially reduced risk of disease or early death compared with those who remained sedentary. So you can significantly improve your chances of a long and healthy life at any time by adopting a more physically active lifestyle. One random-controlled trial in people identified as at risk of diabetes showed that the group assigned an exercise programme had, over the 6-year-study period, only 61% of the incidence of clinical diabetes seen in the control group. The same trend for poorer health in sedentary individuals is seen in all groups within the population, young and old, male and female, and the different ethnic groups studied.

Quality of life

Epidemiological evidence in relation to improved quality of life is less extensive, but still convincing. Sedentary individuals tend to be more depressed, more anxious, have lower self-esteem and sleep less well than physically active individuals. The evidence comes not just from cross-sectional studies comparing people with different levels of physical activity. There have also been well-controlled intervention studies looking at the effect of exercise prescriptions on measures such as self-esteem. A few studies looking at sexual function have provided an indication that active, fit individuals have a better time of it. For example, a telephone survey of over-40-year-olds found 50% more

Table 8 Level and strength of evidence for a relationship between physical activity and prevention of contemporary chronic conditions			
Condition	Level of evidence	Strength of effect	Evidence of a dose-response relationship
Cardiovascular disease			
Coronary heart disease	High	Strong	Yes
Stroke	High	Strong	Yes
Obesity and overweight	High	Strong	Yes
Type 2 diabetes	High	Strong	Yes
Musculoskeletal disorders			
Osteoporosis	High	Strong	Yes
Low back pain	Medium	Weak	–
Psychological well-being and mental illness			
Clinical depression	High	Strong	Yes
Mental function	High	Strong	–
Cancer			
Colon	High	Strong	Yes
Rectal	Medium	No effect	
Breast	High	Strong	Yes
Lung	Medium	Strong	–
Prostate	High	Equivocal	Probable
Endometrial	Medium	Strong	Yes

This table provides a simplified summary of the nature and volume of evidence and an estimate of the strength of effect of activity currently indicated by that evidence. The 'level of evidence' is intended to be a general indication of the volume and quality of the available evidence. The 'strength of effect' is intended to indicate how positive, or otherwise, the findings are. Based on Table 36.1, CMO report, UK Department of Health, 2004., and Part E of the Physical Activity Guidelines Advisory Committee report, US Department of Health, 2008.

erectile dysfunction in sedentary individuals compared with those meeting the physical activity guidelines.

In older individuals, lack of physical fitness due to a sedentary life style can be very limiting. The difference in quality of life is clearly going to be substantial between those who can walk some distance and can manage stairs, and those who cannot. In addition, there appears to be a link between physical activity and cognition in older people. In intervention studies, aerobic exercise programmes have been accompanied by significant improvements in 'executive functions', including rapid decision-making, and in short-term memory.

What are the mechanisms underlying the link between physical fitness and disease prevention and increased quality of life?

The link between exercise that stresses bone and improved bone strength is well understood. We know some of the key factors underlying disease prevention in other conditions, for example underused muscles handle glucose poorly (a factor in diabetes), while exercise leads to an improved blood lipid profile (a factor in heart disease). Even in areas such as improved mental health, we have clues. For example, generation of new nerve cells, neurogenesis, is now known to occur in adult mammalian brain. Amazingly in animal studies, it has clearly been shown that exercise can increase the amount of neurogenesis that occurs.

Conclusion

Physical activity and exercise, leading to improved physical fitness, offer major improvements in health and quality of life. A good way of looking at this is to consider human evolution and the selective pressures that would favour physical activity. Our bodies are designed to be active. So instead of wearing out with physical activity (at reasonable levels), our systems function better and malfunction less often. However, in the developed world, physical work no longer plays a large part in most employment and in housework. The challenge now is to get adequate levels of physical activity back into the lives of everyone.

Further reading

Hardman AE, Stensel DJ. Physical activity and health, 2nd edn. London: Routledge, 2009.
Holden CA, McLachlan RI, Pitts M, et al. Determinants of male reproductive health disorders: the Men in Australia Telephone Survey (MATeS). BMC Public Health 2010; 10:96.
Morris JN, Heady JA, Raffle PA, Roberts CG, Parks JW. Coronary heart-disease and physical activity of work. Lancet 1953; 265: 1053–1057.
Physical Activity Guidelines Advisory Committee. Physical Activity Guidelines Advisory Committee report, 2008. Washington, DC: US Department of Health and Human Services, 2008.

Related topics of interest

Exercise physiology – circulatory and respiratory systems

Key points

- Pulmonary ventilation increases 20 times or more during exercise
- Cardiac output increases up to six-fold in exercise with most of the increase due to increased heart rate
- Maximum oxygen consumption (VO_2max) is limited by the ability of the blood to carry oxygen and of the heart to pump blood

Introduction

This section will concentrate on the important circulatory and respiratory adjustments that are needed for aerobic exercise. In fact, this common way of looking at exercise physiology is really quite wrong. To quote Barcroft (writing in 1937): 'The condition of exercise is not a mere variant of the condition of rest, it is the essence of the machine'. Thus, in many ways the norm, in the world in which our bodies evolved, must have been exercise, and in studying exercise physiology we are really studying the situation for which our bodies, including our circulatory and respiratory systems, evolved.

Respiration in exercise – breathing

Pulmonary ventilation increases with exercise intensity from around 6 L per minute up to 100–150 L/min. For light to moderate exercise, the increase is mostly in tidal volume, with respiratory rate increasing at higher exercise intensities. The relation with oxygen consumption is linear for light to moderate exercise with 20–25 L needing to be breathed to extract each litre of oxygen. So, someone exercising at a level where oxygen consumption is 3 L/min will be breathing about 60 L/min, 10 times the resting level. At moderate to high exercise levels, pulmonary ventilation increases faster than oxygen consumption.

Even at VO_2max, pulmonary ventilation is not at the level that can be attained during voluntary hyperventilation and tidal volume never gets close to vital capacity. However, the high cost of supplying the breathing muscles themselves with oxygen and the fatigue of these muscles probably sets limits during real exercise that is less than the maximum possible.

Quiet breathing at rest involves principally the diaphragm during inspiration and elastic recoil of the lung tissues during expiration. During exercise, additional inspiratory movement is produced by contraction of the external intercostals and the scalene muscles. Also, contraction of some abdominal muscles assists by providing a stable base for the diaphragm. Expiration also now involves active muscle action from the internal intercostals and some abdominal muscles. At high pulmonary ventilation, inspiration is also assisted by the so-called accessory muscles, mainly sternocleidomastoid and the pectorals.

Breathing may become coupled to locomotion during exercise. This is true for rowing, cycling and running (and rather obviously swimming). On a cycle ergometer, it is not uncommon to see sudden switches from one breath every three revolutions, to one every two, then even one breath per revolution close to VO_2max.

Respiration in exercise – control of breathing

During exercise, pulmonary ventilation reaches levels far above anything that can be achieved by administering high CO_2 and low O_2 gas mixtures. This observation immediately indicates that the normal control mechanisms (carbon dioxide/pH acting on central chemoreceptors and anoxia acting peripherally) provide only part of the story during exercise. It appears that neural feedback from the muscles themselves plays some part. Both proprioceptors and, importantly, small fibre 'ergoreceptors' sensing local chemical and vascular changes appear, to be involved. The rapid doubling of breathing that occurs immediately at the start of exercise is certainly driven by peripheral or central motor control signals. Finally, the linking of respiratory rhythm to locomotor time pattern also indicates that there must be coupling between motor control signals and the respiratory centre.

Gas exchange and transport

Gas exchange at the lungs works well during exercise. Carbon dioxide, with its high lipid solubility, crosses readily from circulation to alveolar air. Oxygen crosses sufficiently rapidly to maintain complete arterial saturation except in some highly trained athletes with high oxygen consumption, where a modest degree of oxygen desaturation has been observed. Gas exchange in the muscles is aided by the increased diffusion gradient due to the low tissue PO_2 and high PCO_2 that exist when muscle is metabolising hard. Diffusion of oxygen is aided in slow (Type I) and fast, fatigue resistant (Type IIa) muscle fibres by the presence of myoglobin, responsible for their red pigmentation.

Cardiac adjustments to exercise

Cardiac output increases from its resting value of around 5 L/min to as much as 30 L/min in a trained athlete. The increase is nicely linear with oxygen consumption, as this increases from about 0.25 to 5 L/min. How a six-fold increase in cardiac output is compatible with a 20-fold increase in oxygen consumption will be explained below. Cardiac output is the product of heart rate and stroke volume and both increase during exercise. The heart rate increase falls with age, with maximum heart rate in adults estimated usually by the formula 220 – age. So, in young fit subjects, heart rates of 200 per second are seen. The increase in heart rate follows a reduction in vagal drive to the pacemaker at lower levels of exercise. At higher exercise

levels, the sympathetics and adrenaline push the heart rate up further, and speed up the conducting system. Overall heart rate in a young unfit individual may increase three-fold, while in a trained athlete the increase may be four-fold. The stroke volume increases less, by about 50% and mostly at low- to moderate-intensity exercise levels. The increase partly reflects increased venous return and better filling in the normal Frank-Starling manner. The increased venous return is largely a consequence of the muscle pump. There is also increased contractility of the ventricles due to activation of the sympathetic nervous system and release of adrenaline. Over a long exercise period (>20 min), when oxygen consumption is at a steady level, there is usually a continuing upward drift in heart rate accompanied by a drop in stroke volume. The reduction in exercise capacity in patients on β-blockers is largely because these drugs limit heart rate rises.

Muscle and nonmuscle peripheral vasculature

In the periphery, a massive vasodilatation occurs in the active muscles. Partial compensation occurs with vasoconstriction in viscera. Blood flow to essential organs, such as the brain, is preserved and, obviously, blood supply to the heart is also massively increased. This pattern is largely orchestrated by (1) the sympathetic nervous system and (2) the local dilator actions of metabolites diffusing from muscle fibres. Blood flow to the skin during exercise is regulated to allow the heat generated by active muscles to be dissipated. This means, for exercise at any level in a hot environment and for high-level exercise at almost any environmental temperature, substantial cutaneous vasodilatation occurs.

Blood pressure regulation during exercise

During aerobic exercise, diastolic blood pressure stays approximately stable or may fall a bit, while systolic blood pressure rises.

Pulse pressure is up, while average blood pressure is unchanged or slightly elevated. The situation during isometric exercise or high-force exercise is rather different. Here, long-lasting contractions will increase the peripheral resistance in muscle, thus causing a large rise in average blood pressure. Systolic blood pressures above 250 mmHg are not uncommon during resistance exercises such as bench presses.

The baroreceptor reflex still operates during steady exercise and is one of the control factors. Another important factor is feedback from small fibre ergoreceptors in active muscles. These converge with other relevant inputs in the brainstem to regulate sympathetic and parasympathetic outputs to the heart and the circulation.

Factors limiting maximum oxygen consumption

Maximum oxygen consumption (VO_2max) is an excellent measure of aerobic fitness. It depends on the performance of the circulatory and respiratory systems and the capacity of the muscles to use oxygen. At VO_2max, oxygen consumption is up about 20-fold. Breathing will have increased by

about this amount. Heart rate is up only six-fold, but the greater arteriovenous difference in concentration and the additional proportion of blood going to the muscles means that oxygen-carrying capacity is up 20-fold.

VO_2max appears to be principally determined by the ability of the circulation to get oxygen to the tissues. In some highly trained individuals, there appears to be a limitation on oxygen transport in the lungs. Such individuals have a modest desaturation at high exercise levels and if given higher than atmospheric oxygen to breathe, show increased VO_2max. This does not happen in most individuals. The capacity of the muscle to use oxygen appears to be quite a lot higher than the capacity of the circulatory system to supply it. The circulatory limitations thus appear to be (a) the ability of the heart to pump blood and (b) the ability of blood to carry oxygen. The limiting nature of the oxygen carriage is shown by the fact that increasing blood haemoglobin concentration, by blood doping or taking erythropoietin, does lead to significant increases in VO_2max. The limiting nature of cardiac output is demonstrated by the increases in VO_2max seen with aerobic training.

Further reading

Astrand PO, Rodahl K, Dahl HA, Stromme SB. Textbook of work physiology, 4th edn, Chapters 5 and 6. Champagne, Illinois: Human Kinetics, 2003:127-212.

McArdle WD, Katch FI, Katch VL. Exercise physiology, 7th edn, Chapters 12–17. Baltimore: Lippincott, Williams and Wilkins, 2010:253-352.

Related topics of interest

Exercise promotion

Key points

- Exercise is medicine
- Increasing physical activity is a public heath priority
- Best targets are to increase active travel (cycling and walking) and active leisure (sport, dance, etc.)
- Important to provide the necessary medical support for exercise programmes for patients with chronic diseases or the frail elderly.

Background

Over many years, there has been a reduction in physical activity (PA) in all aspects of our lives – at work, at home, in the ways we travel. Our bodies are not suited to a sedentary life style. The lack of physical activity leads to low cardiorespiratory fitness and other indicators of reduced function. This in turn underlies the growth in noncommunicable diseases – heart disease, diabetes, obesity and many more. So now, according to the WHO, noncommunicable diseases are the commonest causes of death worldwide – more than infection, or trauma, or malnutrition. Consequently, the encouragement of more physical activity has become a public health objective in most countries. Typically, people are exhorted to do 2½ h a week of moderate aerobic exercise, and some strength work (**Table 9**). In the US guidelines, people are also importantly encouraged to do more than this as health benefits improve with increasing activity (**Table 9**).

How many people meet the minimum guidelines for aerobic exercise?

When we look at exercise patterns, it is clear that there is a continuum, ranging from individuals who are completely sedentary to those with a very active lifestyle. So, time spent on moderate or vigorous physical activity ranges from 0 to over 40 h per week in a typical large population sample (**Figure 11**). The distribution is interesting. A lot of people do rather little. In the United Kingdom, 43% do not even do the minimum set in the guidelines. A further 26% are doing 1–3 times the guidelines and a quite considerable group

Table 9 Physical activity guidelines for adults in the United Kingdom and United States*		
UK physical activity guidelines*		
1. Be active daily: minimum 2½ h moderate intensity activity per week (minimum 10 min per session; e.g. 30 min per day, 5 days per week)		
2. Or 75 min vigorous intensity activity per week (or moderate/vigorous intensity combined)		
3. Exercise improving muscle strength ≥2 days per week		
4. Minimise extended sedentary periods		
For greater health benefit (from US physical activity guidelines)**		
1. Increase activity to 5 h per week aerobic activity at moderate intensity		
2. Beyond 5 h per week of moderately intense exercise, or 2½ h per week of vigorously intense exercise, more health benefits will be gained		

*Adapted from Department of Health. Factsheet 4. Physical activity guidelines for adults (19–64 years). London: Department of Health, 2011. https://www.gov.uk/government/publications/uk-physical-activity-guidelines. Accessed 14 Nov 2013.
**http://www.cdc.gov/physicalactivity/everyone/guidelines/adults.html. Accessed 14 Nov 2013.

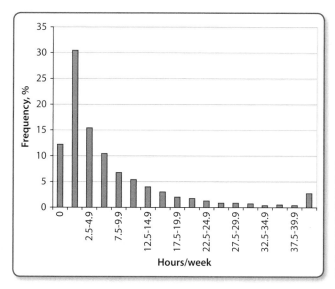

Figure 11 Average time spent doing moderate or vigorous physical activity each week. Note first two bars, i.e. <2.5 h per week, are below the minimum guideline. Data from Health Survey for England, 2008. Excluding people with long-standing illness that limits physical activity. N = 11,231.

(31%) are doing a lot of PA, more than 7½ h per week. Note that these figures refer to the new guidelines. The United Kingdom, and also the United States, Canada and WHO have changed from a guideline of a 30 min period of physical activity 5 days a week to the present one. The same total time is required, but can be achieved in smaller blocks (from 10 min) and not on any particular number of days. Clearly, the new guidelines are easier to achieve. In the United Kingdom, in 2008, only 37% met the old minimum guideline, while 57% meet the new one. Within the population, PA levels are generally higher in males than females and change little with age until falling in the over 60s (**Figure 12**).

What activities can we successfully increase?

Physical activity occurs in four situations:
- At home – housework, gardening, do-it-yourself (DIY), and so on
- At work
- In sporting and other active leisure pursuits
- When travelling – making journeys by foot or cycle instead of car or train

On average, individuals do about the same amount of moderate or vigorous physical activity in each of these categories. Which have the most potential to be increased? It is arguable that we are not going to see a return to heavy physical activity in most occupations. And it is doubtful that we will easily give up our washing machines and other labour-saving aids around the home. That leaves leisure-time exercise and travel. Fortunately, both these areas of activity have plenty of potential.

Access to sports facilities

The provision of accessible sports and exercise facilities is something for which sports medicine professionals have long argued. But sports medicine perhaps has its most important role in ensuring that as many people as possible do feel safe in using such facilities. It is important that suitable reassurance is given about exercise during pregnancy, after illness, etc. Where appropriate it should be possible to organise electrocardiogram and other testing, including exercise stress testing.

It is important also to be aware of the arguments about screening. In some

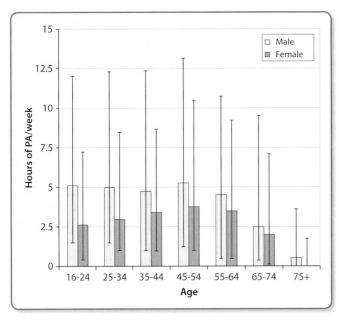

Figure 12 Time doing physical activity by age and sex. Median values for all moderate or above activity, including occupational activity. Error bars are for the 25th and 75th percentiles. Note the large range found, particularly towards high values. Also note that the lower 25th percentiles are all well below the guideline of 2.5 h per week. Data from the Health Survey for England, 2008. Sample sizes were 400–1200. Stratified random sample of the population interviewed at home.

countries, participation in organised sport is only allowed following a medical check-up. While this is appropriate for at-risk individuals, the case for such preparticipation screening for all has not been made. For healthy individuals, a simple screening questionnaire such as the PAR-Q (Physical Activity Readiness Questionnaire) is adequate. It is essential to stress all the time that life is not risk free. And one of the most risky things you can do is not to exercise. There are certainly tragic cases of sudden deaths during sports. But the number of such deaths is very small compared with the premature morbidity associated with lack of exercise. It is noteworthy, however, that the small risk of sudden death during or immediately following a bout of vigorous exercise is higher in those unaccustomed to such exercise. Therefore, good advice is always to build up any exercise programme slowly.

Active travel

Many journeys that we undertake are less the 5 miles. Most of these, in developed countries, are made using motorised transport. But they could almost all (just excepting those that involve carrying heavy loads) be walked or cycled. In addition to the benefits for personal fitness, such a 'mode change' would also improve air quality and cut carbon production. There is particular potential for increasing cycling. This is relatively quick and was, in not so distant times, a much more widely used mode of travel. In order to increase active travelling, a key will be to improve our streets for cyclists and walkers – better pavements and crossings for example.

Exercise is medicine

One problem in the exercise promotion field has been its low profile amongst health practitioners. For example, little is taught about the importance of exercise for health in our training of most health professionals. Can we raise the level of effort put into promoting physical activity? One approach is the 'exercise is medicine' campaign. Giving a prescription for a medicine is standard procedure in health care. So can we present exercise in this way? As we learn more about the way exercise improves how our bodies work, this becomes an easier case to make. The Topic on Exercise and health outlines some of the key facts in this area. It has been pointed out that a drug able to confer the widespread benefits seen in fit individuals would be hailed as a wonder cure (and make some fortunate pharmaceutical company a load of money). So, an important role for sports and exercise medicine professionals is to continually 'sell' physical activity as the 'best buy' in medicine.

To promote exercise for health, one large healthcare provider in the United States (Kayser Permanente) is routinely assessing physical activity during all consultations. If appropriate, brief advice for increasing activity is given. The aim is to reduce the incidence of disorders such as diabetes and cardiovascular disease. Note that this is not just a good strategy for the clients. These conditions are expensive to treat. So, a successful promotion of physical activity will also save the health provider a lot of money.

Exercise prescriptions for at-risk individuals

In the primary care area, it is essential to identify individuals who are particularly at risk due to a sedentary lifestyle. Key factors include: (a) being overweight and (b) poor blood lipid profile. The use of various counselling techniques, often coupled to exercise prescriptions, to get such individuals started has been tried in the primary care area. Results have been variable with problems keeping people exercising over long periods, i.e. in really changing ingrained sedentary behaviour. A Canadian study added simple fitness testing to the usual primary care mix and found maintained increases in activity over 12 months. The effect of having some objective feedback on progress appeared to help in motivation.

Exercise programmes have long been encouraged for patients recovering from heart disease. But such programmes also help with diabetes, arthritis, depression, osteopenia and a range of other chronic illnesses. In these situations, it is important that the development of appropriate clinical exercise programmes with proper medical oversight is encouraged.

Physical activity often falls to very low levels in older individuals. This is an area where the health message about the benefits of physical activity has been getting through. It is difficult to frighten a young person with good health into exercising to improve their health in the future. But for older people, this message is clearly seen as much more relevant. In addition, exercise programmes can help in falls prevention and such programmes have been successfully implemented in many countries.

Why is physical activity promotion so difficult?

Why is it proving so difficult to persuade people to adopt a more active lifestyle? Perhaps we need to take an evolutionary perspective. It is frequently pointed out that our bodies are designed for exercise. And this is certainly the case. But our brains are programmed quite differently. In a primitive environment, it was sensible to rest when one could, and to eat when food was available. Hunting involved serious levels of physical activity. To be successful, one would need to be rested. So, our behaviour patterns have evolved to meet this pattern of life. When food is available – eat. When not needing to hunt or defend territory – rest. In a primitive environment, there is no conflict between a body designed for activity and a brain programmed for rest. The need for regular activity is a survival imperative. In a modern environment, however, these behaviour patterns are disastrous.

Further reading

Blair SN, Sallis RE, Hutber A, Archer E. Exercise therapy – the public health message. Scand J Med Sci Sports 2012; 22:e24–e28.

National Institute for Health and Clinical Excellence. Walking and cycling: local measures to promote walking and cycling as forms of travel or recreation. NICE public health guidance 41. UK: NICE, 2012. http://guidance.nice.org.uk/PH41. Accessed 14 Nov 2013.

Petrella RJ, Koval JJ, Cunningham DA, Paterson DH. Can primary care doctors prescribe exercise to improve fitness? The Step Test Exercise Prescription (STEP) project. Am J Prev Med 2003; 24: 316–322.

Physical Activity Guidelines Advisory Committee. Physical Activity Guidelines Advisory Committee report, 2008. Washington, DC: U.S. Department of Health and Human Services, 2008. http://www.health.gov/paguidelines/guidelines/default.aspx#. Accessed 14 Nov 2013.

Taylor A. The role of primary care in promoting physical activity. In: McKenna J, Riddoch C (eds), Perspectives on health and exercise, Chapter 8. Basingstoke, UK: Palgrave Macmillan, 2003:153-180.

The PAR-Q screening form is available from the Canadian Society for Exercise Physiology. Published on the Internet. Available online at http://www.csep.ca/forms.asp. Accessed 14 Nov 2013.

Related topics of interest

Eye injuries in sports

Key points

- Many sport-related eye injuries may be preventable
- Clinical assessment is of vital importance to assess the severity of the injury
- Vast majority of sport related eye injuries are preventable

Overview

Vision is our dominant sense. Sports-related eye injuries represent a significant eye health hazard globally. However, they are often preventable.

The incidence of eye injuries due to sporting activities has shown a steady increase in recent years. A short survey conducted at Moorfields Eye Hospital, London showed that of nearly 17,000 emergency department attendances, 48 patients (0.28%) had sports-related ocular injuries. It is worth mentioning that none of the victims wore eye protection and, worse, none were given advice regarding preventive measures for future trauma. It is remarkable that the statistics varies in different parts of the world.

Different sports carry varying degrees of associated risk. According to the American Public Health Association, the following sports have been identified as carrying moderate to high risk of ocular injury: basketball, baseball, softball, cricket, lacrosse, field and ice hockey, squash, racquet ball, fencing, boxing, full contact martial arts, air rifle, tennis, badminton, soccer, volleyball, water polo, fishing, football, golf and wrestling. In the United Kingdom, soccer is responsible for most eye injuries, whereas baseball and basketball are responsible for most eye injuries in the United States.

Eye examination equipments

With a few equipment and a good history and physical examination, these injuries can be managed on the given athletic arena. A slit lamp examination may occasionally be necessary. Most eye trolleys should contain the following: ophthalmoscope, a penlight and a light source with a blue filter, fluorescein dye, cotton-tipped swabs, a portable Snellen chart (for those with smartphones, many free apps are available), eye shields, magnifying glass, 18-gauge needles (green needle), sterile saline and a contact lens remover.

Medications include anaesthetic and mydriatic drops, and also antibiotic ointment. A tonopen or iCare for measuring eye pressure would be optional.

Assessment of athletes with eye injuries

The doctor should take a thorough history about the direction and mechanism of injury. After excluding and managing life-threatening conditions, clinicians should then focus on eyes. A good systematic clinical examination can diagnose many eye injuries. Examination starts with assessment of visual acuity by using a vision chart. Pupils should be examined with a penlight and should include assessment of size, reactivity, shape and also extra-ocular movements. At this point, one should check for a relative afferent pupillary defect; this can be done with the swinging flashlight test. Players should always be asked about the presence of double vision after any eye or head injury. A relative afferent pupillary defect is present when the eye with the deficit paradoxically dilates when exposed to the light source.

The penlight can be employed to evaluate the anterior chamber for relative depth and the eyelids for lacerations. Conjunctiva, cornea, and facial and maxillary bones should be assessed as well.

Range of injury

Minor trauma

Blunt trauma is the culprit for most sporting eye injuries. The commonest consequence of such an injury is a periorbital contusion or black eye. Although not serious, this might prevent an adequate examination of underlying globe because of tense swelling of the eyelids.

A direct blow often damages the corneal epithelium, causing an acutely painful corneal abrasion, a major possible complication of which is the development of recurrent corneal erosion. However, the skin might burst causing lid laceration, which needs to be closed with care.

Superficial foreign bodies

Small pieces of foreign material, such as grit or dust may be blown or thrown into the eye. Such material can remain at the surface and become a corneal foreign body or become attached to the inner surface of the upper lid, becoming subtarsal foreign body. Contact lenses may dislodge during game, causing irritation as well as rapid reduction in visual acuity. Only soft contact lenses should be worn during sport. A full evaluation to rule out foreign bodies should include inversion of the upper and lower eyelids. Foreign bodies should be irrigated. If that fails, dislodge it with moistened cotton bud.

Severe trauma

Orbit

Blowout fractures occur when the eye is struck with significant force usually by an object larger than the orbit. This raises the intraocular pressure and the floor of the orbit blows out into the maxillary antrum. There is usually orbital anaesthesia, periorbital oedema and ecchymosis and mainly diplopia due to restricted eye movements.

Anterior segment

Following a blow to the eye, the iris is commonly torn either at pupil margin or at the iris root (iridodialysis). These athletes might complain of having monocular diplopia due to iridodialysis.

This injury results in bleeding into the anterior chamber, or hyphaema. This is evident as a level of blood inside anterior chamber or as diffuse haze in the early period. Such patients should be seen by an ophthalmologist.

Associated injuries might include cataract, dislocation of the lens, damage to the drainage angle, traumatic uveitis and persistent dilation of the pupil from iris sphincter damage.

Posterior segment

A direct blow to the eye may lead to tear in the retina, predisposing to detachment. Damage to the retinal vessels may cause vitreous haemorrhage and traumatic oedema (commotio retinae), which is diagnosed with ophthalmoscopy.

The choroid underlying retina may also rupture and the optic nerve can be damaged by bleeding into the optic nerve sheath or damage in the optic canal.

A devastating consequence of blunt eye trauma is retrobulbar haemorrhage, leading to compartment syndrome. A high index of suspicion should be held in patients with periorbital bruising, visual impairment, proptosis, and pupillary defects in the setting of blunt trauma; these patients should be seen immediately by an ophthalmologist.

Penetrating ocular injury

These are rare in sport and they often carry a poor visual outcome. They may be caused by racquets, sticks, fingers or fish hooks entering the globe. Pain, visual loss, hyphaema, anterior chamber depth loss, and subconjunctival haemorrhage involving all around the cornea are very suggestive for globe rupture. Once globe rupture is suspected, prompt referral to an ophthalmologist is mandatory. An eye shield should immediately be placed; manipulation should be deferred to avoid direct pressure and further damage. Analgesics and antiemetics should be provided to prevent Valsalva maneuvers.

Burns and radiation exposure

Ultraviolet (UV) burns tend to damage conjunctiva and cornea and can happen in water and snow sports as well as mountaineering and athletics at high altitudes. Classic signs include intense pain, photophobia and delay in onset of symptoms, tearing, and lid spasms. Treatment involves systemic and topical analgesics. The best prevention for radiation exposure of the eye is the use of sunglasses that absorbs all forms of UV radiation.

Shatter-resistant polycarbonate lenses should be used for protection.

Trivex lenses are also highly recommended for sports; initially, developed for the military and these lenses became available to the public since 2003. Trivex lenses are stronger, optically better, lighter, and more scratch resistance compared with polycarbonate lenses.

Prevention and protection

Studies shown that more than 90% of sports-related eye injuries are preventable. Prevention of ocular injuries can be considered as falling into four categories as follows:
1. Encouraging safe play by appropriate coaching and training
2. Ensuring that the rules of play are in interest of eye safety
3. Wearing protective eyewear
4. Screening players with special ocular conditions, which render them at risk

The American Society for Testing and Material (ASTM) sets standards for eye protection. These can be viewed at the following website: http://www.astm.org/standards/F803.html

Table 10 Return-to-play guidelines	
Eye injury	**Return to play**
Corneal abrasion	May return to play if no visual loss is present
Corneal foreign body	May return to play if no visual loss is present
Blowout fracture	Should not return back to play
Globe rupture	Should not return back to play
Hyphaema	Should not return back to play
Retrobulbar haemorrhage	Should not return back to play
Retinal tear or detachment	Should not return back to play
Eyelid laceration	May return to play if bleeding is controlled
Penetrating eye trauma	Should not return back to play
Burns and radiation exposure	May return to play if no visual problem is present

Further reading

Cass SP. Ocular injuries in sports. Curr Sports Med Reports 2012; 11:11–15.

Goldstein MH, Wee D. Sports injuries: an ounce of prevention and a pound of cure. Eye Cont Lens 2011; 37:160–163.

Ong HO, Barsam A, Morris OC, Siriwardena D, Verma S. A survey of ocular sports trauma and the role of eye protection. Cont Lens Anterior Eye 2012; 35:285–287.

Related topics of interest

• Prevention of sport injuries (p. 236)

Fatigue

Key points

- The reduction in muscle performance seen in fatigue is in part due to the accumulation of inorganic phosphate due to the breakdown of phosphocreatine
- Reactive oxygen and nitrogen species (ROS/RNS) produced as by-products of oxidative phosphorylation also play a part in reducing force production
- In endurance exercise, fatigue is related to the reduced availability of carbohydrate due to depletion of muscle glycogen
- Central neural factors play an important part in fatigue and the reduction in neural drive to fatiguing muscles may be a useful protection against irreversible cellular damage

The nature of fatigue

Muscular fatigue is often the limiting factor in sports and exercise performance. The fatigued athlete is also more likely to get injured. So establishing the basis of fatigue has occupied much research. Additionally, excessive fatigue is a problem about which health professionals are often consulted. This section will cover central and peripheral mechanisms of fatigue directly related to exercise. The more generalised phenomenon of chronic fatigue and tiredness will not be addressed. Aspects of chronic fatigue are seen in unexplained underperformance syndrome (UUPS) and are discussed in a later topic on UUPS.

Fatigued muscles show characteristic falls in peak force and in speed of contraction. Power, the product of these two, is profoundly reduced. The time course of individual twitch contractions is also prolonged due to a slowing of relaxation. The causes of these changes are multiple and will first be considered for different durations of exercise. But one aspect of fatigue is worth pointing out. It is not due to ATP depletion. With severe exercise, ATP levels can drop substantially in fast (Type II) fibres (although well maintained in Type I fibres). However, the crossbridge ATPase has a sufficiently

high affinity for ATP that even the levels of 20% normal seen in some fast fibres are still high enough to ensure normal cross bridge function. Such low levels will be associated with raised magnesium, and the combined effect may be some reduction in calcium release and so in force of contraction.

Fatigue in short bouts of exercise

For maximal efforts up to 1 h or so the two principal factors in fatigue appear to be (1) accumulation of end products from muscle contraction, notably inorganic phosphate ions and (2) production of ROS/RNS mainly as a by-product of oxidative phosphorylation in the mitochondria. Accumulation of phosphate, one of the products of ATP splitting during crossbridge cycling, will directly inhibit further ATP splitting. In addition, there is evidence that accumulation of phosphate also interferes with excitation–contraction coupling, reducing calcium release during excitation.

Fatigue in endurance exercise

For endurance exercise, accumulation of phosphate and other ions appears to be less important. Here, the problem is running out of glycogen. Supplies of glycogen and glucose are limited. Parallel carbohydrate metabolism is also needed for lipids to enter the TCA cycle and be oxidised. To counter this, athletes preload with carbohydrate before endurance events and drink carbohydrate fluids during them.

Slow phase of recovery after fatiguing exercise

We recover quickly from the immediate fatigue following exercise, but only up to a point. After strong exercise there is a lingering fatigue for several days. During this phase, maximum muscle contractions are possible but require more effort. Electrical stimulation experiments show that muscles respond normally to high-frequency (>50 Hz) stimulation, but have reduced force generation at lower frequency. Hence, the term 'low-frequency fatigue' is used for this phenomenon. This is actually not a very good term as it implies that low-frequency stimulation produces the fatigue, which of course is not the case: maximal high-frequency stimulation is the usual trigger. Westerblad and Allen proposed the term 'prolonged low-frequency force depression' (PLFFD), instead. The mechanism of PLFFD may be microtrauma leading to interference with excitation–contraction coupling. If this is the case, then it is similar to the muscle weakness seen following eccentric contraction (part of the diffuse onset muscle soreness, DOMS, phenomenon).

Central fatigue

It is well recognised that during a fatiguing voluntary contraction if you shout encouragement to the competitor, there is usually an increase in force. This phenomenon can be studied more precisely using the twitch interpolation technique, where a maximal shock is applied to the muscle motor nerve during a voluntary contraction. Such experiments show that voluntary activation often fails to evoke a maximum contraction, and this is more often true in fatigue. A more subtle aspect of changing motor control in fatigue is that the motor unit firing frequency falls, but usually only by enough to allow for the fall in tetanic fusion frequency caused by the slowing of relaxation time in a fatigued muscle. The causes of these changes in motor control during fatigue are not well understood, but presumably depend in large part on feedback from sensory receptors in the muscle.

It is possible that the fall in neural drive to fatigued muscle is a useful safety measure. Continuing to contract a muscle fibre to the point, where ATP is very low, or ROS/NOS accumulate too much, could well cause irreversible cellular changes and cell death. Central fatigue effectively eliminates this danger.

Further reading

Allen DG, Lamb GD, Westerblad H. Skeletal muscle fatigue: cellular mechanisms. Physiol Rev 2008; 88:287–332.
Jones D, Round J, de Haan A. Skeletal muscle from molecules to movement. Edinburgh: Churchill Livingstone, 2004.
Westerblad H, Allen DG. Cellular mechanisms of skeletal muscle fatigue. In: Williams C, Ratel S (eds), Human muscle fatigue, Chapter 3.Abingdon: Routledge, 2009:48–75.

Related topics of interest

- Muscle properties relevant to sports and exercise (p. 195)
- Unexplained underperformance syndrome (p. 326)
- Training (p. 323)

Female athlete – exercise during pregnancy

Key points

- Exercise is beneficial during pregnancy
- Care is clearly needed, for example avoiding contact sports
- Pregnancy can be the trigger for previously sedentary individuals to develop a more active and healthy lifestyle

Exercise is recommended during pregnancy

Pregnancy should not mean confinement. Guidelines from the American College of Obstetrics and Gynecology and the Royal College of Obstetrics and Gynecology reflect current best practice in recommending that significant levels of exercise should continue during pregnancy in order to maintain cardiovascular fitness and muscle condition. Clearly any serious pre-existing medical condition must be taken carefully into account, as must any problem developing during pregnancy. Overall, the benefits of maintaining fitness outweigh any risks from continuing to exercise.

Certain changes are, however, necessary. In the second and third trimester, exercising lying supine is to be avoided as the uterus can press on the vena cava and reduce venous return to the heart. Contact sports should be avoided, as should scuba diving. Extra care should also be taken to avoid hyperthermia owing to the teratogenic risk from high body temperature. For competitive athletes, a break from competition is inevitable, as performance will be diminished as weight is gained. However, training can continue, with routine obstetric evaluation.

There are clear benefits from maintaining fitness. Labour is on average shorter in physically active mothers. Also in gestational diabetes, exercise can contribute to normalising blood glucose levels. There is also some evidence that pelvic floor exercises during pregnancy can reduce the risk of postnatal incontinence.

A good time to stress the healthy living message

Pregnancy offers a golden opportunity to improve maternal health. It is notoriously difficult to persuade sedentary individuals to start exercising regularly (just as it is hard to persuade smokers to stop and to persuade those with a bad diet to eat their fruit and vegetable). Becoming pregnant is an event that stimulates people to look hard at their lifestyle and try to make healthy changes. So it is a good time to point out the advantages for mother and baby of taking regular exercise (and stopping smoking, etc.). We certainly need to try this as, at present, quite the opposite usually happens. For example, a recent survey in the United States found that on average pregnant women take only around half the exercise of age-matched nonpregnant women.

Postpartum exercise is also recommended

After birth, assuming no problems, a full exercise programme can be undertaken immediately. Not too many new mothers will want to rush straight out to the gym, so a gradual resumption of full training will be the norm. There is no evidence that high levels of physical activity affect lactation as long as maternal nutrition is adequate.

Further reading

Artal R, O'Toole M. Guidelines of the American College of Obstetricians and Gynecologists for exercise during pregnancy and the postpartum period. Br J Sports Med 2003; 37:6–12.

Nascimento SL, Surita FG Cecatti JG. Physical exercise during pregnancy: a systematic review. Curr Opin Obstet Gynecol 2012; 24:387-394.

Petersen AM, Leet TL, Brownson RC. Correlates of physical activity among pregnant women in the United States. Med Sci Sports Exerc 2005; 37:1748–1753.

Royal College of Obstetricians and Gynaecologists. Exercise in Pregnancy. RCOG, Statement. No4.2006. (http://www.rcog.org.uk/womens-health/clinical-guidance/exercise-pregnancy).

Related topics of interest

• Exercise promotion (p. 112)

Female athlete – the triad

Key points

- Female athletes in weight-sensitive sports may have menstrual disturbance and bone mineral loss associated with undereating
- Key cause appears to be very low body fat mass and consequential low circulating levels of the hormone leptin
- Reduction in training levels and/or increased eating leads to recovery of normal menstrual function but is not paralleled by a full recovery of bone mineralisation
- Athletes need to be educated about the risks of osteopenia and informed so that early signs of menstrual dysfunction are noted and appropriate action taken to prevent bone mineral loss

Overview

The last 100 years have seen increasing participation in elite sports by women. However, an unexpected problem has emerged in weight-sensitive sports (e.g. distance running and lightweight rowing) and areas where slim body shape is important (e.g. ballet and gymnastics). This is menstrual dysfunction associated with a reduction in bone mineral density. These two changes are linked to not eating enough to match energy required for training and so having greatly reduced energy availability. The condition, the female athlete triad, thus has three components: reduced bone mineral density, menstrual disturbance and disordered eating (**Figure 13**)

Undereating to reduce body weight appears to be the fundamental cause, leading to a fall in adipose tissue mass. This might appear a good thing that improves performance or allows competition in a lower weight class. However, we now know that adipose tissue has important endocrine functions. In particular, adipose tissue secretes leptin, a polypeptide hormone. If adipose tissue mass falls, so does leptin secretion. Leptin plays an important biological role in control of reproduction and lack of leptin stops reproduction when food is scarce. In female athletes with very low fat mass there is hypothalamic 'switch off' of GnRH (gonadotropin-releasing hormone) and so of reproduction.

The leptin story continues to develop. It is now known that leptin has effects on bone resorption and formation that are independent of other hormonal factors. It has been found in animal models that leptin can block the bone loss that occurs (a) in a bone-unloading experiment and (b) following ovariectomy. So it appears that some of the female triad effects on bone mineralisation may be due directly to leptin insufficiency, and not just due to falls in oestrogen levels. In addition, leptin appears to have an important role in maintaining an effective immune system. Lymphocytes have leptin receptors and individuals lacking leptin have very low levels of several cytokines. Adipose

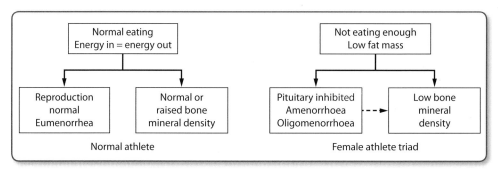

Figure 13 Components of the female athlete triad.

tissue also secretes several other hormones, known collectively as adipokines (they have similarities to cytokines). It is possible that altered secretion of other adipokines may also play a part in the athlete triad.

Once bone mineral density falls, it never appears to recover. Also, many female athletes are in the age (15-25 years) range where bone mineral is laid down at the maximum rate. They may therefore end up with a lower than expected peak bone mass (at age 25-30) and so in later life have a lower bone density. This greatly increases the risk of fracture as a one standard deviation change in bone mineral density means a two to four times increased risk of fracture.

Epidemiology

Incidence of menstrual disorders is higher in athletes and dancers than in the general population. It is clearly associated with low body weight, particularly low body fat levels. For example, it is more common in lightweight than heavyweight rowers. Menstrual problems are not common in swimming or power events. In distance runners an incidence of amenorrhoea of up to 65% have been reported and in dancers an incidence of 69%. This compares with 2–5% in the general population. Surveys of bone mineral density in athletes and dancers usually show higher than average values due to the response of bone to the mechanical stresses of exercise. However, a proportion of athletes in weight sensitive areas of endeavour have lower bone mineral density. Overall in such groups up to 13% have been found with osteoporosis and 22–50% with osteopenia. Finally, eating disorders are seen in 25–31% in this group of athletes, compared with 6–9% in the general population. Note that clinical anorexia or bulimia are rare. The number of athletes or dancers who show all three features of the triad at a clinically diagnosable level is in fact small, only around 4%, not very different from the 3% found in control populations. This is puzzling given the probable association of the three aspects of the triad due to the underlying pathophysiology. In fact, 4% is about what one would expect if each aspect of the triad

were an independent entity. Clearly, we still have a bit to learn about the epidemiology of the female athlete triad.

Clinical features

The key clinical features have already been described: menstrual disturbance, very low fat mass and disordered eating. Useful definitions are given in **Table 11**. As noted above, it is unusual to see all these features at clinically significant levels. So the usual presentation is amenorrhoea or oligomenorrhoea. Lack of energy may also be an issue that leads an athlete to seek medical help. Low fat mass does not lead to requests for medical help.

Cases may present not directly from the triad features, but because of a stress fracture, e.g. of the tibia. Finally, help may be sought from younger athletes and dancers because of very delayed menarche.

The golden rule is that any female athlete presenting with very slim body shape and menstrual problems should be investigated for other features of the triad, especially if there is any history of stress fracture, or undiagnosed skeletal pain that might have been a fracture.

Investigations

Endocrinological. Full history related to menstrual pattern and age of menarche. Blood test for FSH and LH, thyroid-stimulating hormone and free thyroxine. Check urine chorionic gonadotrophin. Conduct progesterone challenge.
Bone health. Dual-energy X-ray absorptiometry scan or quantitative computed tomography
Eating/Diet. Nutritional survey to calculate current energy intake and intake of calcium and vitamin D. Assessment for presence of eating disorder, e.g. SCOFF questionnaire.

Differential diagnosis

If presenting symptoms are principally menstrual irregularity or absence:
- Pregnancy
- Polycystic ovarian syndrome

Table 11 Definitions for components of the triad	
Menstrual disturbances	
Eumenorrhoea	Menstrual cycles at intervals near the median for young adult women (28 ± 7 days)
Amenorrhoea	Cessation of menstrual periods for at least 3 months or less than 3 cycles per year
Oligomenorrhoea	Cycles at intervals greater than 35 days or less than 6 cycles per year
Luteal phase deficiency	Shortening of the luteal phase to less than 10 days
Eating, energy	
Anorexia nervosa	Body weight <85% expected for age and height; disturbed body image; amenorrhoea
Bulimia nervosa	Recurrent episodes of binge eating; recurrent inappropriate attempts to compensate for overeating to prevent weight gain (e.g. vomiting); perception of self-worth excessively influenced by body weight and shape
Eating disorder	Disordered eating that does not meet the criteria for any specific eating disorder. For example, all the criteria for anorexia but with regular menses
Energy availability	Energy intake in diet less energy expended in exercise
Bone mineral density	
Osteopenia	WHO. T-score 1–2.5 standard deviations below average for young healthy women
Osteoporosis	WHO. T-score 2.5 standard deviations or more below average for young healthy women OR ACMS. Z-score more than 2 standard deviations below the age matched average
Low BMD	ACMS. Z-score 1–2 standard deviations below the age matched average
WHO, World Health Organization; ACMS, American College of Sports Medicine; BMD, bone mass density.	

If presenting symptoms are principally tiredness/lack of energy:

- Unexplained underperformance syndrome
- Hypothyroidism

Treatment

Only one treatment works: restoring energy balance and increasing fat stores. However, this is not an easy option for a competitive athlete or an aspiring dancer. It is essential when explaining this that suitable support is on hand in the form of psychology and counselling. One can imagine how shattering it is for a young person to be told that, for their health, they may not be able to train at a level that gets them into the first eight or into the top ballet company. However, it may not be the end of a career. Sometimes, the necessary adjustment to energy balance is quite small and has little affect on performance. In developing a modified training programme and working on an improved diet, it is also important to talk to coaching staff and to close family so that they understand the treatment programme and are fully supportive. Crucial to effective treatment is a team approach. As well as medical input it is important to have a dietician to help with nutritional aspects and a psychologist to deal with eating disorders and behaviour change.

In athletes who have been amenorrhoeic for some time it is worth pointing out that they will start ovulating before the first period. So fertility may return before they realise and they should be prepared for this.

There have been attempts to treat the female triad by giving oestrogens, either in the form of oral contraceptive (OCP) or HRT. Taking OCP does cause periods to restart, but this is not an indication of problem solved. Improvements in bone density have not been seen in most studies. This is probably because any contribution of oestrogen lack to bone loss in premenopausal women is small. The key problems are (a) undernutrition and (b) lack of leptin. Replacement therapy with leptin, something that is done for lipodystrophy, has not been attempted for the female athlete triad. Bisphosphonates are generally not considered suitable for young women due the long action with unknown consequences, with possible effects on the foetus particularly worrying. It is useful to supplement calcium and vitamin D.

Return to sport

Many triad sufferers do not stop training or competing, although they may need to reduce exercise levels. In team sports, coaches may leave athletes out for a spell while they get themselves back to healthy levels of energy availability. In general, as soon as menstruation has restarted there is no reason not to be fully engaged in sport or dance.

Prevention

Athletes and coaches need to be informed so that they can spot early signs. Education about the serious long-term, partly irreversible, effects of bone loss is required.

Further reading

Hill LS, Reid F, Morgan JF, Lacey JH. SCOFF, the development of an eating disorder screening questionnaire. Int J Eat Disord 2010; 43:344–351.

Nattiv A, Loucks AB, Manore MM, et al. American College of Sports Medicine position stand: The female athlete triad. Med Sci Sports Exerc 2010; 39:1867–1882.

Nazem TG, Ackerman KE. The female athlete triad. Sports Health 2012; 4:302–311.

Witkop CT, Warren MP. Understanding the spectrum of the female athlete triad. Obstet Gynecol 2010; 116:1444–1448.

Related topics of interest

Fitness testing

Key points

- VO$_2$max is the accepted measure of aerobic fitness and is the best indicator of cardiovascular and other health risks
- A wide range of submaximal tests is available and these allow safe estimation of VO$_2$max
- Trends in VO$_2$max can give reliable indications of fitness trends, for example when physical activity has been increased as part of an exercise prescription

Why measure fitness?

It is often useful to have a good measure of aerobic fitness and the usual one is VO$_2$max, the maximum oxygen consumption. Fitness is an excellent predictor of future health. Fitness measures also have a role in monitoring rehabilitation and can be used to assess when return to competition is possible. Finally, fitness measures can be useful in monitoring the effectiveness of physical activity programmes, for example as part of an exercise prescription, and can help motivate subjects.

Maximal tests

For young healthy individuals, VO$_2$max can be measured directly using a maximal exercise test. However, before such a test the subject's history needs to be checked to ensure there are no health issues that might make such a test dangerous. A simple questionnaire such as the PAR-Q is generally sufficient.

Maximal tests can involve stepping, running on a treadmill or cycling. The subject starts exercising at an easy level, then the work rate is stepped up until a maximum heart rate is obtained and the subject cannot perform the next work rate. Measurement of expired gases and their volume allows VO$_2$max to be determined. There are several well-established protocols that are given in exercise physiology texts. VO$_2$max can also be estimated without actually measuring VO$_2$. An example is the shuttle test where subjects do repeat sprints between markers with speed increasing each time until the participant cannot keep up. The relation between final speed and VO$_2$max has been determined for test populations and these relations can be used to provide a good estimate for VO$_2$max.

Submaximal tests

A reasonable estimate of VO$_2$max can also be obtained using submaximal tests and such tests are normally used with older subjects and where the highest accuracy is not required. Many different submaximal tests have been described. Most submaximal tests involve modifications of maximal tests and use stepping, treadmill walking/running or cycling and are carried out in the gym or the exercise laboratory, or in many cases in a treatment room or even at home. These tests depend on measuring heart rate at defined submaximal work levels. An estimate is then made of the subject's maximal work rate based on their age-related maximal heart rate. VO$_2$max is estimated from the relation between work rate and oxygen consumption determined for the appropriate population and exercise modality.

Some tests involve making two or three heart rate measures at rising work rates, then graphically extrapolating to maximum heart rate to estimate maximum work capacity. Other tests use a single exercise level and heart rate and interpolate into previously determined data on oxygen consumption in relation to heart rate. A popular method uses stepping or cycling and calculates VO$_2$max using the Astrand-Rhyming nomogram. Quite simple step tests can give good results and when linked to a computer can give an instant printout of VO$_2$max. For example, such a test has been used in a large primary care survey in Canada. VO$_2$max can also be estimated from standard exercise patterns and heart rate. For example, the Rockport test involves walking as quickly as possible for 1 mile, then estimating VO$_2$max from the time taken and the final heart rate. Such tests are suitable for relatively unfit individuals.

What does a given VO$_2$max mean?

Key here is to compare with population norms. Generally, we need to allow for gender and age. Average data are given in **Table 12**. Thus, approximately 50% of people fall within 10–15% of the average. A measured VO$_2$max is 15% lower than the average (shown in brackets), this indicates low fitness, probably in the lowest quartile. Remember that individual submaximal tests only provide an approximate indication of VO$_2$max, typically with confidence limit of around ±15%. Where these test are useful is in following trends in a given individual. Careful repeats by the same person usually vary only by about ±4%, and with repeat measurements it is possible to pick up trends of only a few percent in fitness.

In fact, if the main interest is to follow trends, then this can be done just by monitoring the heart rate at the end of a fixed piece of exercise, for example heart rate at the end of 2–3 min of stepping. So with a heart rate monitor and a metronome one can track fitness. Typically, a 5 beats per minute reduction in exercise heart rate represents around a 10% increase in fitness. And this is the sort of change that can be achieved in a short physical activity training programme.

Table 12 Average VO$_2$max (mL O$_2$.min^{-1}.kg body wt^{-1}) for European populations.					
Age range	16–24	25–34	35–44	45–54	55–64
Males	42 (36)	39 (33)	36 (30)	33.5 (29)	31 (26)
Females	39 (33)	36 (31)	34 (29)	31 (26)	28 (24)

Data averaged from Health Survey for England (HSE 2008), Danish Health Examination Survey (DANHES 2007–2008) and Ekblom B, Engstrom LM, Ekblom O. Secular trends of physical fitness in Swedish adults. Scand J Med Sci Sports 2007; 17:267–273. Total number sampled is 13,268.

Further reading

American College of Sports Medicine (ACSM). ACSM's health-related physical fitness assessment manual, 3rd edn. Philadelphia; Lippincott Williams and Wilkins, 2010.

Par-Q and you. Canadian Society for Exercise Physiology, 2002. Published on the Internet. Available online at http://www.csep.ca/forms.asp.

Petrella R, Koval JJ, Cunningham DA, et al. Can primary care doctors prescribe exercise to improve fitness? The Step Test Exercise Prescription (STEP) project. Am J Prev Med 2003; 24:316–322.

Related topics of interest

Forearm and wrist conditions

Key points

- May be related to acute traumatic event or due to overuse syndrome
- Common, as even in sports where handling is not permitted, a fall on an outstretched wrist may cause injury
- Athletes should be taught to fall by protective rolling in order to reduce the risk to their hands and wrists

Conditions

Scaphoid fracture

- Caused by fall on outstretched wrist
- **Pain in radial aspect of wrist.** On examination, there will be pain in anatomical snuffbox and on telescoping the thumb
- Rate of nonunion is high in cases of missed diagnoses or inadequate cast immobilisation (normally require 8–12 weeks)
- In athletes it is important to make a definitive diagnosis in order to avoid unnecessary cast treatment and promptly progress to surgery if required
- **Management**:
  - The fracture may not be visible on initial X-rays (scaphoid views). If clinically suspected the patient should have further imaging such as MRI (magnetic resonance imaging)/CT (computed tomography) or be placed in a cast and re-X-rayed at 2 weeks. If the fracture line is still not visible but tenderness remains at 2 weeks, further imaging (MRI or CT or bone scan) should be arranged
  - Displaced fractures require an operation (percutaneous/open screw fixation). Operative treatment for undisplaced fractures should also be offered to this population group to allow early range of movement and strength training

Hook of hamate fracture

- Common in athletes with implement in hand (golf stick, bat, racquet)
- Caused by either direct force over hypothenar eminence or shear force from implement
- Pain in proximal hypothenar eminence
- Fracture may not always be visible on X-rays and further imaging with oblique views or CT scan will be needed to make diagnosis
- **Management:** Undisplaced fractures can be treated with cast immobilisation for 6 weeks. Displaced fragments can either be excised or fixed depending on their size

Handlebar/cyclist's palsy

- Seen in cyclists due to the compression of ulnar nerve in Guyon's canal at wrist
- See mostly motor disturbance with hand weakness, lack of coordination. Depending on location of compression, sensory signs may occasionally be present
- **Treatment:** Cycling gloves, changing hand position frequently whilst riding and ensuring adequate bicycle fit will help settle symptoms

Triangular fibrocartilage complex injury

- Can be acute, chronic, or acute on chronic injuries
- Associated with gymnasts, hockey players, racquet sports, boxers
- Can be seen with fractures of distal radius and ulna styloid fractures
- Pain and tenderness on ulnar side of wrist and on resisted supination
- Diagnosis made with MRI arthrogram. Also need to exclude distal radioulnar joint instability
- **Management:** This varies depending on chronicity. Acutely may be treated with rest and rehabilitation. If does not settle may need arthroscopic or open repair

Keinböck's disease

- Avascular necrosis of lunate bone possibly due to repetitive trauma
- Insidious onset with patient presenting with pain over mid-dorsum wrist and restriction in wrist range of movement
- Radiographs may be normal initially and MRI scan is necessary for definitive diagnosis

- **Management:** It will depend on grade. Radial shortening procedures may alter disease progression in early stages and allow return to sport. Unfortunately at latter stages of disease, wrist fusion or carpectomy may be only solution to pain

Distal radius fractures

- Fall on outstretched wrist (in flexion or extension) or may be seen as part of an overuse syndrome in the form of a stress fracture
- Patients require AP and lateral radiographs to diagnose
- Colles – dorsally angulated, Smiths – volarly angulated fracture
- **Management:**
  - Undisplaced/minimally displaced fractures can be treated in a below elbow cast for 6 weeks. Displaced fractures are usually manipulated in the emergency setting under haematoma block. If adequate reduction is achieved, then cast treatment can be pursued
  - Displaced and intra-articular fractures require manipulation under anaesthesia and fixation with either wires or with a plate

Gymnast's wrist

- Physeal injury due to repetitive stress to distal radius and ulna epiphysis
- Patients will present with wrist pain. Most pronounced after a session of training or competing
- Radiographs show widening of the physis and sclerosis or irregularity of metaphysis. Similar to finding in rickets; hence, sometimes called 'pseudorickets'
- **Management:** Rest and splintage will see the resolution of symptoms in most cases. Wrist strengthening programme should be sought prior to return to sport.

Dorsal wrist impingement

- Overuse syndrome commonly seen in gymnasts due to hyperextension with axial loading
- There is impingement initially of dorsal wrist capsule and later, of bony impingement of dorsal lip of distal radius on carpus

- **Management:** Rest, ice, antiflammatory treatment may be sufficient initially, followed by wrist strengthening and gradual return to sport. A corticosteroid injection may sometimes be necessary if symptoms persist and occasionally surgical treatment (cheilectomy) may be required

De Quervain's tenosynovitis

- Stenosing tenosynovitis of first dorsal wrist compartment (contains abductor pollicis longus (APL), extensor pollicis brevis (EPB))
- Common in grasping sports with ulnar deviation, e.g. golf, squash and badminton
- Pain, swelling and tenderness over first dorsal compartment of wrist. Pain on ulnar deviation with thumb in palm (Finkelstein's test)
- **Management:** Most cases can be treated with rest (wrist splint), anti-inflammatories and avoidance of aggravating activity. If symptoms persist good results have been seen with corticosteroid injection into the sheath. If recalcitrant, surgical release may be necessary

Intersection syndrome

- Caused by repetitive extension. Seen in rowers, weightlifters
- Inflammation where APL and EPB crossover extensor radialis longus and brevis
- Pain felt on dorsum forearm 5 cm proximal to wrist
- **Management:** Most cases can be treated with rest, anti-inflammatories. Corticosteroid injection into second dorsal compartment may be required. Rarely surgery to debride and release area is needed

Wrist dislocation

- High-energy injuries
- Lunate or perilunate dislocation most common
- Immediate X-rays required to make diagnosis
- **Management:** Emergent reduction and possible ligamentous/bony fixation based on injury pattern

Exertional compartment syndrome

- Has been described in motorcyclists and weight lifters
- Caused by increase in intracompartmental pressure during exercise/repetitive movements. Resolves when activity is stopped
- Other causes of pain (nerve impingement, stress fractures) need to be excluded by investigations
- Diagnosed by measuring compartment pressures pre and post/during exercise
- **Management:** As symptoms usually recur once activity is resumed, surgical fasciotomy is required to treat patient definitively if return to sport is expected

Return to sport

- Patients should refrain from contact sports until wrist/forearm strength and range of movement is similar to other side
- Most inflammatory conditions usually settle with 3–4 weeks of symptomatic treatment
- Most fractures take 6 weeks to heal. If treated operatively patients will be able to begin rehabilitation earlier. This may be a consideration when deciding upon treatment options for the athlete

Further reading

Miller MD (ed.). Review of orthopaedics, 5th edn. Philadelphia: Saunders, an imprint of Elsevier, 2008

Rettig AC. Athletic injuries of the wrist and hand. Part I: traumatic injuries of the wrist. Am J Sports Med 2003; 31:1038–1048.

Rettig AC. Athletic injuries of the wrist and hand: part II: overuse injuries of the wrist and traumatic injuries to the hand. Am J Sports Med 2004; 32:262–273.

Related topics of interest

- Hand injuries (p. 143)
- Nerve entrapment syndromes – upper limb (p. 203)

Gender verification

Key points

- Principle aim is to prevent males competing as females
- Problems arise with women who have a disorder of sexual development
- Current regulations look at testosterone levels and conduct investigations if serum levels exceed 10 nmol/L

Overview

What a minefield. The main aim of programmes of gender verification has been to stop males masquerading as females in order to gain unfair advantage, given that most males will out-perform most females in most sports. There are few documented cases of straightforward cheating of this sort, but it clearly has happened. The best-known case was Dora Ratjen who won the women's high jump in the 1936 Olympics for Germany, but was uncovered as Heinrich Ratjen, a male, when competing in the 1938 European Athletics Championships. The problem for sports bodies has been the small number of individuals whose gender identity is not identical to their biological sex.

Definitions of gender and sex

According to the World Health Organisation (WHO): 'Sex' refers to the biological and physiological characteristics that define men and women. 'Gender' refers to the socially constructed roles, behaviours, activities, and attributes that a given society considers appropriate for men and women. 'Male' and 'female' are sex categories, while 'masculine' and 'feminine' are gender categories. So gender is a personal and societal issue. If you think of yourself as female and society treats you as such, then your gender is female. As such, gender verification is straightforward. What sports organisations are actually talking about is determination of biological sex. And this is now recognised with, for example, the IAAF no longer referring to 'gender verification' in the new rules that are discussed in the following text (and the title of this topic

should perhaps have been changed).

For some groups, the situation is not too complex. Males who simply pretend to be females for competitive advantage, but otherwise live their lives as masculine individuals, are obviously cheating and need to be detected and banned from competition. Transvestites who are biological males but choose to dress and live in a feminine way are also banned. On the other hand, individuals who have had sex-change treatment are free to compete as their chosen gender, although a 2-year pause is recommended post-treatment.

Genotype versus phenotype

Recent problems have arisen around individuals whose sexual biology is non-standard such as genetic males (with a Y chromosome) who are phenotypically female due to complete androgen insensitivity. Some history is instructive here. The infamous 'beauty parades' were superseded in 1966 by checking for the Y chromosome or later for a functional SRY gene. Introduction of chromosome testing was accompanied by some high profile retirements from international athletics. Notable were the Press sisters, Irena and Tamara, who between them had won five gold medals in the 1960 and 1964 Olympics. A long campaign involving medical specialists led to the abandonment of chromosome testing in 1999. A key figure in the campaign was Maria Jose Martinez-Patiño, a Spanish hurdler who was genetically XY, but due to androgen insensitivity was in every other way female. Sports organisations were by now doing drug testing that involved athletes being watched as they produced a urine sample. Drug test staff were required to check during the sample collection whether competitors had the appropriate external genitalia. It was hoped that this would detect any fully equipped males attempting to compete as females.

Unfortunately, a quick look during a drug test is not necessarily going to be conclusive. So accusations of cheating by males have continued. The most recent example was the case of Castor Semenya, the young South

African 800m runner. She shot to prominence in 2009 by winning the World Championships by a clear 2 s, but was accused by fellow competitors of being male. Her case has prompted a substantial rethink regarding how we assess eligibility, and how such cases should be handled. It was especially unfortunate that an intensely personal matter like gender identity was, in the case of Castor Semenya, paraded across the world media.

New regulations based on testosterone levels

The IAAF has now come up with extremely detailed new regulations that have been picked up by all the Olympic sports. These regulations now look only at testosterone levels. The idea is that the key to gender advantage is having a testosterone level in the male range. The convenience is that testosterone is already checked as part of doping control. Any female competitor with a serum testosterone above 10 nmol/L will be referred to a medical team for assessment. If they have androgen insensitivity, they will be allowed to compete. If not, then they will be advised to have the reason for the high androgen levels investigated. It is argued that this may be important for health reasons. For example, it may be due to polycystic ovarian syndrome, or it may be due to an underlying disorder in sex development (DSD) that will affect fertility. Some conditions may be treatable and if following treatment testosterone levels fall to female levels, then competition can be resumed. The new regulations were used for the 2012 Olympics and Castor Semenya ran in the 800 m and gained a silver medal.

The new regulations appear to deal effectively with much of the problem. An interesting analysis of the case of a Dutch sprinter, the late Foekje Dillema, who was banned in 1950, certainly argues strongly for such a rule. The case of Foekje Dillema was recently re-examined with the approval of her family. DNA methodology looking at skin cells taken from her clothing revealed that she was 46,XX/46,XY mosaic. That is, her skin consisted of equal numbers of cells with XX genotype and XY genotype. Sexual development in such individuals can take several paths. From family history it appears that Foekje Dillema was phenotypically female. We will never know if her testosterone levels were above or below the new eligibility level. However, the Dutch athletic authorities have now reinstated all her results and records.

There are, however, outstanding issues. Although the new rule works well for most DSD cases, it does not cover the significant group of females with androgen insensitivity. They do have testosterone levels in the male range but are allowed to compete as the androgens have no effect and so do not cause advantage, for example, by increasing muscle development. However, some difficult judgements may be required in cases of partial androgen insensitivity. But the strongest criticism has come from those who see all gender verification as unethical. Their argument comes back to the definitions of gender attempted earlier in this topic. Simply put, if a person declares themselves female, then they are female and the rest of us need to respect that. In addition, it is argued that testosterone is far from the only indicator of athletic performance. Its level varies widely in males and females. Should males with unusually high levels be banned? All in all, I am sure we have not heard the last word on the contentious topic of gender verification.

Further reading

Ballantyne KN, Kayser M, Grootegoed JA. Sex and gender issues in competitive sports: investigation of a historical case leads to a new Viewpoint. Br J Sports Med 2012; 46(8): 614–617. doi:10.1136/2 of 4 bjsm.2010.082552

IAAF Regulations Governing Eligibility of Females with Hyperandrogenism to Compete in Women's Competition, 2011, IAAF. http://

www.iaaf.org/mm/Document/AboutIAAF/Publications/05/98/78/20110430054216_httppostedfile_HARegulations%28Final%29-Appendices-AMG-30.04.2011_24299.pdf

Statement of the Stockholm consensus on sex reassignment in sports, 2003. IOC Medical Commission. http://www.olympic.org/Documents/Reports/EN/en_report_905.pdf

Gene doping

Key points

- The methods of gene manipulation being developed for gene therapy will potentially allow manipulation of genes that affect sporting performance
- As gene therapy becomes more effective and widespread some form of control will need to be developed
- Particularly difficult areas are likely to be (a) treatment of injuries and (b) changes imposed on children by parents

A new challenge

Increased knowledge about molecular genetics has led to the development of gene therapy, the treatment of disease by altering the genetic material in cells. The methods used for gene therapy will also be capable of altering the genes in cells in normal individuals in such a way that sporting performance will be enhanced. This process is referred to as 'gene doping'. Gene doping presents a major challenge for sport and especially for sports medicine. In this Topic, we will consider the methods by which gene doping can be carried out, examples of possible target genes, issues related to policing, and the wider ethical issues.

How is gene transfer carried out?

First a target gene needs to be identified and sequenced. Progress in this area has been spectacular in recent years. We have the human genome sequence and the functions of individual genes are being identified at a rapid rate. The alternative forms of each gene ('alleles') that exist within the population and give us each our individual inherited characteristics are also being characterised. Once a particular gene sequence is identified as desirable, the next step is to insert it into cells in the body. There are several ways to do this.

DNA with the correct sequence can be injected into tissue and, remarkably, some will reach the nucleus and get transcribed into RNA and trigger new protein synthesis. However, this direct method is very inefficient and unlikely to be clinically useful in gene therapy or effective as a gene doping method. A more efficient way is to use a safe virus as a 'vector'. Viruses work by inserting there own DNA into the host organism's DNA and getting viral proteins synthesised within the organism. It is possible to insert a novel gene sequence into a virus and then inject the virus into the recipient. The virus will 'infect' cells with the new gene. The process is summarised in **Figure 14** (lower part). The process of virally mediated gene transfer has been shown to be quite effective for a number of gene therapy targets.

An alternative approach (**Figure 14**, upper part) is to take cells from an individual, maintain them for a short period in the laboratory in tissue culture, and under laboratory conditions infect the cells in vitro with the desired DNA sequence. The cells can be checked for the production of the desired protein, then reinjected into the individual. This is how the 'bubble children' with severe combined immunodeficiency (SCID) have been successfully treated. Bone marrow cells have been harvested, modified in vitro, then reinjected. Enough new cells could be re-established in the bone marrow to correct the immunodeficiency, apparently permanently.

An example – introducing the EPO gene into skeletal muscle

As described in the Topic on Drugs in sport: blood doping, erythropoietin and altitude training, erythropoietin (EPO) has been abused by endurance sportsmen to enhance aerobic exercise performance. Suppose we introduce some extra copies of the EPO gene into skeletal muscle, a tissue that does

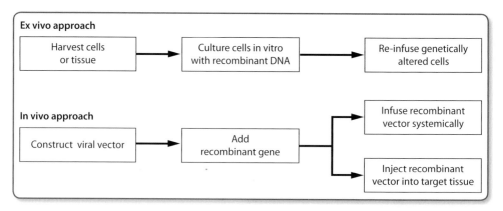

Figure 14 Two basic methods for delivery of genes. The upper panel shows the ex vivo approach. It requires removal of cells or tissues, culture of cells and transfection. Successfully transformed cells are selected and returned to the patient where they home to the original locations of removed cells or tissues. The lower panel shows the in vivo approach. A gene vector construct, suitable for the delivery of genes to the targeted cell or tissue, is generated. The therapeutic gene is incorporated onto the construct and the recombinant vector is delivered to the patient by any of a number of methods.

not normally secrete this hormone. Plasma levels of the hormone would rise just as if recombinant EPO had been injected. The hormone would act on the bone marrow in the usual way to increase red blood cell synthesis and blood Hb levels would rise. In fact this method has been used in experiments on monkeys and high levels of Hb were achieved following a single injection of the viral vector and the levels, and blood Hb, remained elevated for the 6 years duration of the experiment. Note, however, that in early experiments severe problems arose from (a) in some cases such a high haematocrit (70%) that animals had to be bled regularly and (b) in other cases an autoimmune reaction that led to severe anaemia.

When will gene doping become a reality?

Methods for gene therapy are at the early stages of development. Many problems have arisen. Although viral vectors can infect cells, those cells often produce little protein because transcription of the new gene is not properly switched on. In some experiments, too much gene gets switched

on. The key breakthrough will be when reliable methods for switching genes on and off are available. This can already be done experimentally and is being developed for human trials. The trick is to couple the gene to a control element sensitive to an antibiotic. By giving the antibiotic, the gene can be switched on for limited periods. In this way the 'dose' of the new gene can be optimised. Experiments using an EPO gene and such a control mechanism successfully allowed the sustained elevation of blood haemoglobin.

Likely target genes

Hormone genes like EPO or growth hormone may be tried first since any tissue that can release the hormone into the blood stream will be suitable for infection. Local treatment with growth factors may also be tried. For example, one can imagine harvesting muscle myocytes, transfecting them with IGF-1, then reinjecting them into key muscles to get selective growth. At present, we know rather little about different alleles of key genes for muscle performance or metabolism. As that knowledge is garnered, then many more potential drug targets will emerge.

Detecting gene doping

Experts differ in their view about whether gene doping will be detectable. The gene product will be identical to the endogenous protein, so testing for final product will not be sufficient. In this respect, gene doping will be more difficult to detect than traditional drug abuse. On the other hand, it seems likely that viral vectors will need to be used. These specially modified viruses may well be detectable by molecular methods. It has also been shown that recombinant genes can also be reliably detected. This is because these genes dispense with the introns, the noncoding sequences, that are found in all normal genes. So a probe that spans two exons (the coding part of the DNA) will only match a recombinant gene, thus allowing its detection. Enough DNA can be extracted from a blood sample to carry out this test.

Unusual patterns of protein synthesis may also be sufficiently distinctive to point the finger. Simple over production could be indicative of gene doping. Compounds appearing in the wrong tissues (e.g. EPO from muscle, not just the kidney) can be detected. At present, this might require collecting arterial blood samples or taking tissue biopsies, neither of which is likely to be acceptable. But who is to say that imaging methodology, whose advances have been staggering in recent year, will not in the future allow noninvasive determination of a wider range of substances. Even now, phosphorous MR spectroscopy allows detection of many key metabolites in localised tissue volumes.

Some wider ethical questions

The availability of gene modification methods will lead to some spectacular medical advances. However, many difficult ethical questions are going to arise from uses outside the area of serious disease treatment. We may be clear that gene doping to achieve enhanced performance is wrong and may try to police it. In this area, the role of sports doctors is likely to be crucial. This is because no top sports person is going to use such a potentially dangerous technique without medical support. The attitude of sports doctors in such a situation may determine whether gene doping is used or not.

Other areas present a much more difficult set of choices. Consider rehabilitation. It has been shown that certain growth factors can improve healing of muscle or tendon tears. The most efficient method of delivery of such factors is likely to become gene therapy, where a single injection will have a long-lasting effect and the modified cells will be releasing the factors throughout the injured tissue, close to the places where they are needed. This is a much more efficient way to treat an injury than multiple injections of the factor itself. To be able to get back to competition weeks or even months earlier by using gene therapy during rehabilitation will undoubtedly lead to the widespread adoption of such methods. If this is allowed, then how will the line be drawn at where an injury is severe enough to merit such treatment. We could easily see muscle growth factors, delivered by gene therapy, being use for minor training injuries on a wide scale.

Now consider the situation where parents, wishing to see sporting prowess in a child, subject them to gene therapy. Will this child then be banned from all official competition for the rest of their life? Finally, something that everyone will try to stop will be tampering with the reproductive cells. However, the methods for producing genetically altered animals that then pass on the changes to their progeny (e.g. 'knock-out' mice) are well established. Will it be possible to control the desire of parents to have extra-talented children and grandchildren?

These are big issues that will affect many other areas, not just sport. However, the pressures to improve on ones inherited stock of genes are likely to be particularly strong in areas related to sport.

Further reading

Cooper C. Run, Swim, Throw, Cheat. The science behind drugs in sport. Oxford: Oxford University Press, 2012.

Harridge SD, Velloso CP. Gene doping. Essays Biochem 2008; 44:125–138.

Lee S, Barton ER, Sweeney HL et al. Viral expression of insulin-like growth factor-I enhances muscle hypertrophy in resistance-trained rats. J Appl Physiol 2004; 96:1097–1104.

Rivera VM, Gao GP, Grant RL et al. Long-term pharmacologically regulated expression of erythropoietin in primates following AAV-mediated gene transfer. Blood 2005; 105:1424–1430.

Wells DJ. Gene doping. In: Mottram DR (ed.). Drugs in sport, 5th edn. Abingdon: Routledge, 2010:160-172.

Related topics of interest

Groin pain

Key points

- Up to 7% of all sports injuries
- Multidisciplinary approach is recommended
- Adductor strain is the most common cause

Although groin pain affects up to 7% of all sports injuries, the diagnosis of the exact cause remains unclear in approximately 30% of cases. The difficulty diagnosing the aetiology of this condition is attributed to the wide variety of differential diagnosis, complex anatomy of the region and the frequent coexistence of two or more disorders. Therefore, a multidisciplinary approach for its management has been recommended.

Aetiology

Groin pain may originate from muscles, tendons, bones, bursae, fascial structures, nerves, joints, intra and retroperitoneal organs (**Table 13**). In this Topic, we will review some of the most common causes of groin pain in athletes.

Adductor strains

It usually occurs at the musculotendinous junction of the adductor longus.

Table 13 Aetiology of groin pain	
Origin	Cause
Muscular	Adductor longus, iliopsoas, gracilis, pectineus, rectus femoris, rectus abdominous.
Bony	Legg–Calve–Perthes disease, slipped capital femoral epiphysis, femoral neck stress fracture
Articular	Hip joint, sacroiliac joint, pubis symphysis, lumbar spine
Other soft tissues	Joint capsule, bursa, iliofemoral ligament, nerves, blood vessels, lymph nodes, hernias, genitalia (ovary, testicle etc.)

Osteitis pubis

It is a noninfectious inflammation of the pubis. The abdominal and adductor muscles have a central point attachment on the symphysis pubis but act antagonistically to each other, predisposing the pubic symphysis to harmful forces and microtrauma. It is characterised by sclerosis and bony changes about the pubic symphysis. It is most prevalent in kicking sports such as soccer or football.

Hernia

Weakness of the posterior inguinal wall, resulting in an occult direct or indirect hernia.

Iliopsoas-related pathology – iliopsoas strain, snapping and bursitis

These are caused by the overuse and friction of the iliopsoas tendon over the femoral head, acetabular rim or iliopectineal eminence. The tendon is irritated by repeated activity and extensive use of the hip flexors. Can be found in runners, jumpers, hurdlers and footballers.

Femoro-acetabular impingement and intra-articular hip pathology

A disorder consisting of acetabular over coverage and/or decreased femoral head neck offset. Femoro-acetabular impingement (FAI) and intra-articular hip pathology, such as acetabular labral tear or damaged articular cartilage, have been increasingly recognised as a source of disability in high-level athletes.

Clinical features

Adductor strains

Onset of the groin pain may be acute or insidious. The patient usually provides a history of pain at the site of the adductor longus associated with activities involving rapid adduction of the thigh, e.g., by kicking across the body. On examination, there is localised tenderness at one particular point on the pubic bone over the insertion of the muscle. Pain is exacerbated on resisted adduction and passive abduction.

Osteitis pubis

Patients may present acutely or more often subacutely or by gradual onset. The pain is on the anterior aspect of the pubic bone; however, it may radiate to the suprapubic area or into the groin. Pain is exacerbated by kicking, running, jumping and twisting. Squeeze test is very sensitive, in which the patient's knees are flexed to 90°, the examiner's hand is placed between the patient's knees and the patient performs a strong isometric, bilateral adductor contraction; this will exacerbate the bony tenderness.

Hernia

Sports hernia is characterised by insidious-onset, gradually worsening, diffuse, deep groin pain. Manoeuvres that cause increases in intra-abdominal pressure will usually increase pain. It tends to occur in athletes who participate in sports that require repetitive twisting and turning at speed.

Iliopsoas-related pathology

It produces a deep groin pain in which, because of the deep insertion of the muscle, patients find difficult to localise. There might also be a lack of point tenderness. Pain can be elicited by having the patient flex the hip 90° and then try to flex it further against resistance or by passive stretching with hyperextension at the hip.

FAI and intra-articular hip pathology

Loss of clearance between the femoral neck and acetabular rim may compromise maximum hip excursion in multiple planes. This may result in compensatory stresses on the lumbar spine, pubic symphysis, sacroiliac joint and posterior acetabulum. Anterior groin pain with flexion, adduction and internal rotation is common with Cam type impingement (femoral side), whereas trochanteric or the buttock region with flexion abduction and external rotation pain may be associated with Pincer (acetabular side) impingement. It is usually associated with a clicking, catching or locking sensation. On examination, the range of the movement of the hip joint is not usually limited but there may be pain at extreme ranges.

Investigations

Plain radiographs should be obtained in all patients with groin pain. The AP of the pelvis allows comparison with the asymptomatic side to evaluate variations in bony architecture as well as allowing visualisation of the pubic symphysis, sacrum, sacroiliac joints, ilium and ischium. The frog leg lateral is a good lateral of the femoral head and neck.

Magnetic resonance imaging (MRI) is used for soft-tissue injury and for early detection of stress fractures of the femoral neck and osteonecrosis.

Adductor strains

Plain X-rays may show calcification around the origin of the muscle on the pubic bone. Ultrasound imaging can be useful in delineating the lesion as MRI.

Osteitis pubis

Plain radiographs may show widening of the pubic symphysis, irregular contour of articular surfaces or periarticular sclerosis. Increased uptake over the pubic tubercle may be seen with radionuclide bone scan. CT may display abnormalities of the bony structure and MRI will demonstrate bone marrow oedema in the body of the pubis.

Hernia

Ultrasonography can demonstrate the defect in the medial posterior inguinal wall but it is very operator dependent.

Iliopsoas-related pathology

This can be best visualised on MRI, which may reveal a collection of fluid coursing adjacent to the muscle.

FAI and intra-articular hip pathology

Plain radiographs will help exclude degenerative joint changes, osteonecrosis, loose bodies, stress fractures, or other osseous pathology. One should assess for acetabular over coverage or dysplasia, and assess for a prominent femoral neck indicative of hip impingement. Both of these problems may result in labral tears. CT scans can be useful to measure anteversion and retroversion, and they can show the size and shape of the acetabulum and femoral head and neck. MRI combined with arthrography is more sensitive for the diagnosis and description of labral pathology and articular cartilage loss.

Management

Adductor strains

Acute treatment includes RICE (rest, ice, compression, elevation). Following this, the goal of therapy should be restoration of range of motion and prevention of atrophy. Only once the patient achieves a full range of movement, strengthening, flexibility and endurance exercises should commenced, otherwise there is a risk of developing chronic tendinopathy. Patients with chronic adductor longus strains that have failed to respond to several months of conservative treatment have been shown to do well after surgical tenotomy.

Osteitis pubis

This is a self-limiting condition. Treatment involves RICE and NSAIDs. Some clinicians consider corticosteroid injection if patients do not progress with conservative measures. Once the patient is pain free, there should be a staged, progressive return to activity.

Hernia

Nonoperative management usually results in a prolonged clinical course; therefore, once the diagnosis of hernia is made, surgical repair is the main option.

Iliopsoas-related pathology

Managed by RICE, NSAIDs, appropriate stretching and strengthening of the iliopsoas muscle. Surgical release of the Iliopsoas tendon is reserved to those patients who do not improve after conservative treatment has been attempted

FAI and intra-articular hip pathology

Surgical management (open or arthroscopic) has allowed many of these athletes to return to their pre injury level of sporting activities. When both intra-articular and extra-articular symptoms were managed concurrently or at separate settings, 85% and 93%, respectively, returned to full sports without limitations.

Return to sport

Adductor strains

When the athlete has regained at least 70% of his strength and pain-free full range of motion, a return to sport may be allowed. This return may take 4–8 weeks following an acute musculotendinous strain and up to 6 months for chronic strains.

Osteitis pubis

Although it is a self-limiting condition, full recovery may take more than 1 year.

Hernia

Most athletes return to sport within 6–12 weeks following surgery, after specific rehabilitation targeted at abdominal strengthening, adductor muscle flexibility, and a gradual return to activity.

Iliopsoas-related pathology

Return to sport can take between 2 and 6 weeks depending on the severity of the injury.

FAI and intra-articular hip pathology

Following surgical treatment of FAI and labral repair, return to sport may take between 4 and 9 months.

Further reading

Minnich JM, Hanks JB, Muschaweck U, et al. Sports hernia: diagnosis and treatment highlighting a minimal repair surgical technique. Am J Sports Med 2011; 39:1341–1349.

Narvani AA, Tsiridis E, Kendall S, et al. Acetabular labrum tears in sports patients with groin pain. Knee Surg Sport Traumatol Arthrosc 2003; 1:403–408.

Narvani AA, Tsiridis E, Tai CC, et al. Acetabular labrum and its tears. Br J Sports Med 2003; 37:207–211.

Related topics of interest

- Thigh pain (anterior) – quadriceps (p. 316)
- Prevention of sport injuries (p. 236)
- Nerve entrapment syndromes – lower limb (p. 199)

Hand injuries

Key points

- Can involve bone, tendon, ligament or a combination
- Early mobilisation/hand therapy is key to optimal outcome
- Tendency for misdiagnosis and under treatment means many athletes may be left with long-term sequelae

Conditions

Skier's thumb

- Complete or partial rupture of thumb ulnar collateral ligament
- Caused by hyper abduction of thumb causing pain and swelling over ulnar aspect of thumb metacarpal phalangeal joint (MCPJ), with laxity on stressing.
- **Management:** Partial ruptures can be treated in thumb spica cast for 8 weeks. Complete ruptures need operative fixation.

Mallet finger

- Flexion deformity of distal interphalangeal joint (DIPJ) caused by avulsion of terminal extensor tendon.
- May be bony or tendinous.
- **Management:** Tendinous and undisplaced bony mallet injuries can be treated in a mallet splint for 8 weeks. Displaced bony mallet fractures require operative fixation.

Jersey finger

- Avulsion of flexor digitorum profundus (FDP) from its insertion at the volar base of distal phalanx caused by hyperextension of tip of finger, e.g. if caught in other players clothes
- Patient holds the finger in an extended posture. Inability to flex DIPJ
- **Management:** Will require operative repair, ideally in first few weeks. May require fixation of bony avulsion or reattachment of flexor tendon that retracts towards palm

Metacarpal neck fractures

- Most common is neck of fifth metacarpal (boxers fracture)

- Pain and swelling in region of fracture. Clinically one may lose the normal knuckle arch due to shortening of metacarpal, there may be rotational malalignment of finger or palpable lump in palm
- **Management:** Indication for operative management (intramedullary wiring) include malrotation of finger, volar angulation >40°–50°
  - An attempt at reduction with regional anaesthesia can be made in the emergency setting and then splinted with the MCPJ flexed at 90° (Edinburgh splint) to hold the reduction
  - Majority can be treated with buddy strapping for 3 weeks followed by hand therapy

Metacarpal base fractures

- Most common at base of thumb metacarpal fracture
- Extra-articular or Intra-articular: Bennetts (2 parts) and Rolando (3 parts)
- CMCJ dislocation/subluxation must be excluded with fractures at the base of the lesser metacarpals
- **Management:** Undisplaced fractures at the base of thumb can be immobilised in thumb spica cast but must be watched closely for any displacement. Displaced fractures require manipulation under anaesthesia and fixation with either wires or plates

Phalanx fractures

- Look for pain and swelling around fracture site and possible malrotational of finger
- **Management:** If minimally displaced treat with buddy strapping and early (3 weeks) mobilisation. Operative management if displaced or intra-articular. Hand therapy is key to regaining range of movement

Crush injuries

- May cause subungual haematoma, distal phalanx tuft fracture, or nail bed injury
- **Management:** Wound washout/ debridement can be undertaken in the emergency department under ring block. Subungual haematomas can be lanced

Heel pain

Key points

- Heel pain is a very common and limiting problem in sporting patients.
- Plantar fasciopathy is the commonest cause
- While the cause is usually mechanical, other causes (e.g. inflammatory and metabolic) must be excluded

Heel pain can be a very disabling condition in the sporting individual. There are a large number of causes that can be grouped by location of the symptoms (**Table 14**). While the cause is usually local and mechanical, systemic illnesses and inflammatory disorders must be screened for during assessment. This Topic reviews some of the more common causes of plantar heel pain.

Table 14 Causes of heel pain
Plantar
Plantar fasciopathy
Plantar fascial rupture
Calcaneal stress fracture
Neuropathies
Local, e.g. tarsal tunnel syndrome
Referred, e.g. lumbar radiculopathy
Severs disease
Heel pad atrophy
Posterior
Achilles tendinopathy
Insertional
Noninsertional
Retrocalcaneal bursitis
Posterosuperior calcaneal (Haglund) prominence
Other causes
Inflammatory arthropathies
Tumour
Soft tissue/bone
Infection
Soft tissue/bone
Vascular malformations

Plantar fasciopathy

Aetiology

Plantar fasciopathy is the commonest cause of heel pain. The true aetiology is not understood, although studies suggest that it represents a noninflammatory enthesopathy, probably mechanically induced, at the calcaneal insertion. Hence, the term 'fasciopathy' rather than the commonly used 'fasciitis' gives a more accurate description of the condition and guides the clinician away from solely focusing on anti-inflammatory measures. It is an overuse phenomenon in the sporting individual and is usually related to a tight calf muscles.

Certain structural factors may increase the risk of developing the condition such as pes cavus, pronated feet and excessive plantar flexion. Increased age, body mass and spending large periods of time on the feet are also risk factors. Hard play surfaces are believed to pose a risk, and there is emerging interest in the role of individualised footwear and cleat design to minimise lower limb problems and injuries.

Clinical features

Plantar heel pain on initiating ambulation, particularly during the first few steps in the morning that can improve with activity is virtually pathognomonic of plantar fasciopathy. Increased heel loading, with long periods of standing exacerbates symptoms. Participation in sports may be possible, although with suboptimal performance and pain that continues after activity.

Clinical assessment of gait will often reveal an avoidance of heel strike and increased forefoot loading that can be subtle. Forefoot plantar callosities may be present. There is focal tenderness along the plantar aspect of the heel from the insertion along the proximal plantar fascia, often more so the medial side. Dorsi-flexing the ankle and extending the big toe to stretch the facia can worsen the symptoms. Patients will often have tight calves with positive Silfverskiold tests (decreased ankle dorsiflexion with the knee held straight compared with knee flexed, indicating gastrocnemius tightness).

Investigations

The diagnosis is usually clear clinically. During history and examination a careful screen for systemic, inflammatory, infective and metabolic diseases must be undertaken and if suspected these should be thoroughly investigated, with appropriate blood tests and investigations.

Lateral X-rays will show a proximal plantar heel spur in approximately 50% of patients, although a negative finding does not negate the diagnosis or change the management. Where the diagnosis is in doubt, X-rays can be useful be useful to rule out other conditions such as stress fractures, hindfoot joint arthritis and identify periosteal changes in spondylarthropathy. Ultrasound can show a thickened plantar fascia but again is often not used, as the diagnosis is clear. MRI can be very useful for the unclear diagnosis as it gives detailed information on surrounding soft tissue structures. It shows fascial thickening and insertional bony oedema with surrounding soft tissue changes.

Management

First line management should consist of:
1. Heel wedge to prevent contact pain and off-load the fascia
2. A formal eccentric calf gastrocnemius stretching programme. This can be coupled with plantar specific stretching
3. Night orthotic to stretch out the plantar fascia such as a Strassburg sock

Oral anti-inflammatories can help with any inflammatory component of the pain, although these are unlikely to resolve symptoms alone. Local corticosteroid injections may provide temporary relief of pain, although these may also increase the risk of rupture. If performed without ultrasound guidance it can cause nerve injury and fat pad atrophy. Where symptoms remain recalcitrant to first line management, extracorporeal shock wave therapy can be of benefit. Plasma rich protein is also increasing in popularity, although it is more invasive. Both modalities lack long-term evidence, although these are gaining popularity. While surgical release is described for recalcitrant cases, potential complications such as arch collapse may be poorly tolerated in the sporting population.

Return to sport

The level of pain that can be tolerated is the main limiting factor. In milder forms, sport can often be continued, while first line management is commenced. In the more severe form, a short period of abstinence during which stretching is performed, then a stepwise return is prudent.

Other causes

Plantar fascial rupture

Acute sharp plantar pain with or without direct trauma may indicate plantar fascial rupture. A history of dorsiflexion of the foot or local injection may have preceded it. Swelling, ecchymosis, tenderness, difficulty bearing weight and a palpable gap in the fascia may be felt. This is relatively infrequent compared to tendo Achilles rupture and treatment varies. Three weeks of nonweight bearing in a cast or boot, followed by 3 weeks bearing weight, in a walking boot yield good results. Return to sport is from 9 to 12 weeks, although it can take longer.

Calcaneal stress fracture

This classically presents insidiously and is related to impact activity or change to harder walking/playing surfaces. The pain is classically worsens during activity, starting as an ache that becomes severe and then improves with rest. Clinically, mediolateral calcaneal compression can reproduce the pain. Plain X-rays may reveal the fracture, although, an MRI may be necessary. Screening potential underlying causes of osteoporosis is prudent, and, if discovered, these should be treated appropriately. Treatment is rest and mobilising in a walking cast or boot. Surgery is rarely needed for refractory cases. Return to sport can take numerous months.

Nerve pain

Neuropathic pain symptoms such as burning and tingling may present following repetitive activity. The commonest cause is entrapment of posterior tibial nerve branches, particularly the medial and lateral plantar nerves and the nerve to abductor digiti minimi. Work up must exclude more proximal spinal causes. Treatment is initially conservative with rest, stretches and offloading. Surgery is occasionally considered for recalcitrant cases.

Sever's disease
See Paediatrics - osteochondrosis (osteochondritis).

Heel pad atrophy
This presents with a diffuse ache beneath the heel. There may be a history of local steroid injection. Patients may perform excessive impact activity with little support, suffer with neurological conditions and will often be in an older age group. Treatment is based on heel padding.

Peroneal tendinopathy
This presents with posterolateral pain along the course of the tendons (to the fifth metatarsal base for the peroneus brevis and base of the first metatarsal for peroneus longus) and is often preceded by an inversion injury. An association with high medial arch footwear exists without lateral balance. Short periods of immobilisation in a boot may be necessary, and failing that, surgical debridement.

Posterior tibial tendon dysfunction
In the early stages, this presents with posteromedial ankle pain that can spread into the medial foot. Later, the medial arch flattens and lateral pain develops. Clinically single heel raise is difficult or not possible, and in the later stage, when viewed from behind 'too many toes' sign in positive. Mild disease may be treated with a medial arch support. A tenosynovectomy can be performed in the early stage. As the disease advances, a flexor digitorum longus transfers with calcaneal osteotomy to reconstruct the flattened foot often becomes necessary and in more advanced stages when fixed arthritic deformities develop, a triple arthrodesis is performed.

Further reading

Alvarez-Nemegyei J, Canuso JJ. Heel pain: diagnosis and treatment, step by step. Clevelend Clin J Med 2006; 73(5):465-471.

DiGiovanni BF, Nawoczenski DA, Lintal ME, et al. Tissue-specific planar fascia-stretching exercise enhances outcomes with chronic heel pain. J Bone Joint Surg Am 2003; 85:1270–1277.

Digiovanni BF, Nawoczenski DA, Malay DP, et al. Plantar ascia-specific stretching exercise improves outcomes in patients with chronic plantar fasciitis: a prospective clinical trial with two-year follow-up. J Bone Joint Surg Am 2006; 88:1775-1781.

Fahlstrom M, Jonsson P, Lorentzon R, et al. Chronic Achilles tendon pain treated with eccentric calf-muscle training. Knee Surg Sports Traumatol Arthrosc 2003; 11:327–333.

League AC. Current concepts review. Foot Ankle Int 2008; 29: 358–366.

Orchard J. Plantar fasciitis. BMJ 2012; 10:345.

Pepper TE. Plantar heel pain. Foot Ankle Clin N Am 2009; 14:229–245.

Rompe JD. Plantar fasciopathy. Sports Med Arthrosc 2009; 17:100—104.

Thomas JL, Christensen JC. The diagnosis and treatment of heel pain: a clinical practice guideline – revision 2010. J foot Ankle Surg 2010; 49: S1–S19.

Related topics of interest

Imaging – isotope bone scan

Key points

- Involves injection of radioactive substance
- Highlights areas with increased osteoblastic activities or bone turn over
- Although this is largely superseded by MRI for most musculoskeletal disorders, it should be considered when other imaging modalities are negative and there remains clinical concern for occult tumours or fractures particularly in the spine

Isotope bone scans provide physiological and function information on osteoblastic activity. The investigation involves injection of radioactive substance 'coupled' to another substance that has affinity for sites of osteoblastic activity. Once taken up by these sites, the radioactive substance decays and emits gamma rays that can be detected by a camera. This would then permit construction of a skeleton functional image highlighting areas with increased osteoblastic activities or bone turn over. Other factors including blood flow and quantity of mineralised bone also influence the accumulation of the radioactive substance at particular sites.

Single-photon emission computerised tomography (SPECT) is a bone scan tomographic investigation that involves rotating the gamma camera 360° around the athlete. This permits a multiple projection evaluation, resulting in more accurate localisation of the area of the increased uptake.

Isotope bone scans can be particularly helpful in the following situations:

Fractures

Stress fractures

- Isotope bone scanning can be of great use in the diagnosis of stress fractures (sensitivities approaching 100% have been reported) as conventional radiographs are relatively insensitive (initial plain radiography may be normal in over 50% of athletes with stress fractures)
- Due to the increased blood flow and osteoblastic activity, there is increased radioactive substance uptake at the site of the stress fracture. This will show up as intense focal area of increased uptake
- As the stress fracture undergoes healing, this area of increased uptake can become less intense and more diffuse

Occult fractures

- These are subtle fractures that may not be initially seen with plain radiographs
- Acute fractures will result in increased radiotracer localisation at the area of the injury, showing up as intense focal area of increased uptake
- Similarly to stress fractures, as healing progresses, the area of increased uptake loses its intensity
- Vast majorities of fractures are detected by bone scan taken at 24–48 h following trauma; however, in more senior athletes and those who suffer from osteoporosis, it may take up to 72-h postinjury before bone scan becomes positive

Assessment of union

- Isotope bone scanning may also be used to none union as well as indicating the type of none union present (atrophic versus hypertrophic)

Spondylolysis

- This condition is thought to represent a stress fracture caused by repetitive hyperextension loading of weakened or defective pars interarticularis
- SPECT scan is a useful investigation as plain radiographs may not be able to detect the subtle cases
- Furthermore, SPECT scan would allow the clinician to distinguish between those lesions that have healed from those that have not yet healed. This information can be of great importance since athletes with unhealed lesions generally require prolonged absence from sports so that the lesion can undergo complete healing

Paediatric Injuries

- Bone scan can be used to diagnose epiphyseal plate injuries as well as

monitoring the effect of the injury on the growth potential (premature closure of the physis results in decreased uptake)
- Isotope bone scan can also be helpful in the diagnosis of apophyseal avulsion injuries, as these may be difficult to detect with plain radiograph

Infections

- Although not very specific, isotope bone scan is reported to have a sensitivity of over 95% for detecting osteomyelitis
- This accuracy is improved by using labelled leukocytes as these accumulate at the site of the infection

Tumours

- Isotope bone scan is widely used for detection of osseous metastasis in those with known malignancies
- Primary bone tumours may result in 'hot lesion' on bone scan; however, they have limitations as assessment of the tumour extent is complicated by reactive hyperaemia
- Myelomas may not be detected by isotope bone scan
- Most of benign bone tumours (with the exception of osteoid osteomas) do not

accumulate radioactive tracer; therefore, isotope bone scan should not be the investigation of choice

Other pathologies

Osteitis pubis

- This condition is a cause of groin pain in athletes. Plain radiograph appearances may be subtle, whereas as isotope bone scan can demonstrate increased uptake over the pubic tubercle

Shin splints

- Isotope bone scan can diagnose this condition by demonstrating superficial uptake along the medial tibial shaft

Anterior knee pain

- Bone scan can give an indication of the extent of patella over loading in assessment of athletes with anterior knee pain

Complex regional pain syndrome (reflex sympathetic dystrophy)

- This occurs as a result of autonomic dysfunction secondary to injury
- Isotope bone scan may detect this by demonstrating increased uptake

Further reading

Calleja M, Alam A, Wilson D, et al. Basic science: nuclear medicine in skeletal imaging. Curr Orthop 2005; 19:34–39.
Hirschmann MT, Davda K, Rasch H, et al. Clinical value of combined single photon emission computerized tomography and conventional computer tomography (SPECT/CT) in sports medicine. Sports Med Arthrosc 2011; 19(2): 174–181.

Related topics of interest

Imaging – magnetic resonance imaging (MRI)

Key points

- Good for both bone and soft tissue pathology
- Does not involve radiation
- Be aware of abnormal findings that may not necessary be the cause of patients symptoms (treat the patient not the images)

Overview

Magnetic resonance imaging (MRI) is a wonderful imaging tool, which has had a massive impact on the management of sports injuries since being introduced on a large scale into clinical practice in 1980s. It allows imaging of a wide range of structures including cartilage, tendons, ligaments, bone and muscle, yet not involving X-ray radiation) and most cases being noninvasive.

Mechanism

Although the detailed physics of MRI is complicated and beyond the scopes of this Topic, a brief understanding of its mechanism is helpful. MRI involves placing the subject in a magnetic field. The hydrogen atoms, in different body tissues, align in this magnetic field. Then a radiofrequency (RF) pulse is applied to the tissues that cause the hydrogen atoms, in those tissues, to alter their original alignment relative to the external magnetic field. Following this RF pulse, the hydrogen atoms 'dephase' and return to their original relaxed state. As they do so, they release energy (echo). This emitted energy is detected by MRI machine and is converted into images. The time it takes for hydrogen atoms to diphase is called the T2 time and the time taken to return to relaxed state (and release energy) is called the T1 time. Dephasing occurs before release of energy; therefore, T2 time is always a smaller number than T1 time. Different tissues and tissue states, e.g. bone, muscle, fat, cartilage, oedema and tendon, have different T1 and T2 times. This is due to the fact that relaxation of the hydrogen atoms is dependent on size and bindings of the molecules that contain the hydrogen atom. The emitted energy (echo signal) is dependent on several factors. This signal would be high if one allows the majority of the hydrogen atoms to diphase, e.g. if one starts listening relatively late, therefore, giving time for the hydrogen atoms to diphase. If the machine starts listening very early, for a short period of time, the hydrogen atoms may have not 'dephased', and therefore, the signal would be low. The technical term for when the machine starts listening is called 'time to echo' (TE) and is something that can be altered and set on the MRI machine. Therefore, if TE is set to be shorter than T2 time of that tissue, then that tissue would not have a high signal on the MRI.

The echo signal's intensity is also dependent on whether or not the majority of the hydrogen atoms have returned to their relaxed state before another RF pulse is applied. Therefore, if the repeated RF pulse is applied before the hydrogen atoms return to their relaxed state, they would not be very excitable with the next pulse and therefore the next echo signal would not be strong. Again how quickly the next RF pulse arrives is something that could be set on the MRI machine. The technical term for this is 'time to repetition' (TR). Therefore, if the TR is set to be shorter than the T1 time of the image tissue, then that tissue would not be presented by a high signal on the MRI.

It can now be appreciated how by altering the TE and TR parameters on the MRI machine, we can tune it to detect different tissue or pathologies of those tissues. This tuning is performed by having different MRI 'weighted' sequences.

T1-weighted sequences

- TE is set at a short time (approximately 40 ms)
- TR is set as short time (approximately 400 ms)

- Good for demonstrating anatomy
- Bright with:
  - Fat
  - Methaemoglobin (seen in haematoma)
  - Contrast (Gad)
  - Occasionally calcium and slow flowing blood.
- Fluid (oedema) is low signal or dark
- Can be useful to detect meniscal pathology

T2-weighted sequences

- TE is set at a long time (about 120 ms)
- TR is set at a long time (about 1000 ms)
- Good for demonstrating pathology
- Fluid (oedema) is bright
- Fat is also high signal and bright, therefore, often use fat suppression with T2 to improve contrast resolution and show up pathology better.

Proton density (PD)

- TE is set at a short time (shorter than 60 ms)
- TR is set at a long time (longer than 1000 ms)
- Very good for assessment of meniscus

Metal artefact reduction sequences (MARS)

- MRI relies on good uniform magnetic field. Metal distorts this resulting in artefact
- Sequences used in presence of metal include the following:
  - Fast spin echo (avoids gradient echo sequences)
  - STIR sequences (avoid fat suppression which relies on uniform magnetic field)
  - Also increasing receiver bandwidth, using higher resolution and thinner slices to increase number of excitations reduces the effect of metal

MRI may not differentiate solid from cystic structures; therefore, contrast (gadolinium) that enhances solids may need to be administered.

MRI is also prone to artefact:
1. Movement artefact
2. 'Magic Angle Phenomenon' with sequences that use short TE (e.g. T1, Gradient echo and PD) where structures (e.g. tendons) can look artefactually brighter, and therefore, simulate pathology. It occurs when collagen-containing tissues (e.g. tendons)

run at a specific angle (55°) to the static magic angle. Can lead to overcalling of tendon or meniscal pathology)

MRI can be used to visualise a wide variety of tissues and their pathologies in different body parts. These include the following.

Bone

- Fractures:
  - Stress fractures
  - Occult fractures
- Bone bruise:
  - Best detected on STIR or fat suppressed T2 sequences

Ligament

- MRI can be very useful
- T1 sequence good for anatomical detail
- T2 sequence good for detecting ligament pathology

Muscle

- Tears:
  - Intermediate signal on T1
  - High signal on T2
  - STIR and fat suppressed T2 sequences are particularly useful as would permit distinction to be made between fluid collection or haemorrhage from muscle fat
- Haematoma:
  - Intensity and appearance dependent on the stage of haematoma
- Other muscular pathologies that could be detected by MRI include the following:
  - Myositis ossificans
  - Tumours
  - Pyomyositis

Tendon

- Tendinopathy:
  - Acute:
    - Intermediate signal intensity on T1 and T2
    - Tendon thickening
  - Chronic:
    - Thinning and attenuation of the tendon
- Tears:
  - Complete:
    - High signal on T2 involving the full thickness of the tendon extending from one surface to another
    - There may be retraction of the tendon

- Partial:
  - High signal on T2 involving part of the tendon rather than the full thickness

Cartilage

- Articular cartilage:
  - Useful sequences for relieving surface abnormalities include proton density and fast spin echo

- Menisci:
  - Preferred sequences include T1, proton density and gradient echo T2.
  - Tears may be seen as intrasubstance signal that extends either to superior or inferior surface
- Labrum:
  - Pathologies of both glenoid and acetabular labrum can be detected by MRI. Accuracy improves when combined with arthrogram

Further reading

Ho-Fung VM, Jaimes C, Jaramillo D. Magnetic resonance imaging assessment of sports related musculoskeletal injury in children: current techniques and clinical applications. Semin Roentegnol 2012; 47:171–181.

Milewski MD, Sanders TG, Miller MD. MRI-arthroscopy correlation: the knee. J Bone Joint Surg Am 2011; 93:1735–1745.

Related topics of interest

Imaging – plain radiograph

Key points

- Simple, cheap widely available
- First line of investigation for bone injuries and or assessment of joints
- Good for bony injuries/pathologies

Plain radiography is technically simple, cheap and widely available. In many sports injuries, this should be the first imaging investigation obtained. Even a 'normal' plain radiograph can be very helpful by excluding or reducing the likelihood of many conditions. It must, however, be performed competently while paying careful attention to the exposure and positioning. Usually two perpendicular views are adequate although more specialised views may be required to detect specific injuries.

Plain radiography is particularly helpful in the following situations.

Fractures

- In addition to having a very high sensitivity to detecting the majority of fractures, plain radiography also provides information on the anatomy, displacement and characteristics of many fractures
- On occasions, subtle fractures may not initially be seen on plain radiography (however, a follow-up radiograph at about 2 weeks postinjury will usually show resorption of the fractured bone and increased density at margins secondary to callus production). In such cases, if a fracture is strongly suspected clinically, other imaging modalities such as bone scan, computed tomography (CT) and magnetic resonance imaging (MRI) may be required (see topics on bone scan, CT and MRI)
- With stress fractures, plain radiograph may illustrate periosteal new bone formation, callus and a visible fracture line. It may, however, take several weeks before X-rays signs become positive, and in over 50%

of athletes with stress fractures, the initial radiographs can be normal. Therefore, again if there is strong clinical suspicion, other imaging modalities should be utilised (see topic on stress fractures)

Dislocations/subluxations

- Plain radiograph will be able to diagnose the vast majorities of dislocation and subluxation
- In subtle cases, further imaging with other modalities such as CT may be required (CT and MRI will also demonstrate other associated injuries as well)

Avulsion injuries

- These are usually secondary to a powerful muscular contraction.
- Plain radiograph can detect acute avulsion injuries

Other pathologies

- Plain films may also demonstrate other pathologies that are not related to injuries and cause chronic symptoms. These include the following:
  - Neoplastic lesions
  - Metabolic bone disease
  - Infection

Use of contrast

Plain radiography may also be performed in combination with intra-articular injection of contrast (plain film arthrography). Although replaced by CT arthrography and MRI (+/- arthrogram) in many centres, plain radiography with contrast can be useful in evaluating shoulder pathologies (rotator cuff tears, labral injuries, loose bodies, synovitis and capsulitis) and wrist injuries (triangular fibrocartilage complex and ligament tears).

Further reading

Bresler M, Mar W, Toman J. Diagnostic imaging in the evaluation of leg pain in athletes. Clin Sport Med 2012; 31:217–245.

Tung GA, Brody JM. Contemporary imaging of athletic injuries. Clin Sports Med 1997; 16:393–417.

van Dijk CN, de Leeuw PA. Imaging from an orthopaedic point of view. What the orthopaedic surgeon expects from the radiologists? Eur J Radiol 2007; 62:2–5.

Related topics of interest

Imaging – ultrasound (US)

Key points

- Ultrasound (US) is good for soft tissue injuries and image guided injections
- It is safe, mobile, allows dynamic imaging and in combination with X-ray good for assessing many musculoskeletal disorders, where magnetic resonance imaging availability is limited
- It is very operator dependent

Overview

Ultrasonography is a very valuable diagnostic tool in the management of soft tissue injuries as it offers high-resolution imaging of soft tissues. It is safe as there is no involvement of ionising radiation yet, relatively cheap and readily accessible. It permits dynamic imaging as well as real time image guided interventional procedures. It helps to differentiate solids from cystic structures. Additionally, it allows assessment of vascularity of the pathological structure (e.g. of tumours, neo-vascularisation of tendons and areas if inflammation). It is, however, very operator dependent.

Imaging with ultrasound involves transmission of high frequency (3–15 MHz), inaudible sound waves from a probe, through a coupling device gel (which is applied topically to the area of interest). These sound waves are directed into the body, and travel through the different layers, i.e. skin, subcutaneous fat, muscle and bone. The velocity and wavelength with which the waves travel through each layer is dependent on the density of the substance of that layer. At junction between one layer and another layer, at the interfaces, a proportion of the waves are reflected back to the probe. The probe then acts as a receiver, detecting these reflected waves and creating an ultrasound image from them. The bigger the difference between the density of the two structures, the greater proportion of the waves that are reflected at interface of the two structures. This is why it is important to use gel between the probe and the skin, as without gel the large difference between the densities of the probe and the air pocket would imply that almost all the waves

are reflected back and none will go through the body.

Ultrasonography can be particularly helpful for the assessment of the following structures.

Muscle

- Muscle tears:
  - These are well demonstrated by ultrasound
  - There is disorganisation of the normal architecture of the muscle
  - There may be muscle-end retraction
  - There may also be an associated haematoma (see below)
- Muscle haematoma:
  - Acute muscle haematomas will appear as bright, hyperechoic region.
- Myositis ossificans:
  - US can be used to diagnose this condition early by demonstrating calcifications within the muscle at 7–10 days postinjury
- Muscle hernias:
  - Because US is a dynamic investigation, it can be very useful in detecting pathologies that will only become apparent with muscle contraction such as muscle hernias and chronic scars

Tendons

- Normal tendon will appear as regular tightly packed, longitudinally orientated bundles that are bright (echogenic) compared to the surrounding muscles
- The following tendon abnormalities can be detected with US:
  - Tendinopathies, with features such as:
    - Loss of normal structure
    - Blurring
    - Thickening
    - Cystic degeneration
    - Calcification
    - Peritendinous oedema
    - Paratenonitis or synovitis
    - Neovascularisation of the tendons substance
    - There may be an associated tear (see below)

- Tears:
  - They can be partial or full thickness
  - A partial thickness tear will appear as a dark area within the tendon without involving the full thickness of the tendon
  - A full thickness tear will appear as a dark band extending from one surface to the other surface of the tendon. As the size of the tear increases, this dark band will become thicker, eventually appearing as a dark, hypoechoic gap with massive tears
- Newer techniques such as elastography (looks at tissue 'stiffness') are being researched to assess tendinopathy and characterise solid lesions

Ligaments

- US can be a very useful diagnostic tool for the assessment of joint ligaments as it would be able to detect oedema, thickening or absence of the ligament

- Furthermore, as it is a dynamic investigation, the ligaments may be examined under stress
- It is valuable at assessing the ligaments of small joints

Bursa

- Bursitis may be diagnosed by US if there is fluid distension of a known bursa. This would appear as a dark hypochoic area

Soft tissue swellings

- USS can aid in establishing a diagnosis with soft tissue masses by providing information on dimensions and morphological characteristics of the swelling such as:
  - Surface contour and definition
  - Internal structure/contents
  - Relationship to the surrounding structure
- The accuracy of percutaneous core needle biopsy (when indicated) may also be increased by using US to guide the biopsy of these soft tissue swellings

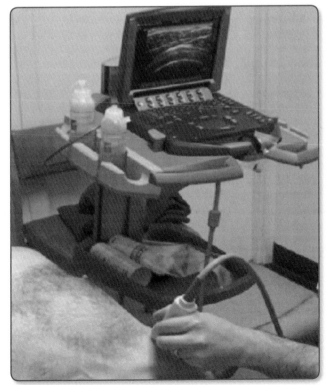

Figure 16 Shoulder ultrasound.

Interventional procedures

- Image guidance with USS may be used in the following procedures:
  - Injection of local anaesthetic and corticosteroids
  - Dry needling procedures
  - Platelet rich plasma injections
  - Biopsy
    - Percutaneous fine needle aspiration
    - Percutaneous core needle biopsy

Further reading

Bresler M, Mar W, Toman J. Diagnostic imaging in the evaluation of leg pain in athletes. Clin Sport Med 2012; 31(2):217–245.

Colquhoun K, Alam A, Wilson D. Basic science: ultrasound. Curr Orthop 2005; 19:27–33.

Yim ES, Corrado G. Ultrasound in sports medicine: relevance of emerging techniques to clinical care of athletes. Sport Med 2012; 42(8):665–680.

Related topics of interest

Imaging of sports injuries – computed tomography (CT)

Key points

- Involves application of X-ray radiation
- Provided three-dimensional (3D) information
- Good for bony abnormality, fractures and head injuries

Since its introduction in early 1970s, computed tomography (CT) has proved to be a very valuable imaging tool. Like plain radiography, CT involves application of X-ray radiation to the body and different body tissues absorbing this radiation at different amounts. However, unlike plain radiography, CT provides 3D information, free of superimposing tissues thus resulting in much higher contrast resolution.

CT involves transmission of radiation from an X-ray tube that rotates around the patient. This radiation is then received by a ring of radiation detectors that are located around the body. The information received by the detectors is then converted to final images with a computer. With a spiral CT, as well as the X-ray tube rotating continuously, the patient is also moved through the X-ray beam. As a result, greater anatomical regions are imaged during a single breath hold, reducing the time taken for the scan and the artefacts caused by movement.

CT provides detail images of bone. This makes it an ideal choice on investigation for evaluating complicated fractures including those that involve articular surfaces. This evaluation of complex fractures is further enhanced by software packages that produce 3D images. CT can also be a very useful aid in diagnosing of 'occult' and stress fractures.

CT can be used in the following injuries.

Head injuries

CT is a vital tool for evaluation of athletes with serious head injuries, revolutionising management since introduction. It can detect:

- Skull fractures
- Intracranial haemorrhage:
  - Epidural
  - Subdural
  - Intracerebral
  - Subarachnoid
- Cerebral contusions:
  - This is 'bruising' of brain parenchyma
- Diffuse axonal injury:
  - Caused by rotational forces resulting in shearing of multiple axons
  - Initial CT may not show any major abnormalities other than petechial haemorrhages

Cervical spine injuries

- CT indicated when:
  - Plain radiography fails to show all of cervical spine in those athletes with cervical spine injuries
  - Fracture or subluxation is seen on plain X-ray, and further evaluation is required

Thoracolumbar spine injuries

CT commonly used to provide anatomical detail of fractures including determination of osseous fragment location in relation to central canal.

Shoulder injuries

- Dislocations +/- fractures:
  - Subtle Hill-Sachs, Bankart's lesions may not be detected on plain radiography, but can be seen on CT images. Accuracy for detecting labrum lesions may be increased CT is performed following intra-articular injection of contrast (CT arthrography)
- Proximal humerus fractures:
  - By providing anatomical detail, CT can be a vital tool for planning the management of the more complex proximal humerus fractures
- Scapula fractures:

- Undisplaced fractures may be difficult to see on plain X-ray, whereas CT is accurate in detecting them. Furthermore, CT will reveal the associated surrounding structure injuries

- Injuries to intra-abdominal organs including retroperitoneal structures
- Haemoperitoneum and its source
- Retroperitoneal haematoma and its source

Chest injuries

- CT can be an extremely valuable tool in management of chest injuries revealing the kind, location and extend of the chest injury

Abdominal injuries

- CT is an important adjunct when evaluating athletes with abdominal trauma
- Supplies information about:

Pelvic injuries

- As well as revealing associated abdominal, pelvic organ and vascular injuries, CT provides vital information when evaluating pelvic and acetabular fractures

Knee injuries

- CT is particularly useful when evaluating tibia plateau fractures

Further reading

Barron D. Basic science: computed tomography. Curr Orthop 2005; 19:20–26.

Laker SR, Concannon LG. Radiologic evaluation of the neck: a review of radiography, ultrasonography, computed tomography, magnetic resonance imaging, and other imaging modalities for neck pain. Phys Med Rehabil Clin N Am 2011; 22:411–428.

Related topics of interest

Infection and sport

Key points

- Moderate exercise can result in a reduced incidence of upper respiratory tract infections (URTIs)
- Vigorous exercise and overtraining can lower resistance to infection
- Up to 40% of traumatic splenic ruptures have occurred in athletes who have been found to have infectious mononucleosis

Sports immunology is a relatively new field that investigates the interaction of physical, psychological and environmental stress on the immune system. There is a complex interaction between exercise and immune function. To understand this, a basic knowledge of the immune system is required.

The body's immune system comprises of two components. The first is the innate system that consists of the body's physical barrier to infection (the skin and mucous membranes) and a non-specific response of phagocytic leukocytes, natural killer (NK) cells and proteins, including cytokines and complement factors. The adaptive system comprises of T and B lymphocytes that recognise specific foreign antigens. Unlike the innate system, the adaptive system develops gradually but exhibits memory of the antigens that it encounters so that it can quickly react to subsequent re-exposure to mount a rapid response.

Moderate physical activity (exercise for 5–60 min within a range of 40–60% of maximum heart rate [MHR])

Numerous studies have suggested that 60–90% of survey responders who exercise regularly report fewer URTIs than their peers. During moderate exercise, several positive changes occur in the immune system, including an increase in neutrophil and NK cells levels and salivary IgA antibody concentrations. Although the immune system returns to pre-exercise levels quickly following this form of exercise, this appears to reduce the risk of infection long term.

Vigorous physical activity (5–60 min of exercise at 70–80% of MHR and prolonged exercise)

A common perception is that overtraining lowers resistance to infections such as URTIs. Epidemiological studies show that URTI risk is increased during vigorous exercise and in the 1–2 week period following competitive endurance races. The immunological changes that occur following vigorous exercise include the following:

- Neutrophilia and lymphopaenia induced by stress hormones
- Decrease in NK cell activity
- Increase in pro- and anti-inflammatory cytokines
- Decrease in mucosal IgA, therefore impairing the ability of the upper respiratory tract to neutralise pathogens
- Blunted major histocompatibility complex (MCH) II expression that results in impaired antigen presentation to T lymphocytes

Upper respiratory tract infections

These are a spectrum of illnesses, which include infectious rhinitis (common cold), pharyngitis and sinusitis.

Epidemiology

The average adult has two to four 'colds' per year, mostly during the winter months.

Aetiology

Viral: Most URTIs are caused by viruses that are transmitted by secretion, contaminated hands or direct droplet transmission through hand contact with the eyes or nose. These include the following:

- **Infectious rhinitis:** It is mostly caused by rhinoviruses
- **Pharyngitis:** It is mostly caused by rhinovirus, coronavirus, parainfluenza virus or respiratory syncytial virus. Other viral agents include herpes simplex and

coxsackievirus and adenovirus Epstein–Barr virus (EBV) and cytomegalovirus (CMV) can also cause pharyngitis, but they also cause other severe systemic symptoms including fatigue, lymphadenopathy, splenomegaly and fever

Bacterial: Beta haemolytic group A streptococcus, chlamydia pneumonia.

Symptoms and signs

Mild fever and fatigue followed by clear rhinorrhoea, congestion, scratchy sore throat, cough, and headache are the most common symptoms. On clinical examination, a low-grade fever may be found. The throat often appears erythematous with exudates and, occasionally, petechiae. Anterior cervical nodes may be swollen and tender. Tenderness over the sinus regions may be present.

Investigations and treatment

Diagnosis of URTIs is usually clinical and does not require further investigation. If a bacterial cause is suspected, throat swabs and cultures may be carried out to isolate the organisms responsible. Symptoms of viral URTIs usually improve within 5–7 days and abate within 10–14 days without need for treatment. Oral decongestants and antihistamines, paracetamol and ibuprofen can all be used symptomatically. Antibiotics are only given if bacterial causes are suspected or isolated. The antibiotic of choice for group A streptococcus infections is Penicillin V, but amoxicillin may also be substituted.

Return to sport

Return to sport can be guided by the 'neck check', described by E. Randy Eichner. If an athlete has symptoms only above the neck (i.e. ear, nose or throat symptoms), he or she may jog slowly for 10 min. If symptoms worsen, the athlete should stop until symptoms improve. If the symptoms do not progress, he or she can continue the exercise at 50% intensity and increase gradually to full training. If symptoms are below the neck (fever, gastrointestinal or respiratory symptoms, fatigue), the athlete should not exercise until they have resolved.

Infectious mononucleosis

Epidemiology

Mainly affects adolescents and young adults in developed countries and young children in developing countries.

Aetiology

Infectious mononucleosis is mostly due to EBV, less commonly CMV.

Symptoms and signs

The most common presenting symptoms include fever and sore throat. Some patients may present with a maculopapular rash, fatigue and left-sided abdominal discomfort due to splenomegaly. There may also be neurological symptoms ranging from encephalitis to peripheral neuropathy. Clinical examination reveals tonsillar hypertrophy with exudates and also generalised lymphadenopathy may be found. Jaundice and haematological abnormalities (thrombocytopaenia or haemolytic anaemia) may also be observed.

Investigations and treatment

Blood tests generally show an increase in white blood cell count with increased numbers of atypical lymphocytes. Serological tests for EBV and CMV IgM and IgG can provide direct evidence of acute or prior infection. A positive heterophile antibody (Monospot) test is diagnostic. Infectious mononucleosis is generally self-limiting and symptoms usually last 2–6 weeks. Treatment is, therefore, mainly expectant.

Complications

Splenic rupture: Up to 40% of traumatic splenic ruptures have occurred in athletes who have been found to have infectious mononucleosis. Most splenic ruptures occur in patients with splenomegaly, but it can happen to patients who do not have an enlarged spleen. Splenic rupture usually occurs between weeks 2 and 4 with an incidence of 1 in 1000 (see Abdominal injuries in sport).

Persistent fatigue: In a few patients, fatigue and lethargy can continue for an indefinite period of time after other symptoms have been resolved.

Return to sport

The American Medical Society for Sports Medicine recommends that athletes should avoid all exercises for the first 21 days after the onset of illness. Following, they can begin slowly to resume their activities, progressing not more than 10% per week in duration or intensity. Full recovery usually takes 2–3 months but can take longer in selected cases. Athletes should refrain from returning to contact sports such as rugby or wrestling until the splenic enlargement has resolved.

Further reading

Brolinson PG, Elliott D. Exercise and the immune system. Clin Sports Med 2007; 26:311–319.
Gleeson M. Immune function in sport and exercise. J Appl Physiol 2007; 103:693–699.

Harris MD. Infectious disease in athletes. Curr Sports Med Rep 2011; 10(2):84–89.

Related topics of interest

- Abdominal injuries in sport (p. 1)
- Skin infections (p. 285)
- Unexplained under performance syndrome (p. 326)

Knee – anterior cruciate ligament (ACL) injuries

Key points

- Acute anterior cruciate ligament (ACL) rupture is always associated with a knee haemarthrosis
- The decision for a surgical reconstruction will be reserved for the young patient with functional instability, the level of sport activity and the personality of that patient
- The long-term risk of Osteoarthritis is unclear, however, a reconstruction of the ACL allows continued sports participation with all its benefits

Aetiology

The incidence of an ACL rupture injury in the United Kingdom is 30 new patients per 100,000 people every year.

The ACL is an intracapsular structure, attached proximately at the posterolateral femur and distally on the tibial spine. The ACL resists anterior displacement of tibia on the femur. Also, as the knee extends, it rotates the tibia externally assisting to 'drive' the tibia under the femur.

The usual mechanism of injury includes, in contact sports such as football and rugby, an excessive rotation force on the tibia or when the knee moves in hyperextension, which usually occurs when a skier falls backwards.

Swelling, caused by haemarthrosis, is present in almost all the patients. Many patients describe an audible 'pop' at the time of the injury.

Physical examination usually confirms a knee effusion. The tenderness is diffused or present posterolaterally in cases of lateral meniscus tears or medially if there is an associated medial meniscus tear.

The anterior draw test may be negative due to muscle spasm, however, the Lachman's test is always positive with a soft or no 'end point'. In experienced hands, the pivot-shift test is also positive. Clinical tests for the other anatomical structures, such as meniscus and other knee ligaments, should be performed too to exclude any complex injuries.

Investigations

X-rays may be entirely normal or may demonstrate, in a young athlete, an avulsion of the ACL from the tibial spine. A Segond's fracture of the lateral tibial edge may be present, which is usually associated with an ACL rupture.

Magnetic resonance imaging scan is currently the investigation of choice to confirm the diagnosis and detect any other associated injuries.

Management
Conservative

This will consist of 4 to 6 weeks rehabilitation programme to absorb the effusion, restore a painless knee joint full range of movement and regain full muscle strength and proprioception, such as long jump, side stepping exercises and 'figure of 8' running.

Following the rehabilitation programme, the patient may be able to return to his sport or will carry on to surgical reconstruction of the ACL, in particular if the knee is unstable on returning to sport or even with daily activities. Functional recurrent instability could be present either as the feeling of the knee keeping 'giving way' or recurrent knee effusions. The patient should be discouraged to continue sport with frequent episodes of instability. Recurrent instability may damage the menisci and the bone articular cartilage, leading to degeneration and osteoarthritis.

Derotation knee braces are still controversial. Some patients have reported improved knee stability using a brace in sports such as skiing or tennis.

Surgery

The decision for a surgical reconstruction will be based on whether the patient is young, with recurrent instability, the level of sporting activity and the personality of that patient.

During surgery, the popular choice among surgeons is an autograft, which is harvested from the patient's hamstrings, patella tendon or quadriceps and will be placed, usually arthroscopically, into the knee joint. Allografts and synthetic ligament materials are also in use around the world. A prolong rehabilitation programme is undertaken following the surgery.

The long-term risk of osteoarthritis is unclear, although many publications have suggested that in knees where the ACL is reconstructed, the knee stability is restored and this reduces the risk of further articular cartilage damage and tearing of the menisci, therefore reducing the probability of degenerative disease and osteoarthritis. Certainly, the reconstruction of the ACL allows the individual to continue sports participation with all its benefits.

Chronic ACL-deficient knee joint

The patient will complain of 'giving way', recurrent swelling, pain and locking. The diagnostic tests, such as anterior draw test, Lachman's test, pivot shift test and meniscus tearing tests, are more obviously positive than the acute rupture of the ACL. Degenerative disease with crepitus and pain over knee compartments on movements may be present. Also, an effusion may or may not be present.

Arthroscopic surgery may be indicated for the torn menisci. ACL reconstruction is indicated when instability is present with daily activities. The rehabilitation programme is similar as for the acute ACL reconstruction.

Return to sport

Following surgery and a prolong rehabilitation programme is undertaken, the patient is allowed to return to competitive sport between 6 months to 1 year. In the hands of an experienced surgeon, the success rate following the surgery approaches 90%.

Further reading

Moses B, Orchard J, Orchard J: Annual incidence of ACL injury and surgery in various populations. Res Sports Med 2012; 20(3–4).

Smith HC, Vacek P, Johnson RJ, et al: Risk factors for ACL injury: a review of the literature. Sports Health 2012; 4:155–161.

Renstrom PA: Eight clinical conundrums relating to ACL injury in sport. Br J Sports Med 2012; 46(12).

Related topics of Interest

Knee – articular cartilage injuries

Key points

- Injuries of the articular cartilage could range from a focal full thickness cartilage defect to an osteochondral fracture that involves the articular cartilage and the underlying bone
- Osteochondritis dissecans (OCD) is a separate condition, in which an osteochondral segment appears fractures as a result of local compromise of its blood supply
- There are a number of treatment option based on how old is the injury, the site and size of the injury and the age of the patient

Aetiology

These injuries could occur from a direct blow or a forceful rotation to the knee.

Acute articular and osteochondral fractures

The patient will report an audible 'snap' at the time of the injury and the knee will become acutely painful. He will probably be unable to apply his full weight on this leg and the knee joint will become swollen soon after the injury. A displaced fragment may produce a locked knee. Aspiration of the knee joint will confirm a haemarthrosis, also the presence of fat cells due to the fracture.

Chronic articular cartilage defects

The individual is experiencing pain, the feeling of 'loud noise' and crepitation during the range of movement (ROM) of the knee joint. Recurrent swelling with activities and sport usually appears adding to the pain. Weakness of the quadriceps thigh muscle will also be observed in many patients. The injury could sometimes mimic a meniscus lesion with pain on rotational knee movements and positive clinical tests of meniscus injury.

Osteochondritis dissecans

This is a condition that is usually affects the knee joint in a young patient aged between 10–18 years old and is predominant in males.

Common sites include the medial femoral condyle (80%), the lateral femoral condyle (15%) and the patella (5%).

A segment of bone adjacent to the articular cartilage is deprived of its blood supply and becomes avascular, which will lead to avascular necrosis. The avascular segment may remain in its anatomical position and is called stable or it may displace and then is called unstable. Complete displacement with the fragment free into the knee joint will form a loose body.

A patient with an OCD will complain of diffuse pain and swelling with sport or other vigorous activities. Locking and 'giving way' will appear in unstable lesions and in the presence of loose bodies. The bulk of the thigh muscles may get reduced. Internal rotation of the tibia and movement of the knee from flexion to extension will increase the pain as a result of the impingement of the medial tibial spine over the commonly placed medial femoral condyle OCD. Therefore, some of the patients may walk with the affected leg kept in external rotation. Patella OCD produces pain behind the patella and crepitus.

Investigations

X-rays will be able in many cases to detect an osteochondral fracture, OCD lesions and loose bodies. Special views for the patella and the femoral notch may be requested.

Magnetic resonance imaging scan will be indicated to confirm the diagnosis in cases that the articular cartilage pathology is not demonstrated with the radiographs, also in an OCD to distinguish between a stable and an unstable lesion.

Management

Acute articular and osteochondral fractures

Accurate reduction and internal fixation of the displaced osteochondral fracture is necessary. In cases with a very small fragment, it could be removed with arthroscopic surgery. Gradual weight bearing, exercises for strength and knee ROM will follow surgery.

Chronic articular cartilage defects

Conservative management of a partial thickness articular cartilage defect may be considered in a patient that is not an athlete. This includes modification of activities, physiotherapy sessions and orthotics if appropriate.

For the young athlete, many surgical options exist, aiming to treat the articular cartilage defect and restore weight bearing. Microfracture, which is a bone marrow stimulating procedure, has return good results in relative small sized defects and in Medical Institutions that they implement a strict rehabilitation programme following surgery. Chondrocyte transplantation and osteochondral grafts have produced promising results for larger lesions in young athletes.

Osteochondritis dissecans

Patients younger than 18 years old with a stable lesion could be treated with a period of 1–2 weeks rest and a knee brace if the knee is acutely swollen and painful. Gradual mobilisation under physiotherapy guidance is introduced for a period between 3 and 6 months.

If the patient is over 18 years old or in an unstable lesion, regardless of the patient's age, then surgery is indicated. Surgical options include reduction and fixation of an unstable fragment or excision of the fragment and drilling or microfracture of the defect. Older patients may have already developed degenerative knee joint changes with a less successful outcome.

Return to sport

Return to sport will be permitted when:
- The patient is pain free
- There is no joint tenderness and effusion
- There is full ROM of the knee joint
- Normal muscle strength is restored
- X-rays confirm healing by the disappearance of the radiolucent line that outlines the fracture
- Fitness levels have been restored

The average time to return to sport if the athlete underwent successful surgery is 12–18 months.

Further reading

Bekkers JE, Inklaar M, Saris DB. Treatment selection in articular cartilage lesions of the knee. Am J Sports Med 2009; 37:1485–1555.

Magnussen RA, Dunn WR, Carey JL et al. Treatment of focal articular cartilage lesions of the knee. Clin Orthop Relat Res 2008; 466:952–962.

Ralston BM, Williams JS, Bach BR Jr et al. Osteochondritis dissecans of the knee. Phys Sports Med 1996; 24:73–84.

Knee – lateral ligament injuries

Key points

- The posterolateral structures together resist excessive varus and external rotation forces.
- Usually combined with other ligamentous injuries
- With posterolateral corner injuries, direct anatomic repair of all injured structures is indicated in injuries diagnosed acutely (2-3 weeks)

The lateral collateral ligament is a component of the posterolateral (PLC) corner of the knee

Anatomy

Seebacher (three) layers

Superficial layer: The iliotibial tract and its anterior expansion, the superficial portion of the biceps and its posterior expansion.
Middle layer: The quadriceps retinaculum anteriorly, the patellomeniscal ligaments and the two patellofemoral ligaments posteriorly.

Deep layer:
Superficial lamina: Encompasses the lateral collateral ligament and ends at the fabellofibular ligament,
Deep lamina: The coronary ligament, the popliteofibular ligament, the popliteal hiatus, terminating at the arcuate ligament.

Sudasna and Harnsiriwattanagit

Identified the popliteofibular ligament in 98% of the knees, a fabellofibular ligament in 68%, and arcuate ligament in 24%.

Biomechanics

The posterolateral structures together resist excessive varus and external rotation forces. They also provide secondary restraint to posterior translation.

The lateral collateral ligament provides the greatest resistance to a varus moment on the tibia. The posterolateral capsule and adjoining structures provide greatest resistance to an external rotation torque on the tibia. The popliteus tendon resists external rotation of the tibia during 20° to 130°knee flexion and varus rotation from 0° to 90°.

The popliteofibular ligament and the popliteus tendon are important in resisting posterior translation, primary varus rotation and external rotation, and coupled external rotation.

Mechanism of injury

Isolated injury of the PLC is uncommon and results from a posterolateral force directed against the proximal part of the tibia with the knee in extension.

Combined PLC and other ligament injury

1. Combined hyperextension and external rotation force
2. Hyperextension moment.
3. Varus bending moment.
4. Tibial external rotation torque.
5. Posteriorly directed force on externally rotated tibia of a flexed knee.

Noyes concept of single, double and triple varus syndromes

Partial to complete loss of the medial meniscus is a significant factor in physiologically varus aligned knees in terms of the early onset of medial compartment wear. Frank Noyes proposed a classification for the anatomic abnormalities of these knees, using the terms primary-, double-, and triple-varus knee syndromes. *Primary varus* refers to the tibiofemoral osseous alignment and geometry at the knee joint including the added varus alignment that occurs with loss of the medial meniscus and damage to the articular cartilage in the tibiofemoral joint. *Double varus:* In varus angulated knees,lateral soft tissue restraints may become slack, allowing for increased lateral joint opening especially with activity (lateral condylar liftoff). *Triple varus:* Chronic excessive tensile forces in the posterolateral ligament structures, or traumatic injury, may further result in a varus recurvatum position.

Clinical diagnosis

Symptoms and signs: Pain, common peroneal nerve symptoms, edema, ecchymosis, induration, and tenderness.

Posterolateral rotatory instability (Hughston): Posterior subluxation of the lateral tibial plateau with external rotation torque in knees with pathologic laxity of the posterolateral corner.

Stance and gait: Varus alignment; varus thrust gait; hyperextension-varus thrust gait, flexed knee gait.

Voluntary posterolateral drawer sign: Patient actively reproduces instability.

Isolated LCL tear: Increase in varus stress at 30° of knee flexion

Injury of PLC with intact PCL: Increased varus, external rotation (dial), and posterior translation at 30° of flexion

Injury of PLC and PCL: Increased laxity at 30° and 90°.

Tibial external rotation (dial) test: External rotation of tibia is performed at 30° and 90° knee flexion in prone or supine position

Posterolateral external rotation test: Coupled posterior translation and external rotation force is applied to the proximal part of the tibia at 30° and 90° knee flexion

Reverse pivot-shift test: Sensation of reduction when the flexed, externally rotated knee is extended with valgus stress. May be positive in up to 35% of normal knees examined under anesthesia.

External rotation recurvatum test (Hughston): Used to diagnose posterolateral rotatory instability in the extended knee. Patient's legs are lifted by the great toes and side-to-side differences in hyperextension, varus, and tibial external rotation are noted.

Plain Radiographs: May show lateral joint space widening; an arcuate fracture of the fibular head; avulsion of the Gerdy tubercle; or a Segond fracture.

MRI: Useful to establish diagnosis and visualize anatomic structures.

Arthroscopy: Increases lateral joint laxity may be seen as a so-called drive-through sign.

Non-operative treatment

Focused physiotherapy for muscle rehabilitation and gait retraining may be useful for incomplete PLC injuries and peri-operatively in chronic injuries. Reconstructive surgery is often necessary in active patients.

Operative treatment

Primary repair: Direct anatomic repair of all injured structures is indicated in injuries diagnosed acutely (2-3 weeks). Direct suture, sutures via drill-holes through bone, or suture anchors may be used for repair.

Augmentation: In severe injuries precluding direct repair or delayed presentation, allograft or autograft tendons may be used for augmentation of attempted repairs.

Advancement and tenodesis: May be used in chronic injuries provided sufficient intact collagenous tissue is available at the injured site.

1. The osseous attachment of arcuate ligament complex (the lateral gastrocnemius tendon, LCL and popliteal tendon) is advanced anterior and distal.
2. The PLC is advanced proximally.
3. Tenodesis of the biceps femoris tendon to the lateral femoral epicondyle.
4. Recession of the popliteus and lateral collateral ligaments into the lateral femoral condyle.

Reconstruction: One or more components of the PLC may be reconstructed using allografts or autografts.

Osteotomy: A valgus tibial osteotomy is performed as an initial procedure to prevent excessive load that may follow staged soft tissue reconstruction in the presence of marked varus alignment not controlled by muscle activity (the Noyes triple varus knee syndrome) and a lateral thrust in the stance phase of gait. In valgising upper tibial osteotomy, the correction should be a 'fine-tuning', with a much more minor realignment.

Rehabilitation

Varies depending on various factors such as time since injury, type of reconstruction or repair and concomitant ligament injuries. Bracing with monitored increase in range of knee motion, focused muscle rehabilitation and gait training are the key.

Further reading

Bulstrode C, Buckwalter J, Wilson- Macdonald et al. (eds) Oxford textbook of orthopaedics and trauma, 2nd edn. Oxford; Oxford University Press, 2010:713-717.

Related topics of interest

- Knee – multiligament injuries (p. 176)
- Knee acute injuries (p. 189)
- Knee – anterior cruciate ligament (ACL) injuries (p. 164)
- Knee – posterior cruciate ligament (PCL) injuries (p. 187)

Knee – medial ligament injuries

Key points

- Medial collateral ligament (MCL) is the primary medial stabilizer in resisting valgus loading and the secondary stabilizer against excessive external tibial rotation.
- These injuries are common and usually occur as a result of valgus force
- Most isolates MCL injuries could be managed non-operatively

MCL is one of the most frequently injured ligaments of the knee.

Anatomy

Warren and Marshall – superficial to deep

Layer 1: Sartorius, sartorial fascia
Layer 2: Superficial MCL, posterior oblique ligament (POL), semimembranosus.
Layer 3: Deep MCL, posteromedial capsule.

Sims and Jacobson – anterior to posterior

Anterior third: Capsular ligaments, extensor retinaculum of the quadriceps mechanism.

Middle third: Deep medial capsular ligament, superficial medial collateral ligament.

Posterior third: (postero-medial corner of the knee; PMC) POL, semimembranosus expansions, oblique popliteal ligament, posteromedial horn of medial meniscus.

Biomechanics

MCL is the primary medial stabilizer in resisting valgus loading and the secondary stabilizer against excessive external tibial rotation.

The MCL maintains relatively constant tension throughout knee range of motion. Strain in the anterior fibers remains constant; while in the posterior and central portions, strain decreases with increasing flexion. The greatest strain is in full extension at the femoral origin of the posterior fibers.

The POL resists valgus stress in full extension.

The PMC is a static and dynamic restraint to anteromedial rotatory instability.

Mechanism of injury

Valgus forces to the knee tear medial structures

Force to the lateral side of the thigh or upper leg, e.g. football tackle

External rotation of tibia with femur fixed, e.g. snow skiing

Forceful shift in direction off the weight-bearing foot, e.g. change in direction while running

Clinical diagnosis

Signs and symptoms: Swelling, stiffness, pain and tenderness to palpation. Meniscal and anterior cruciate (ACL) injuries frequently coexist.

In chronic injuries, a medial thrust may be identified on gait examination and valgus malalignment may be present.
Clinical grading (opening on valgus stress):
Grade 1: 0 to 5mm,
Grade 2: 6 to 10mm
Grade 3: > 10mm
Isloated MCL injury: Valgus laxity at 30 degrees of flexion but not at 0 degree.

MCL and POL injury: Valgus laxity at both 30 and 0 degrees

Plain Radiographs: May show concomitant bone injury, avulsions, osteochondral defects or physeal injury (stress views). Valgus malalignment may be seen on weight bearing views.

Ultrasonography: Sensitive investigation but operator dependent.

Magnetic resonance imaging (MRI): Diagnostic imaging of choice. There is poor correlation between MRI grading and clinical laxity. Treatment should hence, be based on the latter.

Conservative management

Grade 1 and 2 injuries and isolated grade 3 injuries may be managed non-operatively by adequate analgesia, edema control and protective bracing while encouraging immediate range of motion exercises and focused rehabilitation programmes.

Grade 2 and worse MCL tears need bracing. The patient is braced 30-60° and non-weight bearing for the first 2 weeks then progressed to 10-90° in the brace and partial weight bearing for the next 2 weeks then for a final 2 weeks the brace is set to free motion and full weight bearing is allowed.

In multi-ligament injuries in which the PCL is not involved or only has a maximum grade 1 laxity, then a period of bracing first may allow the MCL to heal and not require surgery. When is a major MCL disruption is associated with a complete ACL tear, most should be braced to heal the MCL then have ACL reconstruction

Surgical management

May be necessary in:
1. Grade 3 MCL injuries with associated ACL, posterior cruciate (PCL) or posterolateral corner (PLC) injuries.
2. Distal MCL avulsion that flips over the pes anserinus.
3. Medial meniscus is avulsed from the joint with the MCL, or if the avulsed end of the MCL is 'flipped' into the joint.
4. In knee dislocation, when the joint is irreducible due to the medial femoral condyle prolapsing through a rent in the medial soft tissues
5. Chronic multi-ligament knee injury.
6. Failed conservative management in grade 1 or 2 MCL injuries which present with failed ACL or PCL reconstruction.

Surgical treatment options
Acute repair

Indications
1. When the MCL tear is not an isolated injury and is part of a multi-ligament injury

2. If there is major PCL disruption early PCL reconstruction is usually preferable. At the same time a major MCL injury should be dealt with surgically

Acute surgery allows the possibility of repairing tissues to allow them to heal in correct positions and at correct tensions; and to give the best chance of neural recovery and restoration of proprioceptive sensitivity.

The operation requires a large medial longitudinal incision. The first layer of deep fascia is often intact but stretched and needs to be opened. The failed MCL may be directly repaired and insertion sites advanced (anteriorly and inferiorly for tibial attachment; superiorly and posteriorly for femoral attachment) to attain ligament tension while maintaining isometricity. Sutures or suture anchors may be used for this purpose. Mattress sutures may be used to imbricate lax portions of the ligament to adjacent intact portions.

Occasionally the medial hamstrings are avulsed and need reattachment.

Augmentation in acute and chronic injury

Autograft, allograft tendons or synthetic ligaments (e.g. LARS, Orthomedic) may be used for this purpose. One or 2 graft or polyester ligaments are used attached to the femur in bone tunnels. One is always taken along the line of the superficial MCL to be attached just below the joint line, to make it act like the deep MCL, by double stapling. The second when used reproduces the POL.

Chronic injury

The medial soft tissues are exposed by a medial longitudinal wound. The superficial layer of deep fascia is split longitudinally and and an attempt to separate the superficial and deep MCL layers is made, whenever possible. For laxity above the meniscus slack is taken up in the deep / superficial MCL by placing 'figure of eight' sutures to 'plicate' the lax tissue. The sutures are placed to pull the tissues towards the medial femoral attachment of the MCL. For laxity below the meniscus the MCL tissue needs to be split longitudinally and elevated directly from the bone. It is then tensioned to slide it on the bone before being reattached in the new position with suture anchors placed close to the joint line. Synthetic augmentation is always used in such cases, before double-breasting the deep fascia over the synthetic ligament(s) to further augment the reconstruction.

Rehabilitation

The post-operative rehabilitation should be designed with knowledge of the functional anatomy- the superficial MCL resists valgus stress, but the deep MCL also resists external rotation. The posterior oblique ligament part (POL) resists internal rotation. Hence when weight-bearing for walking or quads exercises is started the foot should be kept in neutral to avoid torsion at the knee.

A hinged knee brace is often used with gradual increase in flexion until quadriceps control is achieved.

Full active and passive extension is achieved as soon as possible. Flexion range depends on other ligament surgery also undertaken at the same operation.

Further reading

Bulstrode C, Buckwalter J, Wilson- Macdonald et al. (eds) Oxford textbook of orthopaedics and trauma, 2nd edn. Oxford; Oxford University Press, 2010:713-717.

Narvani A, Mahmud T, Lavelle J et al. Injury to the proximal deep medial collateral ligament: a problematical subgroup of injuries. J Bone Joint Surg Br 2010; 92(7):949-953.

Related topics of interest

Knee – multiligament injuries

Key points

- These are associated with knee dislocations and vascular injuries
- Acute management includes exclusion of vascular injury, vascular surgical intervention if required, reduction of the dislocated knee and maintains congruency of the knee either by brace or external fixation
- Definitive management requires referral to a specialist unit for repair or reconstruction of the ligaments (may require osteotomy too)

Introduction

Multiligament injuries are often a sequel of knee dislocation. They may be associated with neurovascular injuries, meniscal injuries or fractures.

Mechanism of injury

1. Athletic and sports injuries
2. High-energy trauma
3. Obese individuals sustaining low-energy falls

Classification

Kennedy: This is based on the position of the tibia in relation to the femur.

Schenck: This is an anatomic classification based on the ligaments injured:
i. One collateral and one cruciate
ii. Both cruciates
iii. Both cruciates and medial (III M) or lateral structures (III L)
iv. All four ligaments
v. Wascher: Fracture dislocation:
   V1. One cruciate and collateral with fracture
   V2. Both cruciates with fracture
   V3. Both cruciates and medial (V3M) or lateral (V3L) structures with fracture
   V4. All four ligaments with fracture

Neyret classification and Boisgard modification. Describes direction of dislocation and injured ligaments:
Type 1. 'Simple' bicruciate lesion without dislocation:
   Type 1a. Medial
   Type 1b. Lateral
   Type 1c. Posterior
Type 2. 'Pure' dislocation without peripheral tear:
   Type 2a. Anterior
   Type 2b. Posterior
Type 3. Dislocation with single cruciate lesion:
   Type 3a. Anterior cruciate ligament (ACL)
   Type 3b. Posterior cruciate ligament (PCL)
Type 4. 'Combined' lesions associating peripheral tear and dislocation:
   Type 4a. Medial (lateral dislocation)
   Type 4b. Lateral (medial dislocation)
   Type 4c. Complex (rotational, medial and lateral tear)

Biomechanics

Bicruciate lesions without medial, lateral or posterior dislocation is a result of gaping. Simple translation causes pure anterior and posterior dislocation. Combined gaping and translation causes dislocation with peripheral tear.

The energy level is a factor in whether lesions are simple or combined. With increasing energy, gaping can lead to peripheral then cruciate tearing and, if kinetic energy remains, to translation causing dislocation. On the other hand, high kinetic energy mechanisms may result directly in dislocation, without intermediate lesions.

Clinical diagnosis

The mechanism of knee injury may be obtained from history. Following reduction, the severity of the injury may not be evident. Swelling, ecchymosis, lacerations and fractures are variably present. A thorough neurovascular examination is essential. A preliminary ligament examination should be performed as soon as feasible:

- ACL:
  - **The Lachman test:** The ventral displacement of the tibia with respect to the femur at 30° of knee flexion
  - **The anterior drawer test:** Anterior excursion of proximal tibia to an anteriorly directed force with hip flexed at 45° and the knee flexed at 90°
- PCL
  - The posterior drawer test
  - **The posterior sag:** Position of tibia in relation to femoral condyle. Normal tibia is 1 cm anterior
  - **The quadriceps active test:** Distal limb is fixed in place and the quadriceps activated which serves to reduce the tibia and translate it forward
- **Medial and lateral ligament complex:** See Topic on collateral ligament injuries
- Common peroneal nerve is commonly injured (14–25%)

Investigations
Diagnosis of vascular injury
- Serial ankle brachial pressure index (ABI)
- Arterial duplex
- Computed tomography (CT) angiography
- Arterial duplex ultrasonography (operator dependent)

Plain radiographs
- Identifies ligament, osseochondral defects, capsular avulsions, fractures (tibial plateau, proximal fibula). Stress radiographs may demonstrate occult ligament instability

CT
- Good for pre-operative planning especially in the presence of fractures

Magnetic resonance imaging
- Identifies ligament, meniscus and other soft tissue injuries

Management of multiligament knee injury (see Figure 17)

Urgent reduction of the dislocated knee. Failure of reduction may occur if the medial femoral condyle is 'button-holed' through soft tissue and open reduction may be needed:

1. Hold the knee in congruent reduction in a brace. An external fixator is indicated only in cases of vascular reconstruction
2. Evaluation of neurovascular status before and after reduction
3. Early angiogram or high-quality Doppler ultrasound. Vascular surgical intervention if needed
4. Allowing early motion and soft tissue care, particularly prevention of contractures, in preparation for surgery
5. Plan surgery

Delayed operation around 2 months is ideal for injuries to the medial collateral ligament (MCL), of all severities or when the PCL is normal or has minor increased laxity (grade 1 maximum).

Early surgical repair (2–3 weeks) is undertaken for posteromedial and posterolateral corner injuries. Autograft or allograft ACL and PCL may be undertaken at the same time or as a staged procedure. With delayed presentation augmentation, advancement and reconstruction are planned using autografts or allografts.

Osteotomy can be very effective in controlling dynamic deformity and therefore protect soft tissue reconstructions.

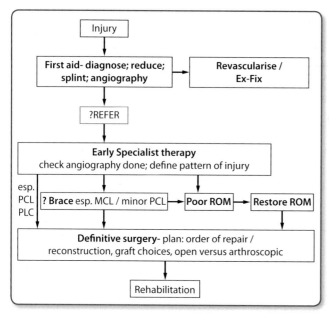

Figure 17 Algorithm for treating multiligament injuries. PCL, posterior cruciate ligament; MCL, medial collateral ligament; ROM, range of movement.

Further reading

Williams A, Narvani AA. Multiple ligament injuries to the knee. In: Bulstrode C, Buckwalter J, Wilson-Macdonald J, Fairbank J (eds), Oxford textbook of orthopaedics and trauma, 2nd edn. Oxford; Oxford University Press, 2010.

Related topics of interest

Knee – other injuries

Key points

- Serious injuries will include fractures, disruption of the knee extensor mechanism and patella dislocation
- Surgical management is likely in most of the cases
- Long recovery is probably expected, before returning to sport activity

Aetiology

Fractures

They involve the distal femur, proximal tibia and patella bone. In most cases, the fracture will involve the articular bone surface, disrupting the congruity of the knee joint.

The individual complains of pain at the knee is unable to bear weight on the leg. The knee joint is usually swollen. Deformity of the leg could also be observed.

Adolescents in contact sports are particular vulnerable to fractures of the epiphysis at the knee region. A shearing force may cause a disruption across the cartilaginous growth plate with the fracture extending to the epiphysis or metaphysic and sometimes in both regions. Permanent damage of the growth plate could lead to a shortened limb or deformity.

Fractures of the distal femoral epiphysis are more common than proximal tibia fractures. They are usually seen in boys 10–14 years old. Apophyseal tibia tubercle fractures could also occur in boys from a violent quadriceps contraction with the foot fixed on the ground.

Fractures of the patella could be transverse caused by an unexpected eccentric contraction of the quadriceps applying force over the patella bone in jumping sports. The patient is usually over 30 years old and the fracture is usually displaced leading to disruption of the knee's extensor mechanism. The individual will not be able to raise the leg straight up. A direct force on the anterior knee could also cause a fracture, which is stellate in shape or comminuted.

Extensor mechanism knee injuries

These injuries include:
- Rupture of the patellar tendon
- Transverse fracture of the patella
- Rupture of the quadriceps

The mechanism of the injury is either a forced flexion of the knee at the same time of quadriceps contraction or a violent quadriceps contraction with the foot planted on the ground.

Which structure of the extensor knee mechanism will be damaged is usually associated with the individual's age group. Young athletes will suffer a patellar tendon rupture; patients over 30 years old will suffer a transverse patella fracture; however, older than 50 years individuals will sustain a quadriceps rupture.

The athlete will feel a loud 'pop', he will not be able to apply weight on the affected leg; also, he will be unable to raise or keep the leg straight up. Swelling is usually present into the knee joint.

Traumatic patella dislocation

This usually occurs with a sudden internal femoral rotation on the fixed tibia. The patella dislocates laterally and may spontaneously reduce.

The diagnosis is easily made if the patella is still dislocated. In cases where the dislocation is reduced, the clinical examination may reveal the presence of haemarthrosis, tender medial patella retinaculum, pain during quadriceps contractions and a positive apprehension test.

Traumatic prepatella bursitis

Direct blow at the anterior knee may cause a collection of blood into the prepatella bursa. A grossly distended warm-felt bursa will be observed at the front of the knee; however, the patient is able to straight raise the leg.

Investigations

X-rays will confirm the diagnosis of a fracture. Further imaging, such as a CT scan, will assist to collect information about the fracture's displacement and comminution. MRI scan may be deemed necessary in some fractures to detect associated soft tissue injuries of the ACL or other knee ligaments.

Ultrasound scan could assist with the diagnosis of a patellar tendon rupture and in particular to detect a quadriceps rupture. A prepatella bursa could also be confirmed and aspirated at the same session.

MRI scan may complete further the imaging of these injuries and assist in the decision-making process.

Management

Fractures

If the fracture is not displaced at all, then it could be treated into a plaster cast. However, many of these fractures are displaced and the congruity of the knee joint is also compromised. Therefore, surgery will provide an accurate reduction and adequate stability through internal fixation. Protective gradual weight bearing of the leg will follow surgery, maintaining the knee range of movement and muscle strength until the fracture is clinically and radiologically united.

Manipulation under anaesthetic of a fracture in an adolescent athlete with open growth physis is usually enough for an acceptable reduction. In more complex cases, failure to reduce the fracture or maintain the reduced position, an open reduction and fracture fixation may be considered.

Extensor mechanism knee injuries

These injuries will be probably treated with surgery to repair the patellar tendon or the quadriceps and re-produce a powerful straight leg raising. Patella fractures are dealt with surgical reduction and appropriate internal fixation. Quadriceps ruptures could sometimes be diagnosed with delay. Surgery may then be more complex involving lengthening or re-enforcing graft techniques, in addition to the repair.

Following surgery for these injuries, a period of protection and the repair will be followed by a lengthy and elaborate rehabilitation programme.

Patella dislocation

Management will include the immediate reduction of the dislocation and aspiration of the haemarthrosis. A period of immobilisation in a cast or a brace, usually in extension, for a period of 3 weeks is recommended by some specialists. Then

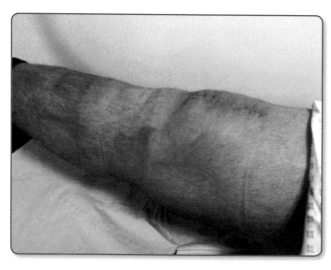

Figure 18 Straight leg raise following quadriceps repair.

exercises for knee flexion are commenced. Rehabilitation with strengthening of the vastus medialis in particular is introduced.

Surgical reconstruction of the medial patella-femoral ligament, as immediate treatment following a first time dislocation, in an athlete, is still under debate. However, recurrent patella instability will lead to surgical management.

Return to sport

It will take over 12 months to return to sport following the treatment of a fracture or repair of the knee extensor mechanism.

An athlete treated for Patella dislocation without surgery may take 6–12 weeks to return to sport, however, following surgery sport participation will be between 4 and 6 months.

Further reading

Kao FC, Tu YK, Hsu KY et al. Floating knee injuries, a high complication rate. Orthopaedics 2010;33(1):14.

Khan W, Johnson D. The management of knee extensor mechanism injuries book. LAP Publishers; 2010.

Tsai CH, Hsu CJ, Hung CH et al. Primary traumatic patella dislocation. J Orthop Surg Res 2012; 7:21.

Knee – overuse injuries

Key points

- These injuries include Iliotibial band friction syndrome (ITBS), popliteus tendinopathy and pes anserinus bursitis
- Biomechanical abnormalities often contribute to the injury pattern
- Nonsurgery treatment plans are the mainstay of management in these injuries

Aetiology

Iliotibial ITBS

The iliotibial band is a tendon within the fascia lata inserting into the Gerdy's tubercle on the anterior lateral aspect of the tibia. The iliotibial band drops posteriorly behind the lateral femoral epicondyle during knee flexion, then snaps forward over the epicondyle during the extension phase. This syndrome is the result of the inflammation of the distal iliotibial band and the bursa that lies underneath it and over the lateral femoral condyle.

Predisponding anatomical factors to the injury include:

- Varus knees (genu varus)
- Feet overpronation
- Leg length difference
- Prominent greater Trochanter at the upper femur

The injury is also called a runner's knee, and it is usually the result of training errors, such as a single run over excessive distance, increasing the running mileage too quickly or excessive hill running.

Pain is at first present in downhill running or going downstairs. Later on, the pain becomes continuous restricting all running and eventually routine daily activities. Tenderness on palpation is present 2–3 cm above the lateral knee joint line at the lateral femoral epicondyle with the knee flexed at 30°. Crepitus locally may also be present on palpation.

Ober's test is positive. The patient lies on the nonaffected side. From a position of 90° of knee flexion, the thigh is passively abducted and extended to catch the ITB over the gr. Trochanter. In this position, the examiner will withdraw his hands that support the leg, which will remain suspended in the air.

Popliteus tendinopathy

Athletes experience pain in the popliteal fossa area with sport, which later on becomes persistent even affecting daily activities.

The pain could be reproduced by resisted knee flexion with the tibia held in external rotation.

Pes anserinus tendinopathy and bursitis

The condition occurs at the anterior medial aspect of the proximal tibia, below the knee joint, where there is a bursa present that can become inflamed and cause localised symptoms. The condition is associated with repeated hamstrings injuries or even tight hamstrings.

The athlete's complaint will be localised 'burning' sensation and tenderness.

Investigations

X-rays could only be helpful in chronic conditions if there is any calcified tendonitis present.

Ultrasound scan could assist the diagnosis; also, procedures such as dry needling or an injection could be performed at the same time.

Magnetic resonance imaging scan could be useful in the different diagnosis between an overuse tendinopathy and other conditions if the diagnosis was uncertain.

Management ITBS (runner's knee)

The management in the acute presentation will include rest, ice and non-steroidal anti-inflammatory drugs (NSAIDs) medication. Reduction of the running mileage or even switch over to a different sport activity is very effective. However, in the average patient, it will take around 6 weeks for a complete pain relief.

A local steroid injection could produce relief in chronic cases. Physiotherapy modalities will concentrate to stretch the iliotibial band and improve the strength and co-ordination of the nearby muscles. Attention to correct any predisposing anatomical factors such as leg shortening, mal-alignment and feet overpronation is equally important.

Conservative treatment is usually successful but in persistent cases surgery, with division of the iliotibial band 3 cm above the knee joint at the level of the anterolateral femoral condyle, may be recommended.

Popliteus tendinopathy

The management will include rest, ice and physiotherapy sessions with localised soft tissue treatments, electrotherapy modalities and stretching the knee flexor muscles. The site could be injected, usually under ultrasound scan guidance, with a corticosteroid agent.

Pes anserinus tendinopathy and bursitis

The management include NSAIDs medication, rest from sport, ice applications, compressions and physiotherapy sessions to stretch the hamstrings. Prescription of orthotics in overpronated feet is advised. Aspiration and corticosteroid injection, probably under ultrasound guidance, is also recommended.

Return to sport

Athletes suffering from ITBS or other acute tendinopathies will be able to return to previous sport activities between 4 and 6 weeks, following an appropriate conservative programme.

Recurrence of the condition and prolong beyond 3 months recovery to sport, could occur, if the treatment plan was not completed.

Further Reading

Falvey EC, Clark RA, Franklyn-Miller A et al. ITBS: examination of evidence behind different treatment options. Scand J Med Sci Sports 2010; 20:580–587.

Ferber R, Hreljac A, Kendall KD. Suspected mechanisms in the cause of overuse running injuries: a clinical review. Sports Health 2009; 1:242–246.

Nielsen RO, Buist I, Sorensen H et al. Training errors and running related injuries. Int J Sports Phy Ther 2012; 7:58–75.

Related topics of interest

• Tendon overuse injuries (p. 302)

Knee – patellofemoral conditions and anterior knee pain

Key points

- The majority of the cases with anterior knee pain are related to patellofemoral joint issues
- Other causes of pain include patellar tendinopathy, a synovial plica, Hoffa's fat pad condition, prepatella bursitis, apophysitis such as Osgood-Schlatter's disease or in rare cases bipartite patella
- Anterior knee pain could be referred from elsewhere such as the hip joint
- Conservative management and attention to anatomical predisponding factors are the foundations of treatment in most of the cases

Aetiology

Patellofemoral joint related pain

It is usually presents either early in adolescence as chondromalacia patellae or later on during the fourth or fifth decade of life. Females are affected more from the condition.

Pain is predominant anteriorly and aggravated by climbing stairs, walking on hills and after a prolonged sitting down position. Crepitus may be present too. Clinical examination reveals patella pain under compression. Small effusion may be present too. In adolescence tests to exclude patella instability should be added during the examination, such as the apprehension test.

Biomechanical factors associated with the condition include:

- Wide Q angle, which is above 15° in males and 18° in females
- High-placed hypermobile patella
- Small patella
- Shallow intercondylar femoral notch
- Valgus knee (genu valgus)
- Overpronated feet

In addition to the above, other factors associated with patella instability include:

- Increased femoral antiversion
- Tight lateral patella retinaculum
- Underdeveloped lateral femoral condyle
- Weak vastus medialis

Patellar tendinopathy (jumper's knee)

Biomechanical analysis suggests that the greatest tensile forces apply on the patellar tendon during the landing phase during running and jumping.

The condition could be considered an overuse injury with a gradual onset of pain at the lower patella pole. Later on localised swelling and crepitus may be present. In advanced stages, patellar tendinopathy causes significant morbidity and performance impairment.

Histology study shows degenerative changes of the tendon instead of any inflammation features.

Prepatella bursitis (other knee bursitis)

Bursitis could be caused by:

- Trauma
- Infection
- Rheumatoid arthritis
- Metabolic disorders
- Tumours

Pain and localised swelling are the presented features.

Synovial plica

Plicae are the remnants of the septa that were a soft tissue diaphragm present in the embryonic knee and absorbed at birth.

The commonest medial plica runs from the medial suprapatellar pouch to the infrapatellar fat pad. Following an injury of the anterior knee, the medial plica may become thick and tight, so it may impinge under the patella and the medial femoral condyle on knee flexion.

The athlete will complain of pain at the front of the knee, usually following a sport activity, sometimes worse in the morning.

Fat pad syndrome

Martial arts sports or multiple knee operations are associated with the condition.

Repetitive injury with the knee in extension, may lead to bleeding, scarring and proliferation of the infrapatellar fat pad. The fat pad could then impinge between the femur and the tibia on knee extension.

In severe cases, the progressive scarring and fibrosis of the fat pad may lead to functional shortening of the patella tendon, which will track down the patella and block the knee flexion (patella baja).

Osgood-Schlatter disease

It is a traction type injury of the apophysis at the attachment of the patellat tendon to the tibia tubercle. Sinding–Larsen–Johanssen disease is a similar condition affecting the attachment of the patellar tendon to the lower patella pole.

It develops in boys between 10 and 15 years old and in girls between 8 and 13 years old, usually at the beginning of their growth spurt.

Patients complain of pain pointed at the tibia tubercle that may appear enlarged. Pain always appear with or after sport activity and is relieved with rest. In severe cases, pain will be present even with daily activities.

Bipartite patella

Bipartite patella (in two parts) is present in 3% of the population, more common in males.

It is not a fracture and usually it is present at the superolateral patella corner with rounded edges.

Diagnosis will be made by other conditions exclusion. The pain presents locally with or after activity. The knee joint is normal on clinical examination.

Investigations

Patellofemoral joint X-rays also include a 'skyline' view and may detect a lateral patella tilt, a shallow intercondylar femur notch, a small patella, a highly placed patella, a bipartite patella or a separate patella edge 'fragment' in chronic patella instability.

History and clinical examination is usually accurate for the diagnosis of Osgood-Schlatter disease, otherwise, X-rays will show an enlarged sometimes fragmented tibia tubercle.

Ultrasound scan can be useful in patellar tendinopathy; also, in many cases treatment needling procedures may take place at the same time.

Magnetic resonance imaging scan could be arranged to detect fat pad or synovial plica conditions, to investigate a jumper's knee or to look into other knee pathologies.

Management
Patellofemoral joint related pain

The management of patellofemoral joint related pain will focus on:
- Quadriceps rehabilitation with an emphasis on the vastus medialis. In the normal knee there is a tendency of lateral shift of the patella on the femur, which is avoided by the vastus medialis contraction
- McConnell regime, involving taping of the patella so it can track correctly when the quadriceps muscle contracts
- Correction of the biomechanical factors, such as overpronated feet

Surgery is rarely indicated, in most cases is reserved for patella instability cases and may include a lateral retinaculum release, medial patellofemoral ligament (MPFL) reconstruction or trochleoplasty.

Patellar tendinopathy

The phases of treatment from the acute symptoms are as follow:
1. Rest and cryotherapy sessions (Low temperature chamber exposure)
2. Prolotherapy of the tendon or dry needling if there is a defect during an ultrasound scan
3. Shock wave therapy over the tendon attachment to the patella
4. Strengthening of quadriceps and stretching of hamstrings
5. Progress to eccentric training when pain subsides
6. Attention to orthotics and taping the patella
7. Plyometric sport specific training
8. Patella tendon heater or splint

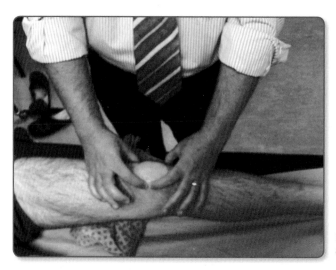

Figure 19 Patella instability apprehension test.

9. Surgery will apply in a few resistant cases. Debridement of the tendon is usually the choice

Synovial plica

The treatment includes rest, cryotherapy and local infiltration of a corticosteroid agent. If the symptoms persist, then arthroscopic excision of the plica is recommended.

Fat pad syndrome

Management is based on rest, soft tissue release and avoidance of repetitive knee extensions. Surgery in refractory cases involves arthroscopic debridement of the fat pad.

Osgood-Schlatter disease

The treatment is symptomatic and self-limiting. Activity is unrestricted unless pain is disabling. Osgood-Schlatter disease pads may protect the tubercle in contact sport

Return to sport

Return to sport will occur when the pain subsides and varies from 2 weeks to 3 months.

Conservative treatment in a jumper's knee will allow return to sport between 3 and 6 months, which will increase to 12–18 months following surgery.

Further reading

Collins NJ, Bisset LM, Crossley KM et al. Efficiency of nonsurgical interventions for anterior knee pain. Sports Med 2012; 42:31–49.

Knee – posterior cruciate ligament (PCL) injuries

Key points

- Look for the skin graze. Direct blow at the proximal part of the anterior tibia can cause an isolated posterior cruciate ligament (PCL) injury
- In many cases, the PCL will be damaged as part of an injury of the knee posterolateral corner (PLC)
- Football goalkeepers and motorcyclists are prone to this injury
- Conservative management is successful in many cases with an isolated PCL rupture

Aetiology

The PCL is an intra-articular but extra-synovial knee structure, whose course runs from the posterior of the tibia upwards and forwards where it becomes wide at the attachment in the medial femoral condyle.

The PCL function is to resist the femur slide over the tibia (keeps femur over the tibia), also to resist hyperextension of the knee joint.

The PCL could be damaged from a direct blow to the upper anterior tibia with a flexed knee, or during a fall on a flexed knee with the foot in plantar flexion. Severe hyperextension is another common mechanism of injury.

The athlete in acute cases will complain of intense pain in the posterior aspect of the knee. He will describe a characteristic 'pop' heard at the time of the injury. Effusion could be mild or not present at all because the PCL is an extrasynovial knee structure. The knee may be kept in a flexed position as a result of muscle spasm to avoid stretching of the posterior capsule. Pain and locking is common in young athletes with an avulsed fracture of the PCL tibial attachment.

In a chronic PCL rupture, the patient will present with pain or the feeling of 'giving way' when he runs downhill or downstairs. Later on, he will complain of pain and crepitus of the patellofemoral joint. When the PCL is torn, the extensor mechanism alone, including the patella, holds the tibia in a reduced position under the femur. The increased patellofemoral pressure will lead to pain and eventually to patella articular cartilage damage and early osteoarthritis.

On clinical examination, in acute injuries, look for the skin graze, or laceration or other skin lesions at the upper anterior surface of the tibia, indicating a direct applied force, suspicious for a PCL injury. During the examination an increased knee recurvatum, a posterior tibia sag and a positive posterior draw test may be observed.

Investigations

X-rays of the knee joint will exclude any bone injury, in particular an avulsion fracture of the PCL tibial attachment often seen in young athletes.

Magnetic resonance imaging scan will confirm the diagnosis, also it will provide information of any other knee soft tissue injury such as the posterolateral knee corner complex (PLC).

Management

In young patients with posterior cruciate ligament tibial avulsions beyond 2 mm, primary surgical reduction and fixation will produce excellent results. The leg will be immobilised in full extension for 6 weeks following surgery.

Treatment of an isolated PCL rupture is controversial. Conservative management is successful in most patients achieving a gradual return to sport with some alterations in training. Rehabilitation is concentrating to quadriceps strength, endurance and sport specific skills. Braces may be used during the early phases of rehabilitation or the first period of return to sport.

Some surgeons debate that after a PCL injury, major kinematic changes occur in the knee joint at the patellofemoral and medial knee compartment. Degenerative changes have been confirmed during arthroscopic surgery at the medial and patellofemoral

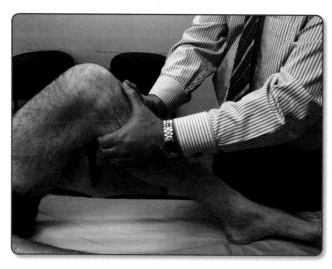

Figure 20 Posterior draw test.

joint (PFJ) compartments, in patients with chronic PCL rupture, even with 'normal' knee X-rays. Therefore, they recommend an early arthroscopic PCL reconstruction. However, the results have not been as good as in anterior cruciate ligament (ACL) surgery, providing at the best 70–80% of normal knee stability.

Surgical reconstruction will be recommended for patients with multiple ligament injuries or in cases of a patient with an isolated PCL rupture with continuous functional instability despite conservative treatment.

Return to sport

It will take 3–6 months to return to sport for an athlete suffered a PCL isolated rupture and was successfully treated by conservative means.

Surgery will prolong the recovery to sport, in most of the cases, beyond 12 months.

Further reading

Gill TJ, et al. Tibiofemoral and PFJ kinematics after reconstruction of an isolated PCL injury. Am J Sports Med 2009; 37:2377–2385.

Sohn DH, Balasubramanian S, Demetropoulos C et al. Biomechanical Verification that PCL reconstruction is unnecessary in the muscle stabilized knee. Orthopaedics 2010; 33:300.

Related topics of interest

•   Knee acute injuries (p. 189)

Knee injuries - acute

Key points

- Acute knee injuries may affect predominantly one structure, although more complex patterns with more than one structure involved may also exist
- Aseptic aspiration of a knee effusion is recommended, which will assist to confirm the presence of a haemarthrosis and provide some pain relief
- Accurate diagnosis of the Injury could be achieved using a methodological intact of history, clinical examination and appropriate diagnostic imaging

Aetiology

- The history intake will describe the mechanism of the injury as 'contact' following a direct challenge or 'noncontact' such as landing from a jump. Patients with an anterior cruciate ligament (ACL) rupture very often feel a 'pop' when the injury occurs.

The time and presence of an effusion is important to clarify a haemarthrosis, which usually appears very quickly following the injury and is highly associated with an ACL rupture.

Rupture of the extensor knee mechanism will result to loss of full active extension, the presence of an effusion and a palpable tendon defect. Quadriceps rupture usually occurs in patients over 40 years old of age.

Patella dislocation usually reduces spontaneously and physical examination will reveal movement reduced by discomfort and an effusion. History of recurrent patella instability may exist and Apprehension test is positive.

Meniscus injuries may produce mild knee swelling, localised joint line pain, also discomfort in the end of knee range of movement and during McMurray and Appley tests. An unstable meniscal fragment may cause locking or 'give way'. Displaced meniscal fragment will produced a 'locked knee', with loss of full extension.

Ligament injuries could be the result of both direct and indirect trauma. The extent of the injury in many cases does not correspond to the presented symptoms of pain or swelling. Posterior cruciate ligament (PCL) and Collateral ligament injuries may not produce knee swelling at all. A skin lesion, such as laceration or a graze, over the proximal tibia could often represent the direction of the applied force that has caused a PCL rupture.

Injuries of the articular bone cartilage could lead to a haemarthrosis; also, in the case of a loose fragment then mechanical symptoms of giving way and locking may appear.

Direct injury at the anterior knee could produce localised blood collection such as a traumatic Pre-patella bursa.

Investigations

X-rays of the knee joint, in an acute injury, should include an anteroposterior and a lateral view. Patella sky-line views, oblique views and tunnel view should be considered to assist with the diagnosis. Fractures could be ruled out with X-ray imaging. Avulsions of the cruciate ligaments from the tibia could be identified. Further other findings include a Segond fracture, which is associated with an ACL injury and a bony fragment next to the medial patella border in cases of recurrent patella dislocation. Loose bony fragments could be detected in cases of a 'locked knee'.

Magnetic resonance imaging scan is currently the investigation of choice to image soft tissue injuries such as meniscus and ligaments.

Arteriograms should be performed in cases of a knee dislocation, where vascular injury must be ruled out.

Ultrasound scans could have some issue in the management of acute knee injuries but they carry a less diagnostic value.

Nuclear Medicine scans and computed tomography scans are rarely necessary in the diagnosis and management of an acute knee injury.

Management

Aspiration of a knee haemarthrosis under sterile conditions is recommended to produce pain relief and assist with the rehabilitation in particular the range of knee movement and quadriceps contraction.

Acute Injuries that involve some form of trauma and serious trauma may require immediate first aid and stabilisation; even hospital treatment deepens on the severity of the injury. Bone fractures will be treated into a cast, or in cases of fragment displacement and dislocations, by surgical means.

Rupture of the extensor knee mechanism should be treated surgically with a primary repair. Following surgery immobilisation in extension for 6 weeks and rehabilitation will ensue.

Arthroscopy will be necessary for the 'locked knee' to address the displaced meniscus tear or to deal with a loose body.

Acute injuries to the muscle, tendons (strains) or ligaments (sprains) could be treated with the 'RISE' protocol:

R: rest the knee joint
I: ice application
C: compression of the injured part
E: elevation of the leg

The RICE protocol will apply for the first 48–72 h, then with the completion of the clinical examination and the diagnostic imaging a more definitely approach to the injury should be considered by surgery or nonoperative means.

Return to sport

Recovery to sport will vary, depending on the nature and severity of the injury, the management of the injury including surgery and the length of the rehabilitation programme. In addition, return to the prior the injury fitness level and 'get in shape' could take a significant period of time. Also, an important factor is to maintain a positive attitude and the will to succeed that will make the path to full recovery in a short a time as possible.

Further reading

Cabitza F, Ragone V, Arrigoni P et al. Management of knee injuries: consensus based indications from a large community of orthopaedic surgeons. Knee Surg Sports Traumatol Arthrosc 2013; 21(3):708-19.

Hagglund M, Walden M, Atroshi I. Preventing knee injuries in adolescent female football players. BMC Musculoskeletal Disord 2009; 10:75

Maffulli N, Longo UG, Gougoulias N et al. Long-term health outcomes of youth sports injuries. Br J Sports Med 2010; 44:21–25.

Maxillofacial injuries

Key points

- Maxillofacial injuries are common in contact sports
- Principles of ATLS applies
- Important to involve maxillofacial specialists as early as possible

Overview

Trauma to the head and neck can range from fairly superficial cuts and bruises to serious and life-threatening injuries, which can result in neurological complications as well as facial scarring and disfigurement. This Topic aims to summarise the assessment of the head and neck as well as highlighting common injuries and complications.

Assessment

- Secure airway
- Ensure breathing is adequate
- Control haemorrhage
- How was the injury sustained
- Did the patient lose consciousness
- Are visual disturbances (flashes, diplopia, blurred vision, pain) present
- Does the patient have clear-fluid discharge from the nose or ears
- Is the patient having difficulty opening or closing the mouth
- Does the patient feel like the teeth come together normally
- Areas of paraesthesia/anaesthesia
- Systematic maxillofacial examination:
  - Assess for asymmetry
  - Check zygomatic complex by looking down from behind the patient
  - Check for abrasions, swelling, haematoma and lacerations
  - Inspect open wounds for foreign bodies
  - Inspect the teeth for mobility, fracture or misalignment. If teeth are avulsed, make sure they are accounted for
  - Palpate for bony injury, crepitus and steps, especially around orbital rims and zygomatic arches
  - Eyes: inspect for the presence of exophthalmos or enophthalmos.

Visual acuity, abnormality of ocular movements and pupil size, shape and reaction to light, both direct and consensual

- Look for intraoral lacerations, ecchymosis or swelling. Bimanually palpate the mandible, and examine for signs of crepitus or mobility
- Place one hand on the anterior maxillary teeth and the other on the nasal bridge. Movement of only the teeth indicates a Le Fort I fracture. Movement at the nasal bridge indicates a Le Fort II or III fracture
- Gently manipulate each tooth individually for movement, pain, gingival and intraoral bleeding, tears or crepitus
- Palpate the mandibular condyle by placing a finger in the external auditory meatus while the patient opens and closes the mouth. Pain or lack of movement of the condyle indicates fracture
- Perform a thorough cranial nerve examination

Maxillary fracture

- Le Fort I fracture is a horizontal maxillary fracture across the inferior aspect of the maxilla and separates the alveolar process and hard palate from the rest of the maxilla. The fracture extends through the lower third of the septum and includes the floor of the maxillary sinus extending into the palatine bones and pterygoid plates. Clinically, the upper dental arch is mobile and bruising can be observed in the upper labial sulcus
- Le Fort II fracture is a pyramidal fracture extending from the nasal bone extending through the lacrimal bone downward through the zygomatico-maxillary suture continuing posteriorly and laterally through the maxilla
- Le Fort III fracture is a separation of all of the facial bones from the cranial base including fractures of the zygoma, maxilla and nasal bones. The fracture line extends posteriolaterally through ethmoid bones,

orbits and pterygo-maxillary suture into the spheno-palatine fossa

Pathology

- RTA
- Assault
- Sport injury

Clinical features

- Deranged occlusion of teeth, lengthening of mid face, panda eyes, epistaxis, CSF, palatal haematoma
- Gentle examination of the maxilla with thumb and index finger may reveal mobile maxilla

Investigation

- Plain X-ray facial view
- Computed tomography (CT) scan +/- 3D reconstruction

Treatment

- Surgery with open reduction internal fixation (ORIF)

Return to sport

- 4–6 weeks after operation

Zygomatic fractures

Zygomatico-maxillary complex fractures are usually a result of direct trauma. Fracture lines can involve the zygomatico-temporal, zygomatico-frontal and zygomatico-maxillary components of the zygomatic tripod. Fractures of the zygomatico-maxillary buttress usually extend through the infraorbital foramen and orbital floor. Concurrent ocular injuries are common.

Clinical features

- Bruising and/or swelling
- Epistaxis
- Flattened face over cheek bone zygomatic arch
- Subconjunctival haemorrhage
- Paraesthesia of infraorbital nerve
- Step or dimple over skin of zygomatic arch
- Step deformity at infraorbital margin on palpation
- Limited jaw opening or lateral movement

Investigation

- Plain X-rays (facial and submento vertex views)

Treatment

- Advice not to blow their nose if you suspect zygoma body fracture, may cause periorbital surgical emphysema
- Surgery with ORIF

Return to sport

- 4–6 weeks after operation

Frontal bone fractures

Usually a result of a blow to the forehead. The anterior and posterior wall of the frontal sinus may be involved.

Orbital fractures

Orbital floor fracture ('blow-out fracture') may occur in isolation or can be accompanied by a medial wall fracture. A teardrop-shaped herniation of the orbital contents into the maxillary sinus is a typical radiographic presentation. The incidence of ocular injury is high, but globe rupture is rare. Usually the globe of the affected eye has dropped and appears lower. The eye movements of the affected eye will be restricted due to the interference with the extra-ocular muscles.

Clinical features

- Pain
- Bruising around periorbital region
- Swelling
- Probtosis enophthalmos
- Paraesthesia of infra orbital nerve
- Diplopia
- Reduced or blurry vision

Investigation

- X-ray
- CT

Treatment

- Patients older than 20 can be reviewed in 10 days with a view to surgery (surgical debridement and repair with autogenous or synthetic graft)

- Under 20 need urgent CT and possible surgery to prevent permanent damage

Return to sport

- 2–3 weeks with non operative management
- 4–6 weeks with surgical treatment

Nasal bone fracture

See topic on ENT conditions in sports medicine.

Mandibular fractures

These can occur in multiple locations of the jaw and the condylar neck. Fractures often occur bilaterally at sites away from the site of direct trauma. Commonly these fractures are seen at weak spots that include areas of unerupted teeth or long roots. These areas are the angle of the mandible and the area of the lower canine. Parasymphyseal fractures often present with condylar neck fractures and are difficult to see radiographically.

Clinical findings of mandibular fractures include pain on jaw movement, and misalignment of the teeth on biting. Mobility of the segments, crepitus and steps can be palpated along the fracture sites.

Intra-oral oedema, haematoma, gingival bleeding or tears may be present. An anterior open bite can occur with bilateral condylar or angle fractures. Trauma to the inferior alveolar nerve may cause paraesthesia and/or anaesthesia of the lower lip and chin.

Clinical features

- Pain and tenderness over fractured area
- Swelling
- Bruising, ecchymosis, laceration, bleeding around individual tooth and sublingual haematoma
- Palpable step deformity over fractured bone
- Deranged occlusion
- Fractured or damaged teeth
- Paraesthesia of lower lip
- Sometimes bleeding from ear

Investigation

- X-ray (OPG and AP mandible views)

Treatment

- Surgery with ORIF
- Tooth extraction if needed
- Immobilisation

Return to sport

- 8–12 weeks post surgery

Jaw dislocation

The patient is unable to close their mouth. Although not especially painful the procedure for relocating the mandible will become progressively more difficult as time goes by.

Clinical features

- Anterior open bite
- Inability to close the mouth

Treatment

- The mandible is relocated by firm downward and backward pressure. This is applied to the external oblique ridges of the mandible, which are located on the buccal surfaces of the lower molar teeth.

Fractured teeth
Presentation

- Pain with extreme hot and cold sensitivity
- Bleeding from the gingivae and exposed pulps of teeth, often in conjunction with soft tissue injuries

Management

- So long as the patient does not have any other more serious injuries, the patient should be referred to a dentist as soon as possible, who should stabilise the teeth and explore the wounds for tooth and foreign body fragments before suturing takes place
- Soft tissue radiographs are very helpful in locating glass and other difficult to see fragments

Avulsed teeth
Presentation

- Teeth can either fracture or be completely avulsed from their sockets and the mouth

- This is most common in high-impact sports injuries with a blunt object and usually affects the upper front teeth

Management

- It is important for the tooth to be kept, gently cleaned, without touching the root surface and placed back into the patient's mouth, into the socket, or kept in saline or fresh milk
- If the tooth is placed back into the socket care must be taken to place the tooth the right way round. Often the contra-lateral tooth will provide a clue

- The patient should be referred to a dentist immediately for follow-up treatment

Soft tissue lacerations

Intra-oral lacerations can be sutured with either 4/0 silk on a curved cutting needle or resorbable materials, which will be resorbed within 7–10 days (e.g. vicryl rapide). In case of deep lacerations, the connective tissue can be sutured with a longer lasting resorbable material such as PDS or Vicryl.

Further reading

Boswell KA. Management of facial fractures. Emerg Med Clin North Am 2013; 31:539–551.

Elias H, Baur DA. Management of trauma to supporting dental structures. Dent Clin North Am 2009; 53(4):675–689.

Related topics of interest

Muscle properties relevant to sports and exercise

Key points

- Muscles produce most power at approximately one third of their maximum force production
- There are three quite distinct fibre types in skeletal muscle: slow twitch fibres (I or S), fast, fatigue-resistant fibres (IIa or FR) and fast-fatiguing fibres (IIb or FF)
- Different fuels are used for exercise of different durations: anaerobic glycolysis for up to 1–2 min; oxidation of carbohydrate and fat as the main fuel from about 1–2 min
- Motoneurons form the final path for neural motor control and a single motoneuron can innervate up to 3000 muscle fibres, all of the same fibre class

Muscle proteins

Muscle is the tissue whose properties dominate all others when we want to understand exercise and sports performance. The basics of muscle biochemistry, physiology and anatomy are well covered in medical and sports science texts, so this Topic will concentrate on aspects particularly relevant to sports and exercise. **Table 15** lists muscle key proteins. Myosin and actin interact through crossbridges (the myosin 'heads') to slide the myofilaments and produce force. These two proteins form 85% of total muscle protein. Troponin and tropomyosin are the key regulatory proteins that bind calcium, so revealing the myosin-binding site on actin and allowing contraction to proceed. Titin is a structural protein comprising 7% of all muscle protein. Its role is not fully defined, but in genetic trawls for performance-related genes, titin has emerged as a candidate. Alpha-actinin is in the list for the same reason, one form of the gene being much more common in sprinters than in endurance athletes.

Power – the force–velocity curve

Muscle is an unusual kind of motor. It generates maximum force at zero velocity. As it speeds up, force falls away, with a clear upper limit on contraction speed. Since power is the product of force and velocity, this means that there will be maximum power at some intermediate velocity since power will clearly be zero both when velocity is zero (isometric contraction) and when force is zero (at maximum velocity). In practice, maximum power occurs at approximately one third of maximum force, which also corresponds to about one third maximum velocity. This optimum is important. For example when cycling it is the reason gears can help. These allow us to adjust the force and velocity of limb movement, thus keeping our muscles operating close to the maximum power part of the force–velocity curve under different loads (e.g. varying uphill gradients).

Contraction and length changes: concentric, eccentric and isometric

Typically, a muscle is activated, generates force, and shortens. Such contractions are termed concentric. Sometimes the muscle contracts against a matching force with no external shortening. This is an isometric contraction. Finally, muscle may be stretched by an opposing force during activation.

Table 15 Muscle proteins	
Protein	Function
Myosin	Contractile protein, thick filaments
Actin	Contractile protein, thin filaments
Troponin	Regulatory protein, calcium binding
Tropomyosin	Interacts with troponin
Titin	Elasticity; filament alignment?
Alpha-actinin	Actin binding to Z-line

This may seem wasteful, but in fact muscles acting as 'brakes' play an important part in locomotion (e.g. on heel strike the ankle flexors contract while being stretched in order to limit ankle extension). Such contractions are called eccentric (meaning 'away from centre,' not crazy). In the previous section it was stated that during isometric contraction muscle force was at a maximum. However, this is not strictly true. It is true for muscle shortening. However, during eccentric contractions higher forces can be developed. This is due to the ability of crossbridges between myosin and actin to support higher passive loads than can be created during shortening. Interestingly, these additional forces do not need any extra ATP (adenosine triphosphate) splitting, so eccentric contractions are metabolically very efficient. However, there is a small price to be paid as eccentric contractions cause microdamage leading to diffuse onset muscle soreness.

Fibre types

Muscle contains three different types of fibre with different inherent speeds and hence power production (**Table 16**). Slow (Type I)

fibres predominate in postural muscles where prolonged contraction is the main requirement. These fibres have relatively slow kinetics, but lower basal energy requirements. The other two classes have faster kinetics. The fastest of them, the Type IIb, are specialised for short, explosive actions (e.g. jumping, throwing) and metabolise almost entirely anaerobically. Different individuals can have very different proportions of the three fibre types, largely through inheritance, but also partly by training (see Training). Perhaps unsurprisingly, sprinters and other athletes in explosive events have a large proportion of fast fibres while endurance athletes are just the opposite, with rather few fast fibres and lots of slow ones.

Muscle metabolism – different fuels for different durations of exercise

At the level of actin and myosin, the energy for force generation comes from hydrolysing ATP. However, cells do not store ATP, so a continuous resupply is necessary during contraction. Resupply comes from

Table 16 Fibre types in human skeletal muscle			
Property	Classification		
	Slow	Fast	
Type	I or S	IIa or FR	IIb or IIx or FF
Maximum velocity relative to Type I	1	4	9
Specific force relative to Type I	1	1.2	1.4
Power	Low	Intermediate	High
Energy utilisation	Low	Intermediate	High
Glycolytic capacity	Low	High	High
Oxidative capacity	High	Medium-high	Low
Myoglobin (giving red colour)	High	Intermediate	Low
Myosin heavy chain isoform*	MHC-I	MHC-IIA	MHC-IIX
Fatigue resistance	Hard to fatigue	Moderate-high fatigue resistance	Easily fatigued
Prevalence in limb muscle of sprinters	20-40%	60-80%	
Prevalence in limb muscle of endurance athletes	60-90%	10-30%	

* Note that there are also significant numbers of 'hybrid' fibres in most muscles with a mixture of MHC isoforms, either I-IIA or IIA-IIX

metabolism of carbohydrate and fatty acids. The fastest method is rapid breakdown of glucose to lactic acid – the process of glycolysis. However, even this takes several seconds to get going and ATP will last less time than this. ATP concentration must not be allowed to get too low as it has many important control functions in the cell. ATP levels are maintained on a second by second timescale by having another compound, creatine phosphate (CP, also called phosphocreatine), which acts as a short-term store. CP can rapidly phosphorylate ADP back to ATP, an action catalysed by the enzyme creatine kinase. This cycle of reactions is given in **Figure 21**.

Glycolysis is fast, but subject to two limits. Only carbohydrates can be used, so this supply depends on muscle glycogen. However, the real limit is set by the acidity of the end product, lactic acid. Lactic acid accumulates locally, lowering the muscle pH, and diffuses into the circulation where it is buffered by bicarbonate. However, this in turn pushes up blood carbon dioxide levels. This means that during continuous heavy exercise, e.g. distance running, another energy store must be available after about 30 s and must be supplying the bulk of energy by 2 min. This role is performed by oxidative phosphorylation of glucose. Glucose is broken down by the glycolytic pathway to pyruvate, then pyruvate enters the mitochondria where it combines with

coenzyme A (CoA) to form acetyl CoA. Acetyl CoA fuels the TCA cycle where the dinucleotides (NADH, FADH$_2$) and CO$_2$ are produced. The dinucleotides move to the electron transfer chain where large amounts of ATP are generated using oxygen as an additional reactant.

Oxidative phosphorylation of carbohydrate can provide enough energy for high levels of activity, but cannot generate ATP as fast as pure glycolysis. So exercise levels for durations of 2 min or more are well below the peak levels that can be maintained for 1 min or less. For very long duration exercise, exceeding about 1 h, carbohydrate stores start to be used up. Muscle glycogen will be mostly gone and only limited amounts of glucose can be removed from the blood if blood sugar is to remain at a high enough level for normal brain function. Some glucose is available from the breakdown of liver glycogen, thanks to glucose synthesis in the liver from lactate and other sources. However, this is not enough to support high levels of exercise.

The fuel for long-term exercise is fat. The body has massive stores of fat (too massive in many of us), enough to keep us running for days. However, it can only be converted into ATP relatively slowly, although training can increase this rate (see Training). Fats (triglycerides) are broken down to fatty acids and glycerol. The relatively small amounts of glycerol can be metabolised as carbohydrate. The larger amounts of fatty acids need to undergo beta-oxidation ending up as acetyl-CoA. Acetyl-CoA then follows the same path as for carbohydrate metabolism, generating ATP via the TCA cycle and the electron transfer chain. The way muscle fuel sources change with time during exercise is summarised in **Figure 22**.

The sequence of fuel use has some clear implications for sports performance. Firstly, it is clearly essential for endurance athletes (events lasting more than 60–90 min) to maximise carbohydrate availability. So 'carbohydrate loading', e.g. having some big pasta meals in the 72 h before an event, is useful. Also, drinking carbohydrate-containing fluids during an endurance event can contribute significantly to performance duration.

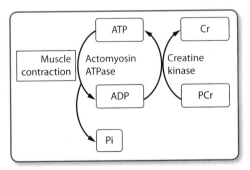

Figure 21 Reactions involved in maintaining ATP levels in the first few seconds of muscle contraction. ATP, adenosine triphosphate; ADP, adenosine diphosphate; Pi, inorganic phosphate; Cr, creatine; PCr, creatine phosphate

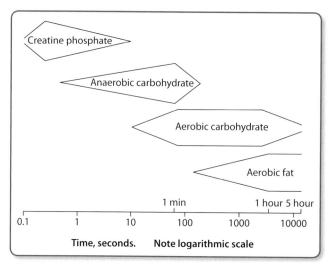

Figure 22 Succession of fuels used during exercise of different duration.

Motor control

Although the properties of muscle tissue itself are crucial, several aspects of performance in sport and exercise depend importantly on the way this tissue is controlled. The motor unit comprises the currency of motor control. This consists of a single alpha motor neurone plus all the muscle fibres to which it connects. A single motoneuron action potential will excite every one of these fibres, so the motor unit is the smallest control element available to the nervous system. A motor unit may consist of just ten fibres in muscles specialised for fine control (e.g. extra-ocular muscles), but is typically 1000–3000 in the large limb muscles. All the fibres in a single motor unit are of the same type (S, FR or FF).

The motoneurons themselves are the final path for central nervous system motor control. Voluntary contractions involve motor cortex and the pyramidal (corticospinal) tract. Involuntary reflex control involves mainly inputs from muscle and joint proprioceptors and from the vestibular system, crucial for maintaining basic postural stability. There is also important protective feedback from high threshold nociceptors in muscles and joints that limit muscle force (for example during eccentric contractions). Locomotion is largely involuntary, involving automatic circuits at brainstem and spinal levels.

Motor learning is an important part of all sports and exercise training. A key structure here is the cerebellum, but basal ganglia and cerebral cortex undoubtedly are also involved. Finally, a key issue in motor performance is motivation and 'psyching oneself up'. Here, cortical and limbic circuits must be crucial.

Further reading

Jones D, Round J, de Hann A. Skeletal muscle from molecules to movement. Edinburgh: Churchill Livingstone, 2004.

Mougios V. Exercise biochemistry. Champaign, IL: Human Kinetics, 2006.

Related topics of interest

Nerve entrapment syndromes – lower limb

Key points

- Can occur at any point from the distal extent of the nerve to the lumbar spine
- Presents with altered sensation and reduced muscle function based upon the location of the lesion

Aetiology

Nerve entrapment is broadly defined as the compression of a nerve as it passes through or by another anatomic structure. These are commonly appreciated and easily diagnosed in the upper limb but less so in the lower limb. Lower limb peripheral nerve compression may be frequently appreciated in some cases such as piriformis syndrome and Morton's neuroma; however, other causes of nerve compression may be overlooked.

Entrapment is most commonly occurs within a fibro-osseous tunnel or fascial opening and can be grouped into external or internal factors. External factors can include leg crossing, pressure from prolonged positioning, boots, casts or braces. Internal factors consist of:

- Trauma
- Muscle hypertrophy
- Local inflammation
- Adjacent compressive tumour
- Post traumatic haematoma
- Local ischaemia
- Prolapsed intervertebral disc
- Recent surgery

Additionally, medical conditions, e.g. chronic inflammation or fluid retention, can exacerbate entrapment. The presence of other disorders such as diabetes mellitus, rheumatoid arthritis, vitamin B deficiency and neurological disorders, e.g. multiple sclerosis and motor neurone disease, must also be considered.

In terms of localised compression the greatest mechanical deformation occurs in the superficial area of the nerve. Small veins are found within the substance of the nerve and although venular nerve flow can be compressed by pressures of 20–30 mmHg slowing conduction, in experimental studies pressures of 120–150 mmHg are required to block conduction.

The duration of compression is also a factor. Mild and brief compression produces an interruption in axoplasmic flow but no major structural change occurs and the nerve normalises following pressure release. In cases of severe acute compression on microscopy, there may be invagination of the myelin sheath. With chronic compression, segmental demyelination is seen resulting in slowing of the action potentials and distal Wallerian degeneration.

Three clinical stages of nerve compression have been described. These tend to be worsened by positional oedema typically during sleep:

Stage 1: Occurring nocturnally with intermittent paraesthesia and sensory deficits.

Stage 2: Occurs with continued compression with more consistent symptoms that fail to resolve during the day.

Stage 3: Occurs with altered nerve microcirculation and oedema leading to morphologic changes such a segmental demyelination. Clinically, these patients have constant pain, which does not disappear even if pressure is relieved.

Specific nerve entrapments

Piriformis syndrome consists of entrapment of the sciatic nerve at the level of the greater sciatic notch by the piriformis muscle. Iliacus syndrome typically involves entrapment of the femoral nerve at the level of the pelvis and groin. The femoral nerve beneath the inguinal ligament through a rigid tunnel called the lacuna musculorum. The obturator nerve may commonly be trapped where it exits the pelvis at the obturator foramen. Lateral femoral cutaneous nerve entrapment can occur either as the nerves passes beneath the inguinal ligament or pierces the fascia lata.

Proximal tibial nerve entrapment typically occurs within the popliteal fossa as it passes over the Popliteus muscle and passes under the arch of soleus. Common peroneal nerve compression occurs due to external compression from a brace and compression due to hypertrophy of the short head of biceps femoris and the lateral head of gastrocnemius. More distally the superficial peroneal nerve can become entrapped as it exits the deep fascia of the peroneal/lateral compartment. Distal compression of the deep personal nerve can occur as the nerve passes beneath the superior and the Y shaped inferior extensor retinacula and beneath the extensor hallucis longus tendon at the level of the talonavicular joint. Compression theoretically occurs within a tunnel beneath the extensor hallucis brevis or due to osteophyte formation, an os intermetatarseum in the proximal first tarsometatarsal space and tight fitting sports shoes. An unusual cause of nerve compression occurs when runners tie a key beneath their laces. Tarsal tunnel syndrome occurs due to nerve compression beneath either the flexor retinaculum more commonly affecting the tibial nerve on the posteromedial side of the ankle and the deep peroneal nerve, termed anterior tarsal tunnel syndrome as discussed in the previous paragraph.

Other than those discussed above nerve compressions in the foot are complex and difficult to diagnose. Baxter's neuropathy is considered to be compression of the inferior calcaneal nerve formed from a branch of the lateral plantar nerve. Jogger's foot consists of medial plantar nerve; compression can occur in the narrow space between flexor digitorum longus (FDL) and flexor hallucis longus (FHL). Sural neuropathy can lead to paraesthesia on the outer aspect of the foot where the nerve bifurcates into medial and lateral terminal branches. Compression can occur by a thickened fibrous arch of superficial sural aponeurosis at the junction of the tendo Achilles and the gastrocnemius. This can develop following an ankle inversion injury. Morton's neuroma is a common pathology in which the digital nerves become chronically entrapped beneath the intermetatarsal ligament.

Clinical features

Careful history taking is required in all areas of sports medicine and this is particularly so for nerve entrapment. Patients may report sensory changes such as dysaesthesias and subjective alterations in function and strength. Examination must be performed based upon the awareness of both dermatomal and peripheral nerve distribution and precise motor testing for strength, e.g. testing ankle dorsiflexor tibialis anterior with the foot in inversion to isolate tibialis anterior from the peroneal tendons. Precise history taking and clinical examination are paramount in the assessment of peripheral nerve entrapment.

In piriformis syndrome, pain is aggravated by sitting, squatting and walking, and relieved by lying supine. Local tenderness over the piriformis muscle may be found. Peripheral nerve deficits are rarely found. The saphenous nerve entrapment leads to decreased sensation and paraesthesia on the medial aspect of the leg. In lateral femoral cutaneous nerve compression patients report a burning pain and numbness and tingling on the lateral aspect of the thigh and local pressure over the nerve aggravates the symptoms. Proximal tibial nerve compression results in weakness of plantar and invertor musculature with sensory loss below the knee and in the sural nerve distribution.

The common peroneal nerve compression results in dysaesthesias of the lateral aspect of the leg and foot together with a foot drop resulting in a slapping gait. The dysaesthesias may be exacerbated by plantar flexion and inversion of the ankle. With isolated superficial peroneal nerve compression the pain may be exacerbated with activity and on careful examination there is sparing of the first web space. Local examination may reveal a palpable fascial defect and a muscle hernia.

Other than those discussed above nerve compressions in the foot are complex and difficult to diagnose. Baxter's neuropathy compression of the inferior calcaneal nerve can present with numbness to the lateral side of the foot. In Jogger's foot, a Tinel's sign behind the medial malleolus can indicate entrapment. Sural neuropathy can lead to paraesthesia on the outer aspect of the foot. Morton's neuroma features intermetatarsal pain and numbness radiating into the toes alleviated by removing the shoe. Symptoms may be exacerbated by shoes tight around the forefoot and high heels. These conditions are typical of a Mulder's click: compression of the transverse metatarsal arch elevates the neuroma, which may then be palpated in the web space, and Greiss sign: forced toe extension pulls the neuroma beneath the metatarsal heads and tenderness is found on palpation.

Specific clinical tests

Provocational tests can be performed by either placing the nerve under relative tension, e.g. by plantar flexing, or by inverting the ankle for sural and superficial peroneal nerves. With continued positioning, symptoms may be exacerbated in the nerve distribution. Greiss' test is a provocation test. By dorsiflexing the toes, the digital nerves tighten and are more susceptible to local pressure on palpation of the plantar side of the web space in case of Morton's neuroma.

Tinel's sign was described for nerve regeneration. This consists of percussion over the course of the nerve from distal to proximal. Dysaesthesia may be produced at the site of the compression. The sensitivity of the test varies according to the location of the nerve assessed. The use of a test injection of local anaesthesia at a likely site of compression may alleviate symptoms aiding the diagnosis. The injection can be repeated with therapeutic steroid.

Investigations

The role of neurophysiological testing

Testing may be particularly useful in distinguishing peroneal nerve lesions together with excluding proximal involvement, e.g. the L5 nerve root. The discriminating factor is the innervation of the short head of biceps femoris for which clinical assessment is difficult. Both sensory and motor conduction studies are required for diagnosis. A superficial peroneal sensory nerve action potential is tested and a loss of amplitude would imply axonal loss, affecting the nerve distal to the root ganglion. Motor conduction studies can be conducted with an electrode placed in the extensor digitorum brevis muscle. Stimulation is then provided both proximal and distal to the fibular head this check the conduction flow past the fibular neck the commonest site of injury. A conduction velocity of less than 40 m/s is considered to be abnormal.

The role of imaging

Imaging is useful for the determination of causes of compression. Plain radiographs are specific for bone tumours, whereas magnetic resonance imaging can reveal perineural inflammation, muscular hypertrophy and soft tissue tumours and other forms of compression.

Management

Stage 1 conditions may be managed nonoperatively with physiotherapy consisting of tendon and nerve gliding exercises, brace wear and pain and inflammation control. The use of systemic nerve modulators such as gabapentin and tricyclic antidepressants can be considered. Stages 2 and 3 typically require surgical decompression.

Further reading

Beltran LS, Bencardino J, Ghazikhanian V, et al. Entrapment neuropathies III: lower limb. Semin Musculoskeletal Radiol 2010; 14:501–511.

Flanagan RM, Digiovanni BF. Peripheral nerve entrapments of the lower leg, ankle and foot. Foot Ankle Clin 2011; 16:255–274.

Related topics of interest

Nerve entrapment syndromes – upper limb

Key points

- Nerve entrapment related to a sporting activity and causing pain and weakness is regularly seen in the sports clinic
- Proximal nerves are at risk in activities involving repetitive overhead movements
- Distal syndromes are related to a variety of sports, particularly those involving throwing or pitching
- Treatment is generally conservative (rest, physical therapy), but surgical treatments are available if the condition is serious and persisting

Introduction

The general features of entrapment syndromes have been covered in Topics on nerve injury and on lower limb entrapments, so this Topic will concentrate on specific upper limb conditions. Note also that brachial plexus injury has been covered in the Topic on cervical spine – nerve root/brachial plexus injuries.

Clinical features and sports relatedness of specific syndromes

A summary of the relevant anatomy and of any relations to particular sports is given in **Table 17.**

Suprascapular nerve

Entrapment of the suprascapular nerve causes weakness in external rotation and abduction of the shoulder. It can be a simple entrapment, often associated with

Table 17 Anatomy and sports relatedness of entrapments of the main upper limb nerves				
Nerve	Skin innervation area	Muscles innervated and affected by syndrome	Tunnel	Sports or movements particularly associated with syndrome
Suprascapular	Posterior shoulder	Supraspinatus, infraspinatus	Suprascapular notch or Spinoglenoid notch	Overhead throwing, tennis serve, volleyball serve
Axillary	Upper part of upper arm	Teres minor, deltoid	Quadrilateral space	Throwing, also crutch use
Median	Palmar hand, digits 1–4	Most forearm flexors. Some intrinsic hand muscles	Within pronator muscle	None
			Carpal	Wheelchair sports
Ulnar	Medial hand, digits 4–5	Some forearm flexors; intrinsic hand muscle	Cubital	Throwing
			Guyon's canal	Cycling; wheelchair sports
Posterior interosseous (deep branch of radial)	None	Forearm extensors	Arcade of Frohse (between superficial and deep parts of Supinator muscle)	None

Nerve injury – overview

Key points

- Neurapraxia is an injury that produces only functional nerve block with full recovery
- Axonotmesis and Neurotmesis are injuries where nerve degeneration occurs
- Good recovery can be expected from axonotmesis, but neurotmesis, where nerves are wholly or partly severed, has poor recovery
- A good knowledge of peripheral nerve anatomy and innervation patterns is essential in interpreting sensory loss and muscle weakness in terms of specific nerve injury
- A range of investigations is needed, including sensory testing, nerve conduction studies and imaging
- Return to full sports participation may be problematic, especially for conditions where the normal sports activity has provoked the injury (e.g. most entrapment syndromes)

Introduction

Nerve injuries are relatively uncommon, but when they occur present particular challenges and carry the risk of significant morbidity. Injury may be due to direct trauma, or to severe stretching or to repetitive movements leading to entrapment syndromes.

A perspective

Consider the problem of wiring up all the sensors and motor units in a highly mobile limb. Wiring must run internally and be highly flexible. It cannot be protected in rigid conduits. During normal limb movement the wires (nerves) must be able to stretch, by as much as 4%, and to slide past adjacent tendons. Sliding must be very low friction as movements such as throwing occur at high velocity.

But our wires – the nerve axons – are fragile and effectively not extensible. The trick is for them to follow a wavy course within the nerve trunk. As the nerve stretches, they straighten; conduction is not impaired. At least 6% stretch is possible without irreversible conduction changes – so normal movements are safely within this value. Nerves actually fail, i.e. fascicles break, at about 18% strain.

Repetitive stretching within the range that does not produce axonal breakdown is normally fine. However, any local inflammation can cause irritation of the nerve trunk. This in turn can cause spontaneous firing, interpreted in the brain as paraesthesia or pain. Irritation combined with pressure can eventually lead to axonal damage, triggering neuropathic pain (sensory fibres) and motor weakness (motor fibres). Finally, our 'wires' need fuel. They are not passive conductors, but depend on energy-requiring action potentials for signalling. Prolonged pressure can interfere with the blood supply and cause ischaemic conduction block. The signs will be numbness, motor weakness and perhaps pain.

Add to the mix that sport often involves fast, large range, repetitive movements for which the body has not evolved. Have we been throwing spears long enough for our peripheral nerve anatomy to have adapted? Probably not. So the surprise is that we see so few neurological problems.

Classification of injuries

Neurapraxia

It is a temporary interruption of conduction without loss of axonal continuity, i.e. there is functional block of nerve conduction. There are sensory and motor problems distal to the site of injury. All nerve connective tissues are intact and there is no degeneration. Full recovery occurs, but may take 2 weeks. There are often strong paraesthesias (e.g. projected burning or stinging in brachial plexus neurapraxia) following the injuring event.

Axonotmesis

It involves loss of the continuity of the axon and its covering of myelin, but preservation of the main connective tissue framework of the nerve. There are sensory and motor deficits distal to the site of lesion. Degeneration occurs distal to the site of injury and no nerve conduction occurs from 3 to 4 days after injury. Axonal regeneration occurs and recovery is possible without surgical treatment.

Neurotmesis

It is a severance or disruption of the nerve. Neurotmesis may be partial or complete. As with axonotmesis there is degeneration distal to the site of injury and nerve conduction is lost distal to the lesion after 3–4 days. Sensory and motor problems are severe.

Response of nerves to injury

Acute injury will produce abnormal high-frequency firing. Hence, the sensations from banging one's 'funny bone' – actually the ulnar nerve in the cubital fossa. Such firing can continue for some time and may be felt as stinging and burning, as in brachial plexus injury.

If axonal continuity is lost, then two processes occur. The distal part of the neurone, now deprived of essential nutrients transported from the cell body in the sensory ganglion or the ventral horn, degenerates. The proximal stump, however, starts to grow back at 1–4 mm per day.

In the absence of disruption to the connective tissue matrix of the nerve, this regrowth can be quite successful in reconnecting peripheral targets. During regrowth, growth cones and adjacent new axons show quite high mechanical sensitivity. This proves useful clinically. Lightly tapping along the course of a nerve in the region of regrowing axons will elicit tingling sensations projected to the distal innervation zone of the nerve (Tinel's sign).

If there is physical damage to the nerve, then regeneration is difficult. Regenerating axons may become trapped in scar tissues and form a painful neuroma. If a route is clear and fibres can follow the remains of the old nerve path, they will seldom make accurate reconnections. Hence, the prognosis from severe nerve injury is poor, although with nerve grafting and other reconstructive surgery, enough recovery can occur that activities of daily living are possible. However, return to high-performance sport is unlikely.

Clinical features

Key difference between nerve injuries and muscle or joint injuries is that signs may be most obvious a long way from the site of injury. So the knowledge of peripheral nerve anatomy is useful in interpreting signs. One needs to know which skin areas and which muscles are innervated by the main limb nerves.

Much can be learnt with the humble von Frey hair (usually, these days a bit of nylon fishing line about 3 cm long stuck to a handle). Sensory loss may be apparent on testing. Remember that areas of substantial sensory loss on the skin of the arm or leg may not have been noticed by the patient (although any sensory loss on the palmar skin of the hand is always noticed). Pain will often be present, as may allodynia (pain from light tactile stimuli). Regions feeling painful, or areas of allodynia do not, unfortunately, map at all precisely to individual nerve territories. Muscle weakness needs to be assessed to see if any pattern of weakness fits with the innervation pattern of specific nerves.

Investigations

Imaging

Imaging can be useful in several ways. It can aid in the tricky business of differential diagnosis, checking whether pain and tenderness are due to a musculoskeletal injury. Some nerve entrapments are due to cysts, and these will be clear with imaging. Both magnetic resonance imaging and ultrasound can be useful for these investigations. Ultrasound has particular value in looking at nerve entrapments, as it is possible to observe patterns of nerve movement during provoking limb movements.

Specific provocation tests

There are a number of tests that can help with diagnosis. Tinel's sign has already been mentioned, for assessing level of regeneration. Various stretching manoeuvres have also been developed to look for problems with particular nerves. Phalens test, a maintained (30–60 s) maximum wrist flexion, is used to diagnose carpal tunnel syndrome, as it stresses the median nerve in the carpal tunnel. Straight leg raises can provoke sciatic pain in some lower leg conditions. Various upper limb tension tests can ascertain whether the median, and perhaps other, upper limb nerves are hypersensitive, and can sometimes usefully reproduce symptoms.

Electrophysiological investigations

Nerve conduction studies can confirm diagnoses and give a quantitative estimate of severity. Electromyographic (EMG) studies can show early signs of denervation (fibrillation potentials and positive sharp waves).

Management

Neurapraxia

Should be fine with rest. If not, then it is not neurapraxia.

Axonotmesis; neurotmesis

These are usually associated with trauma and nonnerve injuries will need to be dealt with first (e.g. fractures). After other injuries are stabilised, it is important to assess the degree of sensory and motor loss. It can be difficult to distinguish axonotmesis and neurotmesis. This will become clear if regeneration is moving distal as this will only happen with axonotmesis. However, this may take weeks to be apparent. It may be possible with imaging to decide quite early on whether there is serious nerve disruption, indicative of neurotmesis. This is useful as early surgical intervention improves the outcome for nerve repair.

Entrapment syndromes

These are associated with pressure or overuse and need a different approach to that for neurotmesis or axonotmesis. In a sports context, we can expect to see these conditions early, as pain or weakness will interfere with training and/or performance. So there should be minimal sensory loss or muscle weakness, although there may be a lot of pain. An investigation to find the likely provoking activity is crucial, followed by a period of rest from that activity. What is ultimately required is a strategy for continuing in sport. This may require changes in technique, or changes in the time pattern of training (more breaks, for example). But in practice it may be very difficult, when entrapment symptoms appear, to continue the sporting activity at the pre-entrapment level. Finally, when recovery is limited following rest and physical therapy, some entrapment syndromes can be improved with surgical release procedures.

Further reading

Birch R. Surgical disorders of the peripheral nerves. London: Springer, 2011:1–645.

Neal S, Fields KB. Peripheral nerve entrapment and injury in the upper extremity. Am Fam Physician 2010; 81:147–155.

Related topics of interest

Osteoarthritis and sport

Key points

- Association between sports and osteoarthritis (OA) is difficult to study, nevertheless there appears to be a definite link between sports and OA in abnormal or injured joint
- Participation in sports that involve high impact or torsional loading of the joint, even in absence of joint abnormality or injury, is also shown to increase risk of OA
- Possible deleterious influence of sport may not outweigh the many benefits of exercise in most individuals

Benefits of exercise to health are numerous and well documented. Providing entertainment, enjoyment and satisfaction, sporting activity is associated with improved physiological well-being and reduced incidence of osteoporosis and cardiovascular diseases. Furthermore, sport provides a profession for many athletes.

OA is the commonest disease of the joints and is reported to affect up to 25% of the people over the age of 55 in the western society. As well as having the potential to impose a great amount of suffering for the individual patients, it is a huge burden to the society. It is also a growing problem because it is associated with aging and people are living longer.

The impact of OA is so great that the question' is sporting activity associated with OA?' is one that all sports clinicians will be faced with.

This Topic will highlight some of the difficulties with answering this question, and aims to provide some ammunition for sports clinicians when they are advising athletes on sports participation and risks of OA.

Difficulties with studies on sports and OA

The influence of sporting activities on the development of OA is complex to investigate because of the following reasons:

1. Sports cover a huge range of activities that range from walking to activities that subject joints to tremendous forces such as American football
2. How is OA diagnosed, e.g. by clinical or radiological assessment
3. Is any influence of sporting activity on development of OA a direct influence or as a result of an injury that has occurred as a consequence of the sport
4. If sport is linked with OA, does this association outweigh the numerous positive influences of sports in physiological and psychological well being

The link

Studies that have investigated the link between OA and sports suggest that the risks of joint degeneration is dependent on two important factors:

- Joint abnormalities or history of joint injury
- Type/level of sporting activity

Joint abnormality or history of joint injury

Presence of joint abnormality or history of joint injuries is the most crucial risk factor for developing OA. There are a significant number of studies that suggest that all those joints that are unstable, malaligned, incongruent, dysplastic, have damaged cartilage, have sustained ligamentous damage and have abnormal proprioception are at increased risk of developing OA. Those athletes with muscle weakness and neurological deficits are also at higher risks for developing degenerative joint changes. It appears that in presence of such abnormities and injuries, participation in even low impact sporting activity leads to increased risks for developing degenerative changes. This is thought to be due to sporting activity preventing optimal healing of the injured joint and causing further damage. It has been suggested that continued joint loading in the immediate period following joint injury may interfere with chondrocyte restoration of their matrix. Similarly, incongruency of the joint caused by different mechanisms leads to amplified shear forces on some parts of the cartilage and therefore increasing the risks of developing degenerative changes.

Level of impact and torsional loading

In normal joints, those that have none of the above-mentioned abnormalities and which are not injured, level of impact and torsional loading becomes a very important factor. There are a number of studies that have shown that, in normal joints, although repetitive running may lead to altered articular cartilage composition and osteophyte formation, it does not lead to joint degeneration. Sporting activities that involve intense impact and torsional activities on the other hand, do lead to increased risks of OA. These sports include American football, rugby, single tennis, squash, soccer and basketball. The mechanism for this increased risk of OA in high impact and torsional loading sports in apparently normal joints

may be presence of unrecognised joint injury and damage.

Therefore, essentially, the athletes can be divided into four groups:
1. Athletes with joint abnormalities/injuries who participate in sports, which subject the joint to minimal or low impact and torsional loading
2. Athletes with joint abnormalities/injuries who participate in sports, which subject the joint relatively high impact and torsional loading
3. Athletes with no joint abnormalities/injuries who participate in sports, which subject the joint to minimal or low impact and torsional loadin
4. Athletes with no joint abnormalities/injuries who participate in sports, which subject the joint to relatively high impact and torsional loading

Table 18 Summarises the risk of OA in these four groups of athletes.

Table 18 Risk of osteoarthritis in different type of activities		
	Low impact/torsional loading	High impact/torsional loading
Normal joint/ no injury	Does not usually lead to increased risk of OA	Increased risk of OA
Abnormal joint/injury	Increased risk of OA	Increased risk of OA

Further reading

Buckwalter JA, Martin JA. Sports and osteoarthritis. Curr Opin Rheumatol 2004; 16:634–639.
Conaghan PG. Update on osteoarthritis part 1: current concepts and the relation to exercise. Br J Sports Med 2002; 36:330–331.

Lievense AM, Bierma-Zeinstra SMA, Verhagen AP, et al. Influence of sporting activities on the development of osteoarthritis of the hip: a systemic review. Arthritis Rheum 2003; 49:228–236.

Related topics of interest

• Prevention of sport injuries (p. 236)

Paediatrics – osteochondrosis (osteochondritis)

Key points

- An overuse injury during childhood
- Usually self-limiting
- Commonly traction related

Introduction

Osteochondrosis are disorders of the development of the ossification centres in the skeletally immature that eventually undergo recalcification. The aetiology is unknown but genetic, mechanical (repetitive trauma or overuse), vascular and hormonal associations have been suggested. They represent the most common group of overuse injuries during childhood.

Osgood–Schlatter disease

This is the commonest of these disorders, more often seen in boys around 12 years of age. The repetitive traction by the patellar tendon applied to the tibial tuberosity (anterior surface of apophysis) can cause a partial avulsion of the secondary ossification centre followed by a repetitive cycle of healing and bone accumulation. This occurs without involvement of the tibial physis. The ossification centre expands proximally and blends with the tibial epiphysis by age 17. If the intervening gap fills with fibrous tissue rather than bone, it can progress to a painful nonunion.

The diagnosis is clinical. Pain around the tuberosity occurs during or after an activity, especially jumping. There is localised tenderness of the tibial tuberosity. In older adolescents separated ossicles in the patella tendon substance, adjacent to the tubercle, may be radiographically evident. Differential diagnosis includes tibial tubercle avulsion, patella tendonitis (jumper's knee) and Sinding-Larsen-Johansson disease.

Treatment is nonoperative except very rarely after skeletal maturity when a painful ossicle may need excising. Explanation of the pathology and natural history assists management. Complete rest does not bring resolution of symptoms, modification of activity and physiotherapy usually control symptoms until spontaneous resolution. Physiotherapy programmes include quadriceps and hamstring strengthening, stretching and balancing. Concentric contractions followed by eccentric exercises and progressive loading aids return to sport. Ice applications and nonsteroidal anti-inflammatory drugs may be helpful after activity. Corticosteroid injections are not indicated. In severe cases of an avulsion, complete rest between 3 and 4 weeks from activity is necessary. Plaster-casts or rigid braces are rarely required. Complete resolution occurs in 1–2 years in most patients.

Sinding-Larsen–Johansson disease

This is caused by persistent repetitive traction at the cartilaginous junction of inferior pole of the patella and the proximal patella tendon (traction apophysitis). This is seen in athletic teenagers complaining of activity-related anterior knee pain, which is aggravated by jumping. In some cases, a separate ossicle from the inferior patella may develop. Occasionally, similar symptoms occur at the superior pole of the patella and the quadriceps tendon. Prognosis and management is similar to Osgood–Schlatter disease, and can take up to a year to settle.

Sever's disease

This is a traction apophysitis of the calcaneum in young athletes between 8 and 15 years old. The repetitive plantar flexion and impact just prior to the fusion of the calcaneal apophysis secondary to the Achilles tensile forces may cause inflammation and microfractures.

Pain usually occurs at the end of or after sport and the patient may limp or toe walk. There is tenderness at the site of Achilles tendon insertion at the calcaneal apophysis. There may be gastrocnemius muscle tightness with reduced ankle dorsiflexion with the knee extended.

The diagnosis is clinical with radiographs only to exclude other pathologies. Radiological appearance of calcaneal apophyseal fragmentation is normal.

Treatment is conservative with attention to footwear: well fitted with firm heel counter and possibly orthotic support. Physiotherapy with gastrocnemius stretching and ankle dorsiflexor strengthening, activity modification and anti-inflammatories are the mainstay of treatment until spontaneous resolution.

The differential diagnosis includes seronegative arthropathies, Achilles tendonopathy and Brodie's abscess.

Navicular bone apophysitis

This is also a traction apophysitis secondary to the tibialis posterior tendon's pull at the medial and inferior aspect of the navicular bone, usually affecting the accessory navicular bone. This condition usually presents in adolescence, and is self-limiting.

Kohler's bone disease

This is an osteochondrosis of the navicula, presenting with spontaneous pain and limp in 3–9 years old children, more commonly boys. This is a clinical diagnosis with possible swelling and localised navicular tenderness. Radiographs may show sclerosis, flattening and fragmentation of the navicula. Treatment is nonoperative, with modification of activity and anti-inflammatory drugs. Cast immobilisation may be helpful in young children. Usually resolves over a number of months.

Freiberg's disease

This is a painful forefoot condition affecting the epiphysis of the second and third metatarsal heads. It is more common in adolescent girls, especially ballet dancers, but can affect adults with degeneration of the metatarsophalangeal joint. Symptoms include pain and swelling over the metatarsal heads, which is exacerbated by weight bearing and activity. Condition is bilateral in less than 10% of cases.

Plain radiographs may confirm deformity, sclerosis and fragmentation of the epiphysis with an often flat articular surface of the metatarsal head.

If the diagnosis was made prior to growth plate closure, the deformity may be reduced by activity modification, stiff-soled, flat-heeled shoes and a rocker sole to off-load the metatarsal heads. Surgical management may be indicated in adults.

Osteochondritis dissecans

The aetiology is unknown, but repetitive trauma may be contributory. It is a misnomer as there is no inflammatory component to it and is not really considered an osteochondrosis. It most commonly affects the knee but can occur in other joints. This condition is beyond the scope of this topic (see Paediatrics - sports injuries).

Scheuermann's disease

This condition affects vertebral end plates, where increased compression forces, anteriorly, can lead to angular deformity and kyphosis.

The aetiology is unknown. Patients present with thoracic back pain, stiffness and kyphosis usually around 12 years of age.

Radiographs confirm vertebral end-plate irregularity, with anterior wedging of at least 5° in at least three adjacent vertebrae.

Repetitive flexion activities should be reduced. Physiotherapy programmes will minimise tightness of fascia and strengthen abdominal and spinal muscles. Braces may be used in more severe progressive kyphosis. Operative intervention is reserved for the skeletally mature with severe curvature, pain, rigidity and unacceptable appearance.

Humeral medial epicondylar apophysitis

This affects throwing athletes, such as pitchers and bowlers. Repetitive throwing leads to stress and traction across the medial epicondylar growth plate. Symptoms include medial elbow pain that may be severe in avulsion fractures. Radiographs may reveal medial epicondylar fragmentation.

Prevention of avulsion fracture is best with activity modification. Anti-inflammatory drugs and ice relieve symptoms. Widely displaced avulsion fractures should be reduced and fixed.

Panner's disease

This is abnormal ossification, necrosis and degeneration of the capitellum with lateral elbow pain in children younger than 10. Radiographs may reveal fragmentation and fissuring of the capitellum. It is self-limiting and usually resolves with conservative measures.

Iselin's apophysitis

This is a traction apophysitis occurring at the tuberosity of the fifth metatarsal. The apophysis appears between 9 and 14 and is located within the insertion of peroneus brevis tendon. Presentation is usually insidious onset of pain over the lateral foot, with history of overuse activities and no trauma. It is commonly misdiagnosed as an avulsion fracture on X-ray. Treatment is conservative, with activity modification and stretching of the peroneal muscles. This is effective until skeletal maturity.

Perthe's disease

This condition involves an avascular event of the femoral capital epiphysis in susceptible individuals, usually boys, between the ages of 4 and 10. It is not strictly an overuse injury or an osteochondrosis, but occurs in more active children and should be recognised.

Table 19* Summary of different conditions			
Condition	Presentation	X-ray findings	Treatment
Osgood–Schlatter disease	Activity-related pain and swelling over tibial tuberosity	May be normal. Avulsion of tibial tubercle may be evident	Activity modification, ice and NSAIDs
Sinding-Larsen–Johansson	Activity-related inferior patellar pole pain and tenderness	Calcification at the inferior pole of patella and within the tendon	Activity modification, ice and NSAIDs
Sever's disease	Heel pain and at insertion of the Achilles tendon with swelling associated with plantar-flexion	Fragmentation and sclerosis of the calcaneal apophysis are normal findings. Diagnosis is clinical. Radiographs and USS are only helpful to exclude other pathology	Activity modification, well-fitted shoes with heel support/cups, calf stretching and NSAIDs
Navicular bone apophysitis	Pain at the medial aspect of the midfoot	Accessory navicular bone at medial/inferior aspect of the navicular bone	Activity modification, well-fitted shoes with orthotic support and NSAIDs
Kohler's disease	Midfoot pain or swelling and a limp with no previous trauma	Navicular sclerosis, flattening and fragmentation	Activity modification, well-fitted shoes with orthotic support/ immobilisation to speed recovery and NSAIDs

Continued

Condition	Presentation	X-ray findings	Treatment
Freiberg's disease	Pain and swelling over the metatarsal heads, exacerbated by weight-bearing and activity	Sclerosis and flattening of second and third metatarsal heads	Activity modification, metatarsal neck supports and shoes without a heel to assist off-loading the metatarsal heads. Loose fragments warrant referral
Iselin's apophysitis	Pain at lateral aspect of foot	Misdiagnosed as an avulsion fracture	Activity modification, shoe support, ice and NSAIDs
Scheuermann's disease	Back pain, rigidity and hump back deformity	Anterior wedging of vertebrae and end-plate irregularity	Physiotherapy, core stability, reduction of repetitive flexion exercises and orthopaedic referral
Medial epicondyle apophysitis	Medial-sided elbow pain associated with throwing	Fragmentation. May show widening of growth plate between epicondyle and distal humerus	Activity modification, cessation of throwing, ice and NSAIDs. Acute displaced avulsion requires referral
Panner's disease	Lateral-sided elbow pain	Fragmentation and fissuring of the capitellum	Activity modification, ice and NSAIDs
Perthe's disease	Hip or knee pain (referred). Limp	Sclerosis, flattening and fragmentation of the femoral capital epiphysis	Orthopaedic referral necessary

*Adapted and expanded from Atanda A, Shah SA, O'Brien K. Osteochondrosis: common causes of pain in growing bones. Am Fam phys 2011; 83:285–291.

Further reading

Atanda A, Shah SA, O'Brien K. Osteochondrosis: common causes of pain in growing bones. Am Fam phys 2011; 83:285–291.

Malanga GA, Ramirez-Del Toro JA. Common Injuries of the foot and ankle in the child and adolescent athlete. Phys Med Rehabil Clin N Am 2008; 19:347–371.

Related topics of interest

Paediatrics – sports injuries

Key points

- Acute fractures involving growth plates may be associated with growth disturbance (Salter–Harris classification)
- Joint stiffness is less common in children
- Fracture displacement remodels, angulation remodels closer to the growth plate if in the plane of movement of the joint, and rotational deformities tend not to

Cervical spine

Neck injuries are extremely rare in children below 11; there is a significant increase in 15–18 year olds, including most of the fatalities and permanent spinal cord injuries. Children younger than 10 have a relatively high incidence of atlantoaxial type of injury while older children may suffer a subaxial injury. If an injury is suspected on the field a cervical spine collar should always be applied prior to hospital transfer.

Clinical features include localised and referred pain, stiffness, neurological symptoms and signs. Head injury and loss of consciousness may be associated with cervical spine injury.

Radiographs of the C-spine including odontoid peg are required. Magnetic resonance imaging (MRI) (ligaments and nerves) and computed tomography (CT) (bone) may be diagnostic. Lateral flexion/extension radiographs may be useful in assessing stability.

Certain conditions increase susceptibility to significant neck injury even with minor trauma. These include syndromes such as Down's syndrome (atlantoaxial and occipito-cervical instability) and Klippel–Feil (congenital fusion of cervical vertebrae). Advice should be provided to restrict these children from certain sports.

Thoracic and lumbar spine

Acute injuries and fractures of the thoracolumbar spine in children are rare but follow a similar pattern to those occurring in adults. The stress in children primarily concentrates at the posterior elements of the vertebrae at the pars interarticularis, facets and pedicles (in contrast to anteriorly in adults).

Repetitive minor stresses may lead to stress fractures. They present with localised back pain. Although spondylolysis is a stress fracture, it has a genetic predisposition. Early diagnosis is essential to prevent a complete fracture and nonunion that may follow. Spondylolysis must be suspected in young athletes with a history of repetitive extension activities and the presence of pain with extension, in particular on single leg extension testing (e.g. dancers).

Disc herniation may occur in children. They may present with back and leg pain.

MRI can confirm the diagnosis. Conservative management is successful with sport limitation, physiotherapy, core stability exercises, back education, occasional bracing and analgesia. In spondylolysis, surgery may be indicated in symptomatic nonunion.

Shoulder

Fractures

Fractures around the shoulder (including clavicle) can occur during sport from falls and contact injuries.

Clavicular fractures in young children remodel with conservative treatment in a sling. Older adolescents should be treated as adults. Medial clavicular fractures may be mistaken for sternoclavicular dislocation.

Proximal humeral fractures in young children have a high propensity to remodel due to the proximity to the growth plate and therefore can be treated conservatively. Growth disturbance is rare.

Dislocations

Sternoclavicular, acromioclavicular and glenohumeral joint dislocations can occur during sport but are unusual in young children. Older adolescents should be treated as adults. Sternoclavicular dislocations (anterior/posterior) may need intervention if symptomatic.

Repetitive injury

Young swimmers and athletes in throwing sports may suffer from repetitive stresses that can result in a subsequent tightening of posterior structures of the glenohumeral joint, increased mobility of the scapulothoracic region, anterior subluxation of the glenohumeral joint with symptoms simulating anterior instability and rotator cuff impingement. Rotator cuff tears are rare. Multiaxial instability of the shoulder can be demonstrated in some young athletes.

Clinical shoulder examination may confirm a combination of more than one direction of instability. Management of multiaxial instability will include strengthening and balancing programmes of the rotator cuff, since surgery is rarely if ever required.

Limitation of sport will be required until healing or stability is achieved.

Elbow

Fractures

Distal humeral fractures

These are supracondylar and lateral condylar fractures occur most commonly in younger children. If displaced they needs reduction and fixation usually with K-wires (to avoid growth arrest). Epicondylar avulsions generally occur in older children and may require reduction and fixation.

Proximal radius

Radial head and neck fractures may require reduction and immobilisation. Fixation is not usually required.

Proximal ulna

Olecranon fractures in children are uncommon but one should be aware of Monteggia fractures that need to be addressed.

Dislocations

Radiocapitellar

This is one of the most commonly missed, but can be diagnosed using AP and lateral radiographs of the elbow. Usually following a simple fall. Reduction is required. Late reconstruction is necessary if missed.

Pulled elbow

This is caused by traction on the arm in younger children. Radiographs are normal. This resolves spontaneously with a sling, or a supination/pronation manoeuvre.

Repetitive injuries

Sports involving fast striking of a ball, e.g. cricket or baseball, with repetition can cause a number of injuries around the elbow. Typically, it will include a range of traction injuries at the medial epicondyle, a valgus impaction injury on the lateral aspect of the elbow ('little Leaguer's elbow' in American literature), osteochondritis dissecans, loose bodies and premature arrest of the medial physis. Both CT and MRI may be diagnostic. With the Little Leaguer's elbow, treatment consists of arthroscopic removal of loose bodies and if appropriate, multiple drilling of osteochondral defects. This will be followed by a lengthy rehabilitation programme and absence from sport. Resolution of symptoms usually occurs with fusion of the medial epicondylar physis.

Radiographs of the elbow should be routinely taken in elbow injuries, but can be challenging to interpret due to multiple secondary ossification centres. MRI may be helpful in older children. Younger children requiring general anaesthesia for MRI may be better imaged with an arthrogram.

Wrist and hand

Fracture

A fall onto the outstretched hand can cause a forearm fracture. The location of the fracture varies with age: fractures at the junction of the diaphysis to metaphysis are commoner in very young children; near puberty the same injury could cause a fracture through the radial physis. Later on, in young athletes after puberty, the same mechanism may cause either a fracture of the radial and ulna metaphysis or a scaphoid injury.

Torus fractures occur in young children and require minimal immobilisation and protection.

Green stick fractures are specific to children and are unicortical fractures that may angulate requiring reduction and a moulded cast.

Unstable fractures may require reduction and fixation with K-wires, flexible intramedullary nails or plate and screws (depending on the age of the child and the site of the fracture). Disruption of the distal radio–ulnar joint (Gelliazzi-type injury) need to be recognised and addressed.

Repetitive injuries

Repetitive impaction and wrist dorsiflexion can cause premature distal radial physeal closure and subsequent Madelung deformity, e.g. in young gymnasts practicing floor work.

Hip and pelvis

The most common group of injuries occurring in the young athlete are apophyseal avulsion fractures as a result of sudden forceful concentric or eccentric contraction of a muscle attached to an apophysis (**Figure 23**):

- **Anterior superior iliac spine:** Sartorius muscle (common) (**Figure 23b**)
- **Anterior inferior iliac spine:** Rectus femoris muscle (**Figures 23c** and **24**)
- **Iliac crest and abductors**: Lateral abdominis muscle (**Figure 23a**)
- **Ischial tuberosity:** Hamstring muscles (common) (**Figures 23f, 23h** and **25**)
- Greater trochanter. Hip abductors (**Figure 23d**)
- **Lesser trochanter of femur:** Iliopsoas muscle (**Figure 23e**)
- **Pubic symphysis:** Hip adductors (**Figure 23g**)

These athletic injuries usually occur during rapid growth in mid adolescence. Treatment is usually conservative: rehabilitation following a week of rest and return to sport after 2 months. Displaced avulsions (>2–3 cm) may require reduction and fixation to avoid nonunion and muscle weakness. AP pelvic radiographs are usually diagnostic but CT, MRI and US can aid diagnosis and management.

Field sports played on hard surfaces may cause osteitis pubis pain in young athletes. X-rays and MRI will assist the diagnosis. Conservative management is usually successful.

Slipped upper femoral epiphysis (SUFE) usually occurs without trauma. Many

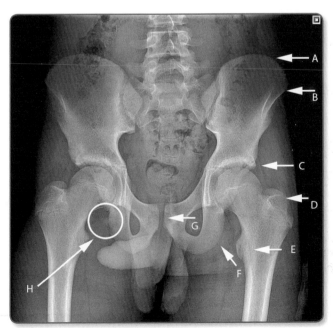

Figure 23 Radiograph demonstrating the possible sites of apophyseal avulsion fractures about the hip and pelvis. Iliac crest (a), ASIS (b), AIIS (c), greater trochanter (d), lesser trochanter (e), ischial tuberosity (f), pubic symphysis (g). The long arrow and circle (h) on the right side correspond to a subtle ischial tuberosity avulsion secondary to a football injury in a 15-year-old boy. ASIS, anterior superior iliac spine; AIIS, Anterior inferior iliac spine.

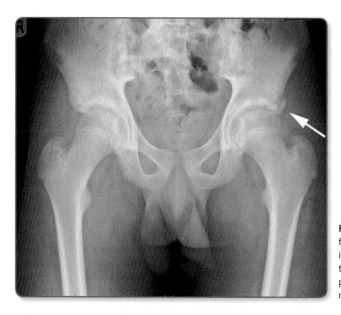

Figure 24 An example of a rectus femoris avulsion off the anterior inferior iliac spine (AIIS). This was treated nonoperatively and the patient was back to sport within 3 months.

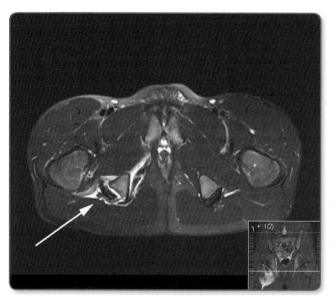

Figure 25 An axial MRI scan (T2 weighted) of the same injury in **Figure 23h** revealing the avulsion of the ischial tuberosity more clearly with extensive soft tissue oedema and bleeding from the injury. This was treated nonoperatively with good results. MRI, magnetic resonance imaging.

patients are obese or prepubescent and may have endocrine pathology. SUFE should be considered in 9–16-year-old patients presenting with hip or knee pain and a limp. AP pelvic and frog lateral radiographs are usually diagnostic. Urgent in situ screw fixation is required. Patients should be bearing no weight for 6–8 weeks.

Contact sport may result in thigh contusions, which are treated with rest, ice and crutches. Significant pain can result from the development of a haematoma. Myositis ossificans (calcification at the site of injured muscle) is a recognised complication that can occur secondary to attempts of rapid rehabilitation and premature return to sport. Calcification can progress to ossification. Management is largely nonoperative with rest, anti-inflammatory drugs and gentle physiotherapy that can take between 6 and 12 months. Surgical excision is rarely indicated. Differential diagnosis should include soft tissue tumours as they can rapidly develop and increase in size.

Knee

Acute: Salter–Harris type fractures, tibial spine (eminence) fracture, patella tendon rupture, patella sleeve fracture, anterior cruciate ligament (ACL) rupture, meniscal injury, osteochondral fractures, patella dislocation.

Chonric: Recurrent patella dislocation, osteochondritis dissecans

Fractures and physeal injuries usually occur in middle to late adolescence. All Salter–Harris fractures of the distal femur and proximal tibia, except types I and V, should be reduced and fixed to reduce risk of growth arrest.

Patella sleeve fractures should be suspected with apparently minor bony avulsions from the lower pole of the patella. This should be distinguished from a bipartite patella that is usually superolateral and evident on X-ray and is a normal variant.

Tibial spine avulsions are more common than ACL ruptures in growing children. Haemarthrosis occurs following a twist or hyperextension injury to the knee. Displaced tibial eminence fractures require reduction and fixation with sutures or screws, avoiding the physis (open or arthroscopic). ACL disruption requires reconstruction if associated with meniscal tear. Otherwise, ACL reconstruction should be considered if symptomatic following rehabilitation. There is a risk of physeal injury and growth disturbance with intra-articular reconstruction. Therefore, it may be preferable in some to defer surgery until skeletal maturity.

Isolated meniscal tears are unusual but may also require repair. Torn discoid menisci may require resection +/- repair. Six weeks of bracing is followed by rehabilitation and can take 6–12 months before fill full return to sport.

Chondral and osteochondral injuries and osteocondritis dissecans occur in young athletes secondary to acute or repetitive trauma. Radiographs may reveal irregular ossification, discreet lesions or loose bodies. MRI identifies bone marrow oedema, presence of damaged articular cartilage and may suggest instability of the lesion. Stable lesions heal with rest from sport. Unstable lesions can be drilled arthroscopically or internally fixed to promote healing. Displaced osteochondral fragments of significant size should, if at all possible, be reduced and fixed.

First patellar dislocations need reduction, immobilisation, then rehabilitation, concentrating on vastus medialis obliquus (VMO) strengthening. Those with abnormal patellofemoral anatomy are susceptible to recurrent dislocation. Patellofemoral osteochondral fractures can occur at the time of dislocation requiring treatment as above.

Patellofemoral pain during growth may be associated with tight iliotibial band and weak VMOs. This may contribute to patellofemoral maltracking and functional pain. Treatment involves physiotherapy with stretching and strengthening.

Ankle and foot

Ankle injuries are common in sporty children. Ligament attachments of the ankle are subphyseal so that injury may cause ligament or physeal damage, as in anterior talofibular injuries or Salter–Harris I fractures of the distal fibula. These require minimal immobilisation and rehabilitation.

Specific ankle fracture patterns occur in children. A Tillaux fracture is a Salter–Harris III avulsion fracture of the anterolateral distal tibial epiphysis. Triplane fractures of the distal tibia occur in three planes. CT may be more informative than radiographs and guide treatment in the form of reduction and fixation for displaced fractures.

Repetitive injuries

Pain at the accessory navicular region can be seen in young athletes (see Paediatrics - sport medicine).

Stress fractures of the distal tibia, calcaneum and tarsal bones may occur in young athletes. Navicular stress fractures are difficult to diagnose. MRI is most useful. Activity limitation and immobilisation +/-

restricted weight bearing for 6 weeks may be necessary to ensure resolution and union. Nonunion is a rare complication.

Tarsal coalition may present as a painful, stiff, flat foot, sometimes following minor injury. Diagnosis should be considered if symptoms persist. Coalitions may be fibrous, cartilaginous or osseous, and are not always evident on radiographs. CT or MRI is diagnostic. Symptoms may resolve with rest and orthotics, but resection of cartilaginous or bony bars may be required. If resection is unsuccessful then arthrodesis may be required. Calcaneonavicular bars have a better prognosis than tibiocalcaneal bars.

Further reading

Caine D, Caine C, Maffuli N. Incidence and distribution of pediatric sport-related injuries. Clin J Sport Med 2006; 16(6):500–513.

Rossi F, Dragoni S. Acute avulsion fractures of the pelvis in adolescent competitive athletes: prevalence, location and sports distribution of 203 cases collected. *Skeletal Radiol* 2001; 30:127–131.

Salter R, Harris WR. Injuries involving the epiphyseal plate. J Bone Joint Surg 1963; 45:587–622.

Related topics of interest

- Elbow – throwing injuries (p. 92)
- Knee acute injuries (p. 189)
- Paediatrics – osteochondrosis (osteochondritis) (p. 211)

Paediatrics – sports medicine

Key points

- Physical activity is necessary for normal growth and development
- Preparticipation physical examination (PPE) policies are in use to detect musculoskeletal and other medical conditions, which will protect the young athlete from harmful physical activities
- Appropriate strength training in the young will increase muscular strength, improve the motor skills and overall enhance sports performance
- Injury prevention programmes have been developed, to assist to understand the sports risks for injury and prevention, therefore, contributing to sport safety

General factors

Physical activities such as 'free play' or group games are necessary for normal growth and development. Modern lifestyles and cultural beliefs have reduced the traditional free 'free play' routine and there is a trend nowadays for children and young people to obtain physical activity and exercise, through physical education (PE) at school or other organised sports programmes.

There is variability in the physical growth in children of the same chronological age:

- A group of 14 years olds may contain children with biological age from 11 to 17 years old, with difference in height, weight and even skill development.
- Girls are taller than boys and may have greater muscular strength, at the age between 11 and 14 years, due to the earlier onset of a growth spurt.
- There is no reason to separate the sexes for sporting activity up to 14 years old, when strength, height and weight will begin to favour the growing boys.

The physiological differences between children and adults are as follows:

- The maximum aerobic power of a child is nearly the same as an adult; however, the anaerobic power is lower until the age of 14–16 years old.
- Children have a higher maximum heart rate at rest and exercise
- The systolic arterial blood pressure is lower at rest and exercise
- The breathing pattern of a child is shallow, with a result of lower absorption of oxygen from the inspired air
- Children are vulnerable to environmental temperature extremes as the sweating mechanism is not fully developed until the adolescence growth spurt. Heat injury may cause a permanent damage to the thermal regulatory system, which will result to long-term heat intolerance
- Children with low fat insulation lose heat quicker during immersion in cold water

Psychological maturation in sport must be adjusted to the child's age. In the first 7 years, motor tasks learning will provide the foundations for later acquaintance of the skills necessary for sports performance. Free play, in this period, will allow the child to practice skills such as running, jumping, swinging and climbing; therefore, the child will improve balance, coordination and position sense (proprioception).

When 6–7 years old, children can organise themselves into groups, play more complex games, seek adult approval for their performance and compare it to their peers. At this age, the child becomes aware of self-esteem, rewards, achieving goals and getting the admiration from others.

Formal games with rules are appropriate after the age of 8–9 years old. Careful encouragement in effort rather than outcome will avoid of developing the stereotype of the children feeling 'a failure' at the end of a performance.

Preparticipation physical examination

PPE is a widely practiced method of screening children and adolescents to detect any medical limitations before sport participation. There are many variations in PPE practices, undermining the value of such medical strategies. Although, PPE presents a legal requirement and they are common in United States and parts of Europe; in the United Kingdom, they are considered by large ineffective and they are not implemented by all Sports authorities.

The Examination objectives usually include:

- The detection of musculoskeletal and medical conditions, which make sport participation unsafe, with specific consideration to the sport that the child was screened
- To screen the child for any underlying illness, using medical and family history and concise physical examination
- To assess the child's development, conditioning and strength for a specific sport

Future considerations to improve the acceptance of PPE policy should consider:

- National PPE standardisation
- Universal endorsement by all different sports authorities
- Sport specific medical protocols and forms
- Appropriate trained personnel only to be allowed to perform a PPE

Strength training strategies

Strength training in children is a specialising method of conditioning that can offer benefits such as increased muscle power and bone mineral density, but at the same time, it could lead to a serious injury if appropriate guidelines are not established.

The most obvious anatomical difference in a child is the cartilaginous growth plate, which is vulnerable during vigorous sport. The same proportional forces that will cause a rupture of ligaments in adults may cause growth plate injuries instead in the immature skeleton. In addition, very intense strength training in children may cause growth plate injury and deformity.

Established training guidelines and safety procedures are based on:

- The quality of instructions by trainers and teachers
- The type and mix of training with an emphasis on the right choice of exercises and learning of skills
- The rate of progression and accepted methods of testing
- The programme design to lead to competitive sport participation

Injury prevention

Injury prevention guidelines will include:

- Careful application and modification of sport regulations
- Supervision by qualified adults at all times
- Coaching staff with a knowledge of child development and different sport routines
- Appropriate sport selection and competition for the individual child
- Safe and free of hazards training environment
- Equipment design for size and skill
- Protective clothing and footwear
- Adequate fluid intake and advice on food choices

Further reading

Bruhmann B, Schneider S. Risk groups for sports injuries among adolescents. Child Care Health Dev 2011; 37:597—605.

Schneider S, Yamamoto S, Weidmann C et al. Sports injuries among adolescents. J Paediatr Child Health 2012; 48(10):E183-189.

Related topics of interest

- Paediatrics – sports injuries (p. 215)

Physiotherapy – acute injury management

Key points

- Appropriate assessment and diagnosis of the athlete immediately postinjury is critical in providing the foundation for successful rehabilitation and return to sport
- Quick and decisive treatment of the injury in the first 48–72 h can optimise tissue healing
- Injury management should commence immediately following injury

Accurate diagnosis is vital in determining the most effective management of acute musculoskeletal injuries. Understanding the mechanism of the injury, biomechanical factors relating to the sport, environmental conditions and past medical history are some of the variables that the clinician must consider when assessing an athlete's acute injury. The first 48–72 h postinjury is considered to be critical in influencing the physiological variables related to tissue healing. The use of special investigations such as musculoskeletal diagnostic ultrasound or magnetic resonance imaging scanning can enhance the accuracy of diagnosis and aid in determining the severity of injury. This will also influence the rehabilitation programme that is designed for the athlete.

Once the clinician has completed their assessment the athlete must be educated about their injury. For efficient and effective management they will play an integral part in optimising their own recovery. The athlete must be empowered to be actively involved in their rehabilitation from the acute phase of injury. They need to know what they can do to assist healing, e.g. applying the Protection, Rest, Ice, Compression and Elevation principles (PRICE).

These principles prevent the initial injury from escalating into a more severe condition by controlling and reducing the extent of the inflammation of the injured tissue and limiting the potential for further trauma caused by moving the tissues too early.

They also help provide the physiological environment to achieve optimal repair and healing. Any injury to the body should be treated by the principles of PRICE during the acute phase. Diagnosis is essential to discover the extent of tissue damage (Grades I–III) and the body tissue injured – bone, ligament, muscle, tendon, fascia, nerve and vessels.

The advice given for 'PRICE' is as follows:

Protection: Protect the injured tissue from further damage. This can be achieved with taping, strapping and orthotic supports. For the foot and ankle, this can be achieved with air cast supports; for the upper limb, this can be achieved with shoulder braces; and for the spine, this can be achieved with corsets and/or collars.

Rest: Minimal movement around the injured area is necessary to prevent further damage. The athlete should try to stop any weight-bearing or upper limb movements for 24–72 h.

Ice: Regular ice packs, every 3–4 h for 10–30 min, reduce excessive inflammatory tissue flooding the injured tissue site. Ice also helps to reduce pain perception.

Compression: A compression support bandage, such as Tubigrip or adjustable neoprene support, helps to keep swelling controlled within the damaged area.

Elevation: The injured limb should be elevated above the heart whenever possible to assist lymphatic damage of inflamed tissues.

The athlete also needs to be aware of what to avoid following soft tissue injury. These factors can be summarised as the HARM factors:

Heat: Do not apply heat in the first 72 h as this can cause more bleeding.

Alcohol: Avoid alcohol as this has a proinflammatory effect on the tissues.

Reinjury: Resting the injured area to avoid further injury.

Massage: Deep connective tissue massage can cause further damage in the first 72 h.

Through being actively involved in their recovery process, the athlete will limit the psychological challenges associated with being injured. The clinician must take a holistic view of the effects the injury can have on the athlete above and beyond the 'injured part'. Reinforcing positive scenarios such as being able to improve other technical aspects of their game while being out injured or improving their core strength or endurance will provide the athlete with some structure to help cope with the psychological aspects of being injured.

After the acute inflammatory stage has been reached, it is important to move onto the next stage of injury management. The next stage is often described as the proliferation/mobilisation phase followed by the remodelling phase. In these phases, it is important to begin the gradual process of moving the injured tissue. Initial rest and protection needs to be followed by movements of the tissue to promote the remodelling phase of healing. Mobilisation techniques can be described as follows:

1. **Passive:** The limb tissue is moved by an outside force, e.g. including CPM and Maitland
2. **Active assisted:** The therapist aids the movements of the limb, which is controlled by the athlete
3. **Active:** The athlete is in control of the direction speed and range of movement

The extent of body tissue damage will dictate the amount of mobilisation allowed. With soft tissue injuries, it is imperative that the extent of tissue damage is diagnosed accurately. For example, a classification of soft tissue injuries is as follows:

Grade 1: A minor soft tissue strain or stretch with tissue integrity maintained.

Grade 2: A moderate to substantial tissue damage, partial rupture/tear of soft tissues.

Grade 3: A full rupture of soft tissue fibre between origin and attachment.

Having established the extent of the injury, a graduated treatment plan can be developed that dictates the timing and progression of mobilisations to the affected area. Progressive movements, which are pain free (or minimal) throughout the range of motion and that do not overly challenge tissue integrity, should be encouraged. Controlled motion acts as a trigger and guide to the remodelling phase.

Once functional tissue range and/or integrity are restored, strengthening/resistance programmes can begin to provide natural protection to the joints. Stabilisation programmes and sports-specific functional restoration provides the injured tissue with protection in the future prior to the return to sports. Rehabilitation programmes should be guided by physiological principles of tissue injury and repair rates.

The role of electrotherapy in the acute rehabilitation of sports injuries

Electrotherapy is rarely seen as the principal treatment modality for the management of musculoskeletal disorders by physiotherapists. It is generally considered as an adjunct to other forms of management such as manual therapy or exercise based therapies. Electrotherapy has the capacity to enhance normal physiological reactions within the body. The following section will highlight some of the more common modalities.

Ultrasound therapy

Ultrasound is a mechanical vibration, which uses high-frequency acoustic energy to oscillate biological tissues and stimulate healing. This helps accelerate tissue healing by stimulating stimulates growth factors within macrophages and mast cells (white blood cells) to clear tissue debris accumulated after injury. Ultrasound can be used pulsed and/or continuously. For acute injuries, pulsed ultrasound is recommended, it is nonthermal, and has an analgesic effect. Continuous ultrasound produces heat and is used for chronic injuries. The frequency and intensity of ultrasound is varied according to the stage of the injury, the size of the area of tissue being treated and the type of body tissue.

Low-intensity pulsed ultrasound

Low-intensity pulsed ultrasound has been used to accelerate fracture healing and in particular nonunion with some studies demonstrating a 38% faster healing rate than conservative casts alone. This form of therapy can be used when metal fixations are in place and can be easily applied by the athletes themselves.

Laser

Low-level nonthermal laser has a relatively short penetration depth in living tissue. The effect of the light energy on tissue can act as a trigger for physiological reactions in a similar manner to ultrasound. Research by Karu et al. and Bjordal et al. suggested that laser was capable of enhancing the inflammatory and proliferative phases of tissue healing.

Interferential stimulation

Interferential stimulation uses low-frequency current produced within tissues, with low-skin impedance. This is created by two medium-frequency currents that cross to produce a 'beat frequency'. The interferential current improves the permeability of muscle and nerve tissue and stimulates the healing process.

Combination therapy

Combination therapy consists of a mixture of interferential stimulation and ultrasound to provide cellular stimulation and tissue fluid flow at lower intensity outputs. Ultrasound can stimulate healing of the ligament, while interferential stimulation reduces general capsular swelling.

Pulsed short wave

Pulsed short wave uses magnetic field energy to stimulate cellular activity. Biological research suggests that the process of cellular mitosis is enhanced by the use of pulsed magnetic energy. The transportation of fluid flow across the cell at the surface of the membrane enhances the resolution of inflammatory exudates.

Iontophoresis

Iontophoresis is used to help the penetration of the anti-inflammatory medicine into injured soft tissues or joints. It is the therapeutic process by which pharmacological agents (nonsteroidal anti-inflammatories) are transported through the skin into the tissues using electrical currents. This technique can help make the application of the anti-inflammatory medication more effective.

Neuromuscular electrical stimulators

Electrical muscle stimulators work between frequencies of 0–50 Hz. Faradic and Russian stimulation currents which are used regularly are of two types. Many companies have produced disease and selective muscle-specific stimulation programmes. The aim is to stimulate weak and atrophied muscles that a patient is unable to activate consciously. In acute injuries or postsurgery, muscle stimulation can maintain muscle activity whilst avoiding placing excessive resistance stress through the joint. In chronic or overuse injuries, muscle stimulators provide a trigger for inhibited and disused muscles.

Surface electromyography for biofeedback

Surface electromyography biofeedback uses surface electrodes that are applied to the muscle belly of selective muscles, and the electrical muscle activity is recorded. The information is converted into visual and auditory signals and the patient is able to alter their muscle activity appropriately by volitional control of their muscles. Electromyography is a useful tool to aid with the re-education of pain-inhibited muscles. Because the athlete can see the activity of the muscle being recorded, they can adjust and alter the behaviour of the muscle. For muscles that are weak at selective joint ranges or during specific movements the athlete can learn to increase the muscle activity while repeating the affected movements. For muscles that work excessively or inappropriately during selective movements, the athlete can learn to reduce the muscle activity.

Transcutaneous electrical nerve stimulation

Transcutaneous electrical nerve stimulation (TENS) is used to provide pain relief. Traditionally, it has been used to control chronic pain; however, it is used in the acute setting quite effectively in the sports medicine environment where oral analgesics could impede athletic performance or disqualify the athlete due to positive drug screen results. The efficacy of TENS is often attributed to two systems firstly the pain gate theory proposed by Melzack and stimulation of the natural opiate systems. High-frequency stimulation of large diameter nerve fibres reduces the perception of pain by closing the 'gate' to pain fibres at the spinal cord level. The pain gate theory proposes that pain is transmitted via the spinal cord by small diameter *c* fibres. TENS machines set at high frequency (80–130 Hz) and high pulse rates (60–80 pulses per second) stimulate large diameter nerves in the spinal cord and inhibit the information transmitted to the spinal column by the small diameter pain fibres. Low-frequency stimulation (<80 Hz and pulse rate <4 per second) of nerve fibres helps to release the body's own pain relieving substances (endorphins or endogenous opioids). Opioids work on the central nervous system to stimulate control of pain transmission and also influence the spinal cord, inhibiting the transmission of messages of tissue damage to the brain. This can produce a low-intensity muscle twitch that can be used on acupuncture or trigger points.

Heat

Heat can be used to promote blood flow, provide analgesia and to relax muscles. It is applied to the damaged tissues only after acute inflammation has resolved (to avoid increasing any exudates). Hot packs and whirlpools provide superficial heating, and deep heating modalities include continuous ultrasound and short-wave diathermy. Superficial heating techniques are useful to encourage the circulation in ligaments and tendons just beneath the skin. Deep heating modalities are useful for fascia and deeper structures.

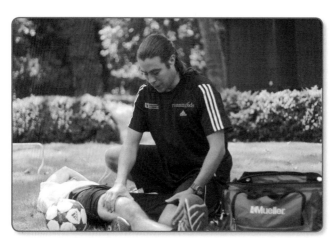

Figure 26 A thorough early assessment of the injured athlete is critical to efficient management and treatment planning.

The role of massage in the acute to chronic rehabilitation of sport injuries

Massage has many proposed benefits, including physiological and psychological. Massage helps to reduce swelling, breaks down scar tissue (adhesions) and improves circulation to facilitate healing. There are many different techniques used in massage and these include kneading, effleurage, picking up, pounding, shaking, rolling, hacking, vibrations and myofascial release. These techniques range from movements designed to promote fluid mobility and circulation within arterial, venous and lymphatic vessels, to techniques designed to aid the mechanical breakdown of fibrotic and/or adhered scar formation that could prevent healing. Deep connective tissue massage techniques should be avoided in the acute inflammatory phase as further tissue damage and bleeding may result. This could result in such conditions as myositis ossificans.

Acupuncture

Acupuncture can assist with improving local circulation and decreasing muscle spasm and pain. This can help by decreasing swelling and improving the range of movement of the affected limb. Clinicians that practice the 'eastern approach' to acupuncture would use systemic points to help restore overall balance to the body's systems and to help promote an optimal healing environment.

Hyperbaric oxygen therapy

The use of hyperbaric oxygen therapy is well established in some areas of clinical medicine; however, current research has produced conflicting results regarding its efficacy in treating soft tissue injury. Whilst it is currently being used by a number of professional football teams to treat muscle, tendon and ligament injury further research is required before evidence based protocols could be recommended.

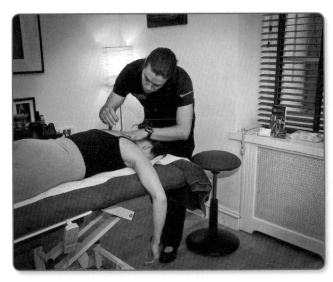

Figure 27 Acupuncture can be used in the acute phase of soft tissue healing both to control pain and stimulate physiological responses.

Further reading

Bjordal JM, Lopes-Martins RA, Inverse VV, et al. A randomised placebo controlled trial of low level laser therapy for activated Achilles tendonitis with microdialysis measurement of peritendinous prostaglandin E2 concentrations. Br J Sports Med 2006; 40(1):76–80.

Heckman JD, Ryaby JD, McCabe J, et al. Acceleration of tibial fracture healing by non-invasive, low-intensity pulsed ultrasound. J Bone Joint Surg 1994; 79-A(11):26–34.

Karu TI, Pyatibrat LV, Afanasyeva NI, et al. Cellular effects of low power laser therapy can be mediated by nitric oxide. Lasers Surg Med 2005; 36(4):307–314.

Melzack R. Prolonged relief of pain by brief, intense transcutaneous somatic stimulation. Pain 1975; 4:59–65.

Watson T. (ed.) Electrotherapy: evidence-based practice, 12th edn. London: Churchill Livingstone Elsevier, 2008.

Related topics of interest

- Knee acute injuries (p. 189)
- Physiotherapy – rehabilitation (p. 233)
- Shoulder – acute dislocation (p. 256)

Physiotherapy – general principles

Key points

- Physiotherapy can improve human performance by optimising many of the physiological variables that make up human performance such as flexibility, strength, control, speed, endurance and power
- Physiotherapy techniques can accelerate recovery from injury by providing appropriate treatment at the correct stage of healing
- Thorough musculoskeletal assessments that record objective measures provide the foundation to build a rehabilitation programme that enables progression to be made on the basis of reproducible data from valid tests

Physiotherapy has a key role in the optimisation of human performance. Many of the variables that make up an optimal sporting performance can be influenced by physiotherapy treatment and management. An important skill of the physiotherapist working with athletes is to consider all of the variables that make up human performance and identify which ones can be influenced through physiotherapy techniques. While physiotherapists are very adept at assessing injury and preparing rehabilitation programmes, their role in optimising performance is becoming an increasingly important factor in professional sport. Many physiological variables can be positively influenced such as muscular strength, flexibility, speed, control and endurance. The physiotherapist is often a clinician in the best position to have a thorough overall perspective of an athlete, as he or she will often spend the most time assessing, treating, rehabilitating, training and communicating with the athlete. This information is often vital to other members of the team such as the coach, team doctor, nutritionist, sports psychologist and exercise physiologist. The overall health and performance of the athlete can be enhanced by collectively improving all of the variables that make up performance.

The ability of the physiotherapist to perform a thorough musculoskeletal assessment that can provide objective measures and a framework for an efficient treatment and management plan is essential for the efficient management of an injured athlete. The physiotherapist is able to analyse the mechanism of injury and consider the biomechanical forces involved and the effects these forces can have on surrounding tissue. Where tissue has been damaged physiotherapists will be able to record observations from their assessment and take various objective measures such as range of joint movement recorded by a goniometer or through video analysis. They will be able to determine strength or endurance recorded by a force dynamometer or functional test. Physiotherapists with formal training in musculoskeletal diagnostic ultrasound are using this form of scanning during standard musculoskeletal assessments to assess soft tissue lesions more accurately. This has the potential to improve diagnostic impressions and enhance the rehabilitation process by being able to more accurately match the phase of healing with appropriate treatment approaches.

Knowledge of the physiological principles of soft tissue healing is essential in determining what stage a rehabilitation programme commences. The graduated treatment plan for the injured tissue/limb is based upon the healing status of the injury, acute to subacute to chronic. The results of the musculoskeletal assessment combined with clinical reasoning models considered by the physiotherapist help to match treatment to the stage of healing. **Table 20** demonstrates the phases of rehabilitation in relation to the progression of physiotherapy treatment and the stage of tissue healing.

Physiotherapy treatment should include continual reassessment at each phase and be goal orientated. Goal setting during treatment is important psychologically to help the

Table 20 Tissue healing classification in relation to phases of physiotherapy treatment			
Phase 1	Early	Control inflammation; protect injured tissue	Haemostasis (6—24 h)
Phase 2	Intermediate	Initiate loading of injured tissue	Inflammation
Phase 3	Late	Progress load and movement	(Initial onset 3 h, max. reaction 2–3 days, resolution 2–3 weeks)
Phase 4	Advanced	Sports specific; return to athletic activities	Proliferation (24–48 h postinjury with peak at 2–3 weeks)
			Remodelling (commences 1–2 weeks postinjury up to 12 months)

athlete maintain a strong mental state and motivation. Educating the athlete regarding their injury is important to ease anxiety and to understand prognosis and expectations.

With a move towards evidence-based practice, physiotherapists attempt to use validated outcome measures to determine the baseline function of a patient at the commencement of treatment. This enables the physiotherapist to repeat the same test or scoring system during treatment to help guide treatment progression and at completion to determine efficacy of treatment and to provide data for analysis (see **Table 21**).

Table 21 Assessment tools used in physiotherapy to acquire objective measures	
Objective measure	Tool
Motion/flexibility	Goniometer, video analysis 2D and 3D
Strength	Oxford scale, dynamometer, isokinetics
Balance/proprioception	Balance error scoring system (BESS)
Tissue integrity	Magnetic resonance imaging, diagnostic ultrasound
Endurance	Repetition count to fatigue, holding time
Functional	Speed agility quickness drills, jump and hop tests, throwing and catching.

Preconditioning programmes

Prior to any sport, it is essential that the athlete is physically prepared for the specific sport and is generally conditioned to tolerate the load the sporting activities demand. It has been suggested that athletes of all sports should have preconditioning programmes that involve specific exercise to optimise physical performance and prevent injuries. Low threshold stabilisation exercises combined with an isolated approach for retraining specific local stabilising muscles has become the leading active treatment option for movement dysfunction. There is significant evidence for this approach in the treatment and prevention of lumbopelvic dysfunction. The second phase of conditioning would be to progress the athlete onto more functional training that involves more complicated movement patterns to enhance neural control systems.

The objectives of a preconditioning programme to assist injury prevention are similar to the first phase of rehabilitation, i.e. exercise prescription would be low load, low effort, avoiding impact and torsion, focus on selective muscle control and improve quality of movement patterns. There are a number of associated exercise therapies that can complement these programmes such as Clinical Pilates, Yoga, Alexander Technique and Gyrotonics. It is important that if the clinicians are referring an athlete elsewhere for these forms of exercise that they discuss

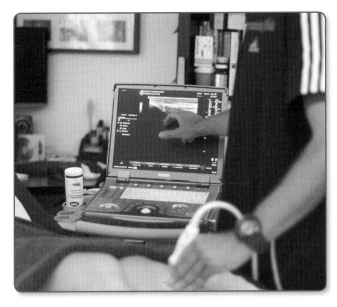

Figure 28 The use of musculoskeletal diagnostic ultrasound by suitably trained physiotherapists during the assessment of athletes with soft tissue injuries has the potential to improve the efficiency of management and treatment.

the needs of the athlete with the instructor first. For example, there are many different forms of yoga and within that many different ways of teaching the exercise. It is vital that the needs of athletes are met and the physiological loading they receive from the exercise is appropriate for any underlying pathology they may have and have functional crossover to the sport they are preparing for.

The principles of treatment for soft tissue injury

Grade I (minor soft tissue strain with soft tissue integrity maintained)
- Initial rest and pain/swelling control methods
- Early motion and early muscle activity
- Proprioceptive training
- Progressive return to sports within 1–3 weeks

Grade II (moderate to substantial tissue damage with partial rupture/tear of soft tissues)

- Initial rest and pain/swelling control methods
- Protection and rest from early motion
- Proprioceptive training
- Progressive muscle exercises – isometric/eccentric/concentric/isokinetic
- Progressive return to sports within 3–9 weeks

Grade III (full rupture of soft tissue fibres between origin and attachment)
- Initial rest and pain/swelling control methods – surgery
- Complete immobilisation and protection/rest from early motion
- Progressive muscle exercises, initial very low effort/resistance
- Proprioceptive training
- Maintenance exercises for noninjured body parts including resistance and cardiovascular work
- Progressive return to sports within 12–36 weeks (3–9 months)

Further reading

Boyle M. Functional training for sports. Champaign: Human Kinetics, 2004.

Davidson KL, Hubley-Kozey. Trunk muscle responses to demands of an exercise progression to improve dynamic spinal stability. Arch Physical Med Rehab 2005; 86:216–223.

Liebenson C. Functional training part 3: transverse plane facilitation. J Bodyw Mov Ther 2003; 7:97–100.

Related topics of interest

Physiotherapy – rehabilitation

Key Points

- Optimal loading
- Combination specific targeted exercise and functional exercise
- Specific retraining specific to athletes needs

Rehabilitation allows us to return an athlete to normal full function. This is where the injured segment has optimal loading and strength of surrounding tissues is sufficient to allow the individual to return to their preinjured level of function. Physiotherapists need to have sound clinical and diagnostic skills to assess the injury and level of function and design an appropriate programme to ensure a full recovery. The examination procedure begins with a thorough examination both subjective and objective, which is crucial to the diagnosis and understanding the mechanism of injury. This is important to allow accurate grading of the injury and to assist in designing the necessary features of the rehabilitation programme. It is vital to be able to marry up the functional capacity of the injured patient and the need for optimal loading of the injured region in a controlled and suitable environment.

Rehabilitation components

Rehabilitation encompasses a range of aspects (**Figure 29**) from local tissue quality to appropriate joint mobility and muscle flexibility, isolated joint control and functional control and sufficient strength and endurance of the injured segment along with good movement patterns and lumbo-pelvic stability to whole body fitness and sports specific retraining.

It is critical that the acute phase of injury is managed appropriately to help reduce the inflammatory response and allow optimal loading of the injured segment. Optimal loading is imperative for tissue healing as it helps to restrict excessive scarring and early mobilisation once safe allows restoration of strength local tissue and enhances tissue quality.

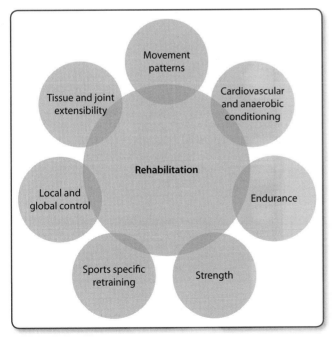

Figure 29 Rehabilitation.

Manual skills

Tissue extensibility and joint mobility are two early goals of a rehabilitation programme. It is imperative once the acute phase has progressed to subacute that the physiotherapist begins allowing appropriate load into the tissue. The use of the clinicians manual skills is important within this phase to ensure there is sufficient length of muscle and fascial tissue and that all surrounding joints glide and mobilise appropriately. The physiotherapist may use a range of techniques from soft tissue work and acupuncture to release muscle spasm to various joint mobilisation techniques that may be matitland or mulligan based or a combination of the two. Muscle energy techniques to restore pelvic mobility or muscle length can be useful in this phase and deeper tissue work can occur around scarred regions as the healing phase progresses. In conjunction with a clinician's manual skills, flexibility can be worked through the muscles either dynamically to target the joints mobility and musculotendinous and fascial components or static stretching to help restore muscle length of tissue.

Exercise and strength work

Optimal loading of an injury will involve specific loading exercises to strengthen the muscle groups involved. The strength training may initially include isometric type muscle contractions where joint movement is precluded either due to pain or to protect the injury site. Isometric contractions have been shown as a beneficial way to ensure local stabilisers around joints maintain their stability function with an injury. This helps to reactivate local muscle such as vastus medialis oblique for the knee or rotator cuff of the shoulder and allow improved stability and movement of the joint.

Isotonic muscle contractions involve concentric and eccentric muscle contractions. Concentric muscle contractions will be introduced next as they shorten the muscle fibres and will generally place less load across the musculotendinous junction. Depending on the injury site, band work or weighted exercises may be used with this like external rotation of the shoulder or straight leg raise with the knee. Eccentric loading then needs to be introduced to allow retraining of shock absorption and braking capacity of the joints and to place a higher load across the musculotendinous junction, which is vital to help prevent recurrence of soft tissue injuries and particularly into lower limb tendons. This can help to rearrange and reorient scar tissue formation. Eccentric exercises have been shown to have had good success with lower limb tendonopathy. However, more recent research has suggested that slow concentric exercises achieve similar results in reducing tendon pain and improving strength-associated tissue, comparing two training regimes.

Exercises that promote the various muscle contractions will be used throughout the phases of rehabilitation. Isokinetic contractions can be used as part of the training programme; however, it is often preferable to test the function and isolated strength of tissues using the varying speeds of isokinetic retraining. It is critical that full strength, endurance and power of the injured region are restored and that the rehabilitation programme addresses all of these components individually. Therefore, it is imperative that when looking at trying to hypertrophy a muscle or strengthen a muscle the exercises are prescribed appropriately to ensure sufficient load is placed through the injured site.

Muscle patterning

An important component of the rehabilitation programme is to ensure that the athlete has appropriate muscle patterning of movement. It may well be that the injury has stemmed from altered biomechanics particularly with an overload injury like tendonopathy or anterior knee pain. It is vital that the physiotherapist address a patients movement patterns to ensure the right muscle groups are firing at correct times to support and drive the movement.

Proprioception

The exercises will often fall into two categories open-chain and closed-chain exercises. It is thought that closed-chain exercises like squats for the knee or scapula push ups for the shoulder will allow better approximation of the joint. Proprioception which is the body's ability to recognise what it is doing in space forms an important component of this. Proprioception is critical to regain to enhance a joints control to avoid overloading the passive system. Stability retraining usually involves progressing through stages of closed-chain exercises to alter the level of stability and feedback into the injured region. This is like going through single leg squats on a stable platform to foam mat, rocker board, wobble board or then to a bosu. It is for this reason that open-chain exercises may be avoided in some early rehabilitation programme like post-ACL reconstruction, as it is more difficult to approximate the joint. It is acknowledged that open-chain exercises while increasing the shear forces across some joints may be better at producing high force and improving the strength of isolated muscle groups so are an important component in specific strength exercises once permitted.

Functional exercises

Functional exercises and sports specific drills will form an important component of the end stage rehabilitation programme. Functional exercises like squats, step ups or lunges for the lower limb are a common component of lower limb sports as are high-level scapula work and eccentric rotator cuff work for the throwing shoulder. Sports-specific drills and exercises to help retrain athletes, as in the case of the thrower high-level scapula work and eccentric rotator cuff work to help control and slow down the arm following a throw is imperative as is teaching the footballer how to pivot and twist following an ACL reconstruction. It is generally considered that a return to sports is allowed once the injured limb returns to 90–95% of the non injured side. This can be tested with some isolated strength testing; however, functional tests like 6-m hop test or a hop for distance test offer good objective outcomes that can be reliably measured.

Further reading

Bleakley CM, Glasgow P, MacAuley DC. PRICE needs updating, should we call the POLICE? Br J Sports Med 2012; 46(4):220-221.

Kraemer WJ, et al. Progression models in resistance training for health adults: American College Sports Medicine Position Stand. Med Sci Sports Exerc 2002; 34: 364–380.

Prevention of sport injuries

Key points

- Strategies to prevent sport injuries of vital importance
- These strategies involve risk identification as well as taking measures to minimise risks and their impacts
- Multidisciplinary approach is important

Overview

Treating sport injuries can often be complex, difficult, expensive and challenging. Therefore, all efforts must be made to prevent these injuries and all individuals working with athletes, including sports clinicians must have an understanding of the different injury prevention strategies. All these strategies involve identification of risk factors as well as attempts to minimise the risks and their impact. There a number of classifications for these strategies in the literature, but one of the most practical ones is presented in the **Figure 30**.

Screening

Screening forms a crucial part of any injury prevention strategy. Those athletes who are particularly at risk of injury and risk factors screening permits an assessment of fitness, general health, condition of musculoskeletal system and efficacy of the rehabilitation programme for existing injuries.

Screening programme may consist of:
- Health questionnaire
- Lifestyle assessment questionnaire
- History
- Physical examination
- Investigations
- Follow-up screening

Physical conditioning

Appropriate physical conditioning and balanced training results in better performance and reduced risk of injury. Training programme must be gradual, allowing the athlete to recover, and

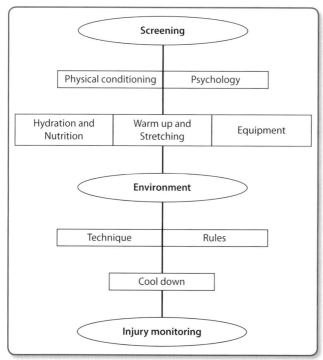

Figure 30 Schemes for injury prevention.

implemented in phases (preparation, precompetition and competition). It must focus on all of the following skills:

- Flexibility
- Strength
- Aerobic capacity
- Anaerobic capacity
- Stamina
- Speed
- Coordination and timing
- Technique and sports-related skills
- Agility
- Proprioception

Warm up and stretching

The proposed benefits of warm-up include:

- Better oxygen delivery to muscle through increased blood flow
- Better release of oxygen by haemoglobin
- Decreased muscle stiffness
- Increased range of motion (controversial)
- Better psychological preparation
  Proposed beneficial effects of stretching include:
- Increased compliance of the tendon unit
- Increased tendon compliance leads to a 'higher ability of tendon to absorb energy'
- Decreased load transfer across the muscle–tendon unit during 'high intensity stretch-shortening cycles' in sports involving jumping and bouncing activities)
- Decreased risk of injury to tendon
- Decreased risk of injury to the muscle

The role of stretching in prevention of injuries does, however, remain very controversial. Although there are a number of studies that have shown the beneficiary effects of stretching, there are also other authors who have not shown any advantages in stretching prior to exercise. It does appear likely that whether stretching has any benefits or not is dependent on the type of the exercise and sport performed by the athlete. Those that pursue sports that involve eccentric contractions and high intensity of stretch-shortening cycles such as basketball, football and long jump require a 'compliant' muscle–tendon unit that is capable of storing and releasing excessive amounts of elastic energy. As stretching has been shown to increase the compliance of the muscle–tendon unit,

such athletes would benefit from stretching. In contrast, those who take part in sports that do not involve high intensity 'stretch-shortening cycles', such as jogging, cycling and swimming, do not require a highly elastic muscle tendon unit. In such athletes, there is no requirement for the tendons to act as energy absorbing structures, and therefore, they may not benefit from stretching exercises. Furthermore, making the tendons more compliant in such athletes may result in decreased ability in decreased performance as rapid tension changes and swift joint motion responses would be more difficult.

Equipment

Correct equipment can play a vital role in injury prevention. Shoes, rackets, skis, gloves and items of clothing, all should be appropriate and compliment the athlete.

The role of protective equipment is to prevent or reduce risk of injury by decreasing the impact of the force on the body part and spreading this force over a large surface area. They may also provide protection of an injured body part during recovery.

These include:

- Helmets
- Eye protection
- Mouth guards
- Shoulder padding
- Gloves
- Elbow guards
- Genital guards
- Thigh guards
- Knee pads
- Shin pads
- Ankle braces
- Taping

Environment

Environmental factors that may play lead to an increase risk of injury include:

- Weather
  - Temperature
  - Rain
  - Icy conditions
  - Fog
  - Snow
  - Wind

- Surface
  - Uneven surface increases risk of injury
  - Hard surface may lead to greater force on musculoskeletal system
  - Inappropriately slippery surface can lead to injuries
- Facilities
  - Availability of first aid equipment
  - Availability of qualified staff
  - Appropriate free space around the playing area
  - Protective padding around the playing field if indicated
  - Field equipment must be regularly checked to ensure it is in working order

Technique

Poor technique can lead to injury. It is, however, difficult to define what 'good' technique is, but it should consist of efficient and comfortable movements with least effort in order to perform the optimal sporting task. Correct technique acquired at an early stage prevents developing bad habits. Poor techniques in jumping, landing, stroke, swing, serve, throw, kick, grip, boxing and posture can all lead to injuries. It is important to emphasise that technique may need to be changed as a result of injury. This is where the role of biomechanist becomes important in management of sports injuries.

Rules

All rules must take the safety of the athletes into consideration and should ensure maximum protection for the athlete. Equally, it is vital that these are followed by all parties concerned including the athletes themselves, coaches, managers, medical staff, referee and the athletes. When rules are not followed heavy punishments must be enforced especially if the safety of any individual is compromised as a consequence.

Cool down

It has been suggested that cool down reduces risk of injury and optimises performance by:
- Allowing gradual drop in heart rate
- Allowing continued oxygen delivery to muscles; therefore, their restoration to the condition that they were prior to exercise
- Enabling removal of lactic acid and other waste products from the muscle
- Promoting flexibility
- Lowering risk of muscle soreness

Cooling down should include gentle aerobic exercise (jogging) and stretching.

Injury monitoring

Data collection of injuries and circumstances associated with the injuries should be an important part of any sport injury prevention strategy. As important is analysis of these data and implementing changes in order to reduce the risk of the injuries occurring again.

Further reading

Walker B. Sports and injury prevention, Chapt 2. Chichester; Lotus publishing, 2007:13-42.

MacKay M, Scanian A, Olsen L et al. Looking for the evidence: a systemic review of prevention strategies addressing sport and recreational injury among children and youth. J Sci Med Sport 2004; 7:58–73.

Witvrouw E, Mahieu N, Danneels L et al. Stretching and injury prevention, an obscure relationship. Sports Med 2004; 34:443–449.

Related topics of interest

Psychology – performance enhancement

Key points

- The benefits of sport psychology
- Sport psychology interventions can be used to enhance performance
- The value of an integrated approach

The benefits of sport psychology

Sport psychologists are consulted primarily for performance related issues. Athletes can spend years physically training for an event yet spend little time in developing strong mental skills. Research has shown that mental training becomes increasingly important in order to progress to higher levels of performance. So the aim of sport psychology is therefore to help athletes develop or strengthen the mental skills required in order to enhance performance. Most psychologists operate according to a cognitive–behavioural model and work on developing focus, reducing anxiety and increasing confidence.

The Cognitive Behavioural model examines how thoughts influence thinking and behaviour. There is a causal relationship between the occurrence of an event and the resultant outcome. However, in between the cause and the consequence, there are thinking processes that are highly influential in performance. Psychological training can help athletes to examine and control their thoughts. Techniques that include focus, imagery, stress management, breathing techniques, self talk and thought stopping can empower athletes to perform optimally as well as to work under pressure.

Sport psychology interventions

Focus is a mental skill that helps athletes concentrate on the tasks at hand. Irrelevant distractions, whether internal (such as unwanted thoughts) or external (such as crowds), can impede success. In addition to focus on the outcome of the event and not concentrate on the process of the event or activity can hinder a successful outcome. A focus on the present by developing a mindset of performing in the moment has been demonstrated to be effective. Whether focus should be broad, narrow or a combination is also part of focus training and developing a strong preperformance routine can facilitate achievement.

Elite coaches and athletes all profess to using imagery as a technique in achieving top-level performance. Imagery is about using the mind to recreate a picture of a sport skill or strategy. It requires the use of the entire sensory system as it involves the integration of visual, auditory and kinaesthetic senses. Developing competency in imagery necessitates being able to control the image as well as the vividness. Imagery can be used to rehearse, motivate, control emotions and learn new strategies. Athletes can visualise internally by seeing themselves through their own eyes do a skill (internal imagery) or by watching themselves as if being filmed by a camera (external imagery).

The managing of anxiety is absolutely vital in dealing with competitive stress. High anxiety levels not only make the athlete more susceptible to injury but also affect concentration and subsequently performance. When the pressure of the event leads to worry and apprehension then confidence can dwindle. Anxiety or stress management can reduce the physical tension and help to relax the mind. Autonomic responses such as heart rate can also be controlled and can be combined with biofeedback methods. There are various methods to achieve this relaxation such as progressive muscle relaxation where athletes learn to distinguish between tension and relaxation. The aim is to gain the skill of relaxing muscles at will. Relaxing under pressure, simulating intense and actual

Psychology – sports injuries

Key points

- Stress increases the likelihood of injury
- There is a psychological response to injury that affects recovery
- Psychological interventions can be integrated within a sport rehabilitation plan

The relationship between stress and injury

Integrating psychological injury prevention and intervention techniques with physiological approaches provides athletes with the opportunity of minimising their chances of injury and of optimising their performance. Integrating a psychological programme within a physical recovery programme will enable athletes to be both psychologically and physically fit upon return to sport.

Athletes in preparing for competition spend a great deal of time in training and attempt to stay injury free in order to obtain optimise performance. However, psychological rehabilitation of injury begins prior to the onset of an injury. Research has consistently shown that athletes or players who have higher stress levels have higher incidence of injury (or are more prone to injury). One of the most robust relationships between psychology and sport is this link between stress and injury. According to the Andersen and Williams model the perception or cognitive appraisal of stressors as well as personality, history and coping mechanisms plays a role in increasing the likelihood of injury.

Stressors, e.g. heavy training schedules or frequent travel, place immense pressure on athletes. How these stressors are dealt with are based on individual factors such as perception, personality, previous experiences and coping styles. Perception is the way an athlete thinks about the situation and this can be altered if it is not productive. Some personality characteristics can have a negative affect on behaviour such as anxiety, anger and perfectionism. Previous history or experiences of injury including the severity and type of previous injury can affect the athlete's thinking. Strategies for coping may be limited or stretched in a competitive situation. Athletes may use emotional coping strategies and/or problem focused strategies. Coping mechanisms will impact on whether a competition is viewed as a challenge, something that is facilitative.

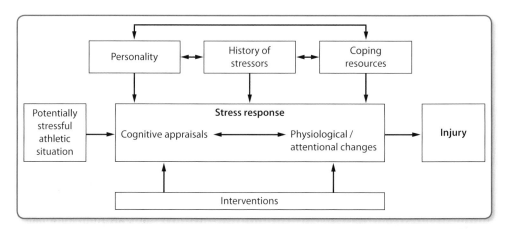

Figure 31 The stress and injury model (From Psychosocial antecedents of sport injury: Review and critique of the stress and injury model by Williams and Andersen (1998) reprinted by permission of the publisher (Taylor and Francis Ltd, http://www.tandf.co.uk/journals).

The relationship between these factors varies with the individual and is dynamic. Consider this example, an athlete negatively appraises the impact of a competition, attention is distracted, muscle tension increased, the athlete has had previous injury that he or she is considering, his or her anxiety is high and coping resources are low, resulting in an distortion of the accuracy of performance and an injury.

Psychological response to injury

Psychological factors are an integral part of the rehabilitative process as the pain and loss of functioning experience by having an injury has a strong psychological component. Research has shown that psychological factors can affect the outcome of the rehabilitative cycle. Injury is a stressor that has strong ramifications for biological, psychological and social functioning. There may be loss of identity as the athlete is not competing or training and this has been shown to parallel the grief process of denial, anger, bargaining, depression and acceptance. Alternatively, how athletes respond may be based on the meaning aligned with the injury, i.e. does it mean relegation or an end of a career. It is difficult for athletes to cope with the lost of identity as an athlete or loss of physical ability due to injury. The cognitive, emotional and behavioural reaction of athletes to injury differs noticeably and is impacted by a variety of individual and situational factors.

Injury can generate feelings of anger, anxiety, depression, embarrassment and frustration. In general, immediately following injury negative emotions increase and then postinjury, emotions fluctuate while athletes adjust to their current state and regain strength. Emotional distress can be clinical, so it is important to keep an eye on potential clinical pathological conditions and if necessary actions.

Cognitive response

Athletes vary in their interpretation of injury, and their perceptions on this contribute substantially to how they adjust psychologically. Injuries perceived as threatening to one's self-identity and well-being are more likely to produce adverse psychological reactions. Typical responses include a sense of low self-worth. Attribution may take place including blaming injury on internal factors such as lack of physical readiness or overtraining. Alternatively, athletes may attribute failure to external reasons such as opponents, coaches or weather. Confidence is often low during this period.

Behavioural responses

Cognitive and emotional responses are closely linked in with how an athlete reacts behaviourally. In fact, adherence and recovery are positively correlated. They are affected positively when athletes feel empowerment within their rehabilitative programme. However, adherence is not the sole factor or determinant for successful outcome. Even if the athlete attends all rehabilitation sessions and sticks to an exercise plan, other emotional problems can, e.g., impair the immune system and result in a slower healing process.

Interventions and prevention

Working with athletes on psychological interventions requires rapport building, education about techniques, implementation through practice and eventually mastery.

Biofeedback involves using physiological information to adjust both physiological and psychological states. This has been found to be effective in recovering and improving range of motion from knee surgery. Relaxation or stress management techniques can be used to calm the client and along with imagery techniques can be used as a way of distracting the athlete from negative thoughts and anxiety, perhaps due to pain. Imagery or visualisation can be used for recovery, emotional control and as a coping strategy. Imagery is effective as part of the healing process and has been shown to assist the mind-body in improving. Imagery can also help the athlete to practice mentally when physically it is not possible. Positive self-talk can be used to help change negative thoughts. Using self-talk generates a positive internal dialogue to offset and challenge negative thinking. Athletes learn to replace negative thoughts with more productive ones. Self-talk can improve emotional state, bolster motivation and encourage adherence to rehabilitation.

Psychology is often looked at being a cure rather than as a preventative approach. However, psychological techniques can be used at any time before, during or following an injury and are integral to the comprehensive training of athletes.

Further reading

Brewer B (ed.). Sport psychology: handbook of sports medicine and science. Springfield, MA: IOC Medical Commission Publication, Wiley-Blackwell, 2009.

Cohen R, Nordin S, Abrahamson E. Psychology and Sport Rehabilitation. London: Wiley-Blackwell, 2010.
Williams JM, Andersen MB. Psychosocial antecedents of sport injury: review and critique of the stress and injury model. J Appl Sport Psychol 1998; 10: 5–25.

Related topics of interest

Pulmonary disorders and exercise

Key points

- Most pulmonary disorders are compatible with exercise provided there is adequate recognition prior to exercise
- Exercise-induced asthma (EIA) is common and occurs in 50–80% of asthmatics and should be distinguished from vocal cord dysfunction (VCD) that can also mimic wheezing during exercise
- Exercise can induce allergic reactions that need to be recognised and preventative measures taken in advance by potential athletes

Background

EIA or bronchospasm and VCD are perhaps the two most common and disabling acute pulmonary disorders that may limit exercise in athletes. Exercise-induced anaphylaxis and urticaria are rare conditions. The aim of this Topic is to review these specific pulmonary conditions that may impact the ability to perform exercise.

Exercise-induced asthma

EIA in which bronchospasm is induced by exercise is common and occurs in 50–80% of asthmatics, 40% of people with allergic rhinitis and 10% of healthy subjects. Symptoms include wheeze, cough, shortness of breath and chest discomfort. Furthermore, postexercise cough is the commonest symptom while wheezing may be absent. Symptoms usually occur 5–10 min after the start of exercise has begun and peak 5–10 min after the cessation of exercise and resolve approximately 30 min after exercise has ended. Cold, dry air is more likely to induce EIA.

Diagnosis is established using exercise and lung function testing with particular emphasis on results that are compatible with an obstructive lung disorder in relation to exercise. Methacholine or histamine challenge test may also assist.

In those who suffer with chronic asthma, it is important to successfully treat the underlying condition. This involves the avoidance of specific allergens such as house dust mite, together with pharmacological treatment. Routine usage of inhaled corticosteroids improves pre-exercise FEV_1 and reduces the propensity to develop EIA. Additional agents include leukotriene modifiers and long-acting beta$_2$-adrenergic agents. Montelukast, a leukotriene receptor antagonist, has been shown to be superior to the long-acting beta$_2$-adrenertic agonist salmeterol in preventing EIA in patients with chronic asthma.

Athletes may also control EIA by performing a period of exercise prior to the actual exercise event. In some cases, initial exercise may be followed by a period of relative refractoriness to EIA if a second period of exercise is commenced approximately 1 h afterwards. Thus, nonpharmacologic options include induction of a relative refractory period and controlling atmospheric conditions (e.g. cold). Avoidance of winter sports and exercising indoors under climate-controlled conditions minimises the occurrence of EIA.

Other pharmacologic options include the use of inhaled beta$_2$-adrenergic agonists such as salbutamol (albuterol) or inhaled sodium cromoglycate (cromolyn sodium) 15 min before exercise. Sodium cromoglycate is not as effective in preventing EIA when compared with beta$_2$-adrenergic agents that may prevent EIA in up to 90% (sodium cromoglycate may prevent EIA in up to 40% of patients). Athletes should, therefore, take the regular daily requirements of these drugs in combination with an extra dose before exercise.

Training goals in an athlete with EIA are no different than for normal subjects and asthmatics should choose their exercise and training activities carefully. It should be remembered that cold, dry air exacerbates asthma and is a major factor in inducing EIA.

Activities that do not generate high minute ventilations such as tennis, handball, karate, wrestling, and golf are preferred, as are water activities such as swimming, diving, water polo. High minute-ventilation activities such as long distance running, cycling, basketball and football or those taking place in a cool and dry climate such as ice hockey and ice skating are more likely to induce EIA.

Vocal cord dysfunction

VCD is characterised by inappropriate vocal cord adduction during the respiratory cycle. This condition is more common in young female athletes. Patients may feel that they are unable to get air in and they may also develop wheezing and shortness of breath. Unlike asthma there is a lack of responsiveness to bronchodilators.

Many patients with VCD are thought to suffer with EIA and they may initially be referred with this condition. Pulmonary function testing as well as exercise testing may be useful to distinguish between these two conditions. Evidence of upper airway obstruction is often elucidated during an exercise test. In addition, the diagnosis can be made using direct laryngoscopy after the signs of VCD have been triggered with exercise.

Treatment is effective both for immediate relief and prevention. Panting or coughing may abort an attack and some patients should be advised to attempt to stop an attack using such manoeuvres. Additional interventions that may help include administration of a short-acting sedative or inhalation of heliox (a mixture of helium and oxygen), which helps by reducing flow resistance, as it is a less dense gas. Other measures include speech therapy consultation to teach diaphragmatic breathing and oral airway relaxation during an attack. Chronic use of sedatives or antidepressants may also be useful in preventing or reducing the incidence of attacks.

Exercise-induced anaphylaxis and urticaria

Exercise-induced urticarial disease may manifest with the development of small papules surrounded by an erythematous region. It is a mast cell disorder and involves increased levels of histamine, tryptase and leukotrienes. There may also be single larger (10–20 cm) macular erythematous and pruritic lesions. Lesions usually appear on the upper thorax or neck but may spread. Classically, they appear in response to exercise, passive warming, and emotional stress. A more dangerous a potentially fatal presentation is exercise-induced anaphylaxis. As well as urticaria, there may be angioedema together with upper airway obstruction and hypotension. Symptoms include shortness of breath, wheezing, dizziness, loss of consciousness, as well as gastrointestinal symptoms and headache. These symptoms may last 30 min to 4 h after termination of exercise.

The diagnosis of exercise-induced urticaria or anaphylaxis is based primarily on history. A history of atopy is also supportive. For patients suspected of having this condition, an exercise test (with emergency equipment readily available) can be performed to elucidate symptoms. A negative test does not exclude the diagnosis, however, as the presentation is variable.

Treatment should be directed at modifying activities. Patients should not exercise alone and should have epinephrine (adrenaline) available at all times. These are usually prescribed as an EpiPen device (a small autoinjector that delivers a single dose of 0.3 mg) with a back up device. Patients should be taught to administer the device as an intramuscular injection. They should also be advised not to exercise within 4–6 h after eating and in the case of women it is recommended that they should not exercise in the perimenstrual period. Patients who develop symptoms should stop exercising and administer epinephrine immediately.

Antihistamines are also effective in preventing this condition and as with anaphylaxis of any kind may be sufficient to prevent the condition if administered early as an intravenous preparation (IV Piriton° 10 mg (UK) or Benadryl° 50 mg (USA) are commonly used preparations). In addition, the patient should have 200 mg IV hydrocortisone administered as soon as possible. As with other allergic conditions sodium cromoglycate (cromolyn sodium), leukotriene antagonists, antihistamines, ranitidine and other H2 antagonists as well as tranexamic acid (an antifibrinolytic agent that is also a potent inhibitor of the complement system) may also play a role in the prevention and treatment of exercise-induced anaphylaxis.

Further reading

Chandratilleke MG, Carson KV, Picot J, et al. Physical training for asthma. Cochrane Database Syst Rev 2012; 16:5.

Helenius I, Lumme A, Haahtela T. Asthma, airway inflammation and treatment in elite athletes. Sports Med 2005; 35:565–574.

Morton AR, Fitch KD. Australian Association for Exercise and Sports Science position statement on exercise and asthma. J Sci Med Sport 2011; 14:312–316.

Related topics of interest

- Chest injuries – chest wall (p. 40)
- Chest injuries – intrathoracic (p. 43)

Shin pain

Key points

- Medial tibial stress syndrome (MTSS) and tibial stress fractures may be considered to be at opposite ends of a spectrum of pathology
- Imaging aids the diagnosis
- The key management principle is rest and activity avoidance

Aetiology

Shin pain is a common symptom of overuse in athletes. The differential diagnosis includes MTSS, tibial stress fractures, compartment syndrome and popliteal artery entrapment, infection and tumour, e.g. Ewings sarcoma, osteoid osteoma and eosinophillic granuloma.

MTSS is one of the most common leg injuries occurring in 4–35% of athletes and military personnel. Differing terms have been applied to the same entity: shin soreness, tibial stress syndrome and medial tibial syndrome.

Detmer has subdivided MTSS into three types:

- Type 1 is a tibial microfracture with bone stress reaction or cortical fracture
- Type 2 is perisotalgia from chronic avulsion of the periosteum at the periosteal fascial junction
- Type 3 is considered to be chronic compartment syndrome

Risk factors for MTSS have been shown to include a previous history of MTSS, a high BMI > 30, females have a relative risk double that of males, the presence of increased pronation with heel strike, increased internal tibial rotation, increased calcaneal valgus, a leaner calf girth, decreased standing foot angle and finally increased hip rotation.

Tibial stress fractures are fatigue fractures, where abnormal or unaccustomed forces are applied to bone of normal quality.

Stress fractures of the tibia are one of the commonest of comprising 46% of cases presenting to a sports injury clinic pa. Bilateral involvement occurs in 16.6% of cases. 51% fractures are found in the middle/distal thirds of the tibia and 22.2% progress to nonunion.

Anterior cortical fractures tend to occur in jumping sports, gymnasts and dancers whereas posteromedial fractures are usually found in runners, footballers and military recruits. Fractures may be considered to occur due to Wolff's law with bone responding to the forces subjected upon it. Bone strain has been assessed during different activities. During mid-stance posterior strain is three times the anterior strain. On jumping, the anterior strain is double the posterior strain found in mid-stance. The tibia may be subjected to increased local forces as calf muscles fatigue. Muscles normally oppose abnormal tibial bending and with fatigue increases by 25% within the tibial shaft. It is notable that within the tibia all muscles lie posterior to the bone's anatomical axis.

Additional risk factors to those causing MTSS include having a narrow tibia together with those causing reduced bone healing and stress compensation: smoking, NSAIDs, female athlete triad etc.

Clinical features

MTSS features pain in the posteromedial border of the tibia, worsening with exercise. The diagnosis is classically made by the presence of a diffuse area of tibial tenderness extending over 5 cm (Yates and White definition) at the insertion of the soleus rather than the tibialis posterior, which typically inserts 7.5 cm proximal to the medial malleolus. At the early stages, the pain comes on with the onset of sporting activity before easing and then returning with prolonged exercise. With continued severity, the pain may be continuous and can continue following cessation of activity.

In tibial stress fractures, pain is localised to the tibia with local rather than diffuse tenderness. Percussion of the tibia may also reproduce symptoms.

Investigations

MTSS: Radiographs may remain normal; however, bone scan reveals periostitis at the medial tibial edge.

Stress fractures: Radiographs reveal faint radiolucent striations on the anterior cortex on plane radiographs present after a couple of weeks. These preclude the dreaded black line (burrows). Plain radiographs are most specific modality and as much as a 50% change in the appearance of the cancellous bone is required to be seen on plain films, whereas correspondingly the most sensitive investigation is bone scintigraphy. Magnetic resonance imaging also has high sensitivity revealing oedematous medullary changes on T1 and STIR sequences and altered marrow signal on T2W sequences. Imaging allows tibial stress fractures to be graded and return to play determined.

Management

Treatment recommendations for MTSS include calf muscle training, antipronation insoles, massage, maintaining aerobic fitness, electrotherapy and acupuncture. No intervention has been shown to be more effective than rest. Surgical intervention consisting of fasciotomy may be considered after the failure of conservative therapy. This has been shown to lead to good/excellent results in 69–92% of patients, although RTP times vary considerably. Only shock absorbing insoles have been shown to reduce the incidence of MTSS.

The management of stress fractures must feature the identification and treatment of predisposing factors together with treating the fracture itself. Simple measures such as rest and the reduction of loading activity by braces and internal fixation are beneficial.

The use of a pneumatic air brace off loads the bone onto the surrounding soft tissues. This increase in soft tissue pressure is thought not only to reduce deforming forces on the bone itself but also to promote healing by encouraging a fluid shift to increase the intravascular hydrostatic pressure. This may stimulate osteoblasts according to the piezoelectric effect. In studies, the use of the air brace lead to a significant reduced time to return to training. In Batt's series, patients returned to their previous activity level in 12 months. Other modalities include the use of pulsed low energy ultrasound therapy. The mechanism by which this improves healing is not completely understood.

Given the risks associated with operative intervention, at least 6 months of nonoperative treatment should be attempted before surgical intervention is considered. Surgical intervention consists of the removal of the thickened fibrous tissue at the fracture non-union site, drilling of the hypovascular sclerotic bone to improve blood flow and stabilisation of the fracture site. This may be traditionally fixed using intramedullary nailing; however, this have consequences for healing by interference with the endosteal blood supply and may lead anterior knee pain. Alternatively, a plate fixation may be used as a tension band, converting tensile forces into compressile. Local wound healing has been considered to be a complication of plate fixation. Internal stabilisation of the fracture may typically alleviate symptoms within 6 weeks although radiographic union lags considerably behind clinical union and may take up to 6 months to occur.

Return to sport

Decisions regarding RTS can be made based upon a graduated resumption of loading and imaging findings.

Further reading

Carmont MR, Mei-Dan O, Bennell KL. Stress fracture management: current classification and new healing modalities. Oper Tech Sports Med 2009; 17(2):81-89.

Meon MA, Tol JL, Weir A et al. Medial tibial stress syndrome. Sports Med 2009; 39:523–546.

Shindle MK, Endo Y, Warren RF et al. Stess fractures about the tibia, foot and ankle. J Am Acad Ortho Surg 2012; 20:167–176.

Related topics of interest

• Compartment syndromes (p. 48)

• Nerve entrapment syndromes – lower limb (p. 199)

Shoulder – acromioclavicular joint injuries

Key points

- Common injury in contact sports
- Treatment is dependent on the grade of the injury
- Grades I/II injuries could be treated nonoperatively; Grades IV, V and VI usually require surgery. Management of grade III injuries is controversial

The incidence of acromioclavicular joint (ACJ) dislocation is estimated to be at three or four per 100,000 per annum in the general population. Up to 40% of sports shoulder injuries are due to ACJ disruption. These injuries are more common in males, in particular those in the second or third decades.

Anatomy

The ACJ is surrounded by a thin fibrous capsule and contains an intra-articular disc. The joint is reinforced by the superior, inferior, anterior and posterior acromioclavicular (AC) ligaments. The deltotrapezius aponeurosis merges with the parallel fibres of the superior AC ligament, making it the strongest and most biomechanically important of the AC ligaments. The AC ligaments provide horizontal stability to the joint and vertical stability at small physiological loads. The coracoclavicular (CC) ligaments (conoid and trapezoid) provide vertical stability to the joint at higher physiological loads. The displacement of the bone ends that occurs after AC dislocation is caused by sagging of the shoulder girdle rather than by superior displacement of the clavicle.

Mechanism of injury

This is most commonly due to a force applied directly over the superolateral border with the humerus adducted. Rarely, a fall onto an outstretched hand and a downward force on the upper extremity can cause ACJ injuries.

Classification

Rockwood's classification based on the extent of disruption of the AC and coracoclavicular ligaments using the radiological degree of displacement of the clavicle relative to the acromion is most commonly used in clinical practice (**Figure 32**; **Table 22**).

Clinical features

- Pain, swelling, bruising and tenderness over the ACJ
- Prominent clavicle may be evident depending on the grade of the injury
- Pain on shoulder abduction
- Positive cross-body adduction test

Investigations

Radiographs:
- AP, scapular 'Y' and axillary views of the shoulder
- Zanca view (AP angled 20° cephalad) removes AC joint overlap with scapular spine
- Stress views performed when suspicion is high but radiographs are negative

Magnetic resonance imaging (MRI)
- This is not widely used, but may provide information about the extent of injury to the ligaments and the deltotrapezius aponeurosis and help determine the degree of degenerative changes in patients who present with delayed symptoms. Additionally, a significant proportion of these injuries are associated with other shoulder injuries that the MRI may help to diagnose.

Management
Type I and II injuries

Nonoperative treatment is preferred in patients with these injuries. It involves simple analgesia, topical ice therapy and rest in a broad arm sling (causes less shoulder

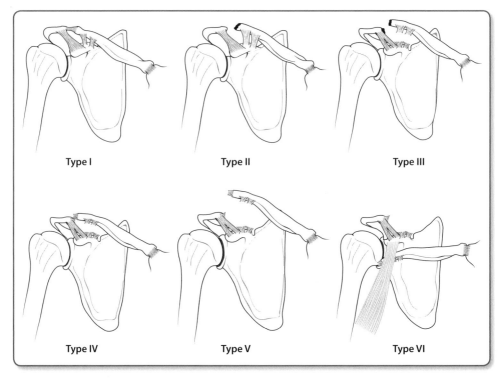

Figure 32 Rockwood's classification of ACJ injuries.

Table 22 Rockwood's classification of ACJ injuries			
Grade	AC ligament	CC ligament	Clavicle displacement
I	Sprain	Intact	None
II	Ruptured	Sprain	None; widening of AC joint (>6 mm)
III	Ruptured	Ruptured	Superior displacement (≤100% relative to acromion)
IV	Ruptured	Ruptured	Posterior
V	Ruptured	Ruptured	Superior displacement (>100% relative to acromion)
VI	Ruptured	Ruptured	Inferior

sagging than a collar 'n' cuff). The sling can be discarded once the acute symptoms have settled, usually 10–14 days after the injury. Physical therapy exercises to restore range of movement and strength are started as soon as pain allows. Contact sports and heavy lifting should be avoided for up to 12 weeks after injury.

Type III injuries

Management is controversial with both nonoperative (described above) and operative treatments being described in the literature. There may be some evidence to suggest that patients with a high level of functional demand on the shoulder, i.e.

overhead athletes may benefit from surgical treatment.

Type IV, V and VI injuries

Operative treatment is recommended in patients who sustain these injuries. A wide variety of operative procedures have been described, but none has been shown to be superior to the others. The different surgical options can be classifies as follows:

- **AC joint fixation:** This technique involves the use of Kirschner wires, screws or plates, i.e. Hook plates to hold the acromion-clavicle–coracoid triad in a reduced position long enough to allow healing of the ruptured CC and AC ligaments
- **CC stabilization:** Screws or sutures (e.g. TightRope) (**Figure 33**) are utilised to connect the coracoid process to the distal clavicle in a reduced position long enough to allow healing of the ruptured CC and AC ligaments
- **Distal clavicle excision and CC ligament reconstruction (Weaver-Dunn procedure).** Excision of the distal clavicle with a coracoid-based transfer of the CA ligament

- **Free graft anatomical reconstruction:** Autograft (hamstrings tendon), allograft or synthetic grafts are used as a free graft for reconstructing the CC ligament

Return to sport

Return to sport is permitted once the athlete is pain free, able to achieve a full range of movement and has regained enough strength to perform their sport-specific activities. With nonoperative management, as far as Type I and II injuries are concerned, return to sports usually takes 1–4 weeks depending on the sport. With Type III injuries, return to sport may be slower than Type I and II injuries. After rehabilitation, the strength and endurance are similar to those of the uninjured shoulder and most patients return to their previous level of employment, sport and recreational activities. Return to sport following operative management usually takes 6 months.

Long-term prognosis

With nonoperative treatment, an aching discomfort may be felt in the area of the

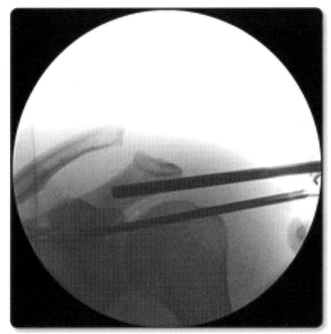

Figure 33a Fluoroscopy images at the beginning of the procedure showing the ACJ separation. The two rods seen are the scope and the radio frequency device used to clear soft tissue under the corocoid.

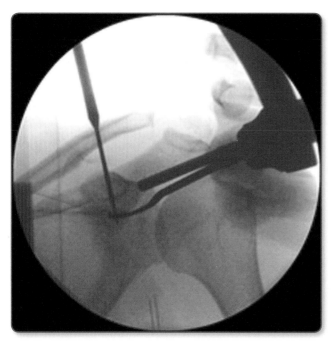

Figure 33b Drill guide is used to drill both the clavicle and corocoid.

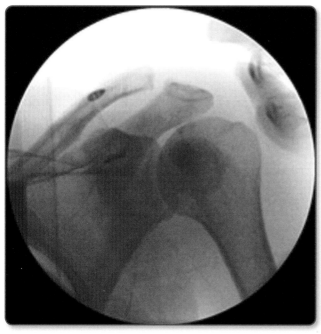

Figure 33c Tight-Rope is passed and tightened. The endo-buttons, one under the corocoid and other over the clavicle can be seen. ACJ separation is reduced.

injured joint for up to 6 months after injury and up to one-third of those with Type I and II injuries have pain on activity at longer term follow-up. This may be due to degenerative changes in ACJ, which is seen in about 35% of the patients who have had ACJ injuries. Osteolysis of the lateral end of the clavicle can occur after a variable period following these injuries. In most cases, symptoms commonly resolve within 2 years. Calcification of the coracoclavicular space appears to be common following both operative and nonoperative management of ACJ injuries. This calcification, however, does not usually affect the final clinical or functional outcome.

Further reading

Fraser-Moodie JA, Shortt NL, Robinson CM. Injuries to the acromioclavicular joint. JBJS (Br) 2008; 90:697–707.

Related topics of interest

Shoulder – acute dislocation

Key points

- Vast majority of shoulder dislocations are anterior but beware of posterior dislocations as these are sometimes missed.
- Look for associated rotator cuff tear in particular in those above the age of 50.
- Different reduction techniques have been described but generally speaking traction techniques are safer than leverage ones.

Overview

The shoulder joint is the most commonly dislocated joint with its stability being sacrificed for range of movement. Over 95% of the shoulder dislocations are traumatic in nature. The vast majority of the dislocations are anterior (95%), but they may also be posterior (4%) and inferior (1%).

Epidemiology

The incidence of shoulder dislocation is estimated to be 17 per 100,000. It is also very common in athletes with over 70% of all anterior dislocations occurring as a consequence of athletic activity. There appears to be a bimodal distribution with peaks in second and sixth decade. In the young active population, it is more common in males than in females.

Predisposing factors

Risk factors include:
1. Prior dislocation or subluxation
2. Increased joint laxity
3. Involvement in sports that are either violent or force the glenohumeral joint into extreme positions
4. Excessive retroversion of the humeral head
5. Neuromuscular conditions such as cerebral palsy

Pathology

Both static and dynamic factors contribute to shoulder stability. Static factors include:
1. Bony articulation
2. Labrum
3. Capsule and its thickenings which form the various glenohumeral ligaments
4. Adhesion–cohesion between the intra-articular fluid and joint surfaces
5. Negative intra-articular pressure producing a vacuum effect

Dynamic stability is provided by the musculature around the shoulder. These include the rotator cuff, the deltoid, the long head of the bicep and the scapula.

As the glenoid only covers around 25% of the humerus, the contribution of the labrum to the stability of the glenohumeral joint is very significant. As well as adding to the depth of the glenoid and increasing the contact area of the glenoid and the humeral head, the labrum also acts as a chock block resisting glenohumeral translation. The labrum also acts as a site for the insertion of the glenohumeral ligaments. In vast majority of the cases with traumatic anterior dislocation, there is disruption of the labrum and the attached inferior glenohumeral ligaments. This is known as 'Bankart lesion' and usually occurs as a result of forced external rotation, abduction and extension of the arm forcing the glenohumeral head out of the joint. This detachment of the labrum and the glenohumeral head makes the glenohumeral joint very unstable.

Another common associated injury with traumatic anterior dislocation is a compression fracture at the posterolateral part of the humeral that occurs as a consequence of impaction of the humeral head into the glenoid edge. This is referred to as the 'Hills Sach's lesion'.

Shoulder dislocation may also be associated with rotator cuff injuries in particular with the more elderly population.

Occasionally, capsule is torn from the humerus. This is known as 'HAGL' lesion (humeral avulsion glenohumeral ligament).

Clinical features

There is usually a history of trauma. With anterior dislocation, this usually involves an indirect force to the arm in extension, abduction and external rotation, whereas with posterior dislocation occurs as a consequence of an axial directed force to an arm that is internally directed and rotated. Commonly patients complain of severe pain with decreased range of movement.

With anterior dislocation, the arm is held in abduction and external rotation.

The arm is retained in adduction and internal rotation with posterior dislocation.

There may be associated neurovascular damage in particular to axillary nerve. There may be a history of prior dislocation.

Investigations

Plain radiography involving two views (anteroposterior and axillary or Y view) will demonstrate the dislocation. This may also reveal any associated fractures; however, these may be illustrated with more detail by a computed tomography (CT) scan. MRI will demonstrate associated rotator cuff injuries and when combined with arthrogram, it will illustrate any damage to the labrum or HAGL lesion. As associated cuff tears are common in those above 50, it is important to exclude them by magnetic resonance imaging (MRI) or ultrasound.

Posterior dislocations are sometimes missed; therefore, it is important to look for them, which sometimes may require CT scan.

Treatment

Acute dislocation will require reduction. Various close reduction techniques are advocated. These include:

1. Patient lies prone, the affected arm hangs vertically from the table with some weights attached to it. This may take twenty minutes before the shoulder is relocated
2. With patient lying supine, while an assistant provides counteraction by pulling a sheet that has been rapped around the chest, the clinician gently pulls and rotates the affected arm to unhinge the dislocated humeral head
3. Clinician abducts and externally rotates the affected arm while the same time disengaging the humeral head with his or her thumb

4. Clinician's foot is placed under the athlete's axilla while applying gentle longitudinal traction to the arm (hippocratic method)
5. With the elbow flexed to 90°, the arm is externally rotated, elbow brought forward. The arm is adducted next and finally internally rotated. This is known as Kocher's method and is an example of leveraging technique. With this technique, there is a risk causing fracture and nerve injury.
6. Longitudinal traction is applied to the arm with extended elbow and forearm in neutral rotation. Next, starting from 0° abduction, the arm is brought slowly into abduction while at the same time applying vertical oscillations to the arm. When arm is past 90° of abduction, the arm is brought into external rotation at same time as continued vertical oscillations (reduction is said to be usually achieved at around 120° of abduction (FARES method)

Reduction of posterior dislocation involves prolonged axial traction on the humerus while manually applying pressure to the humerus head in order to disengage it.

In those above age of 40, it is safer to perform the reduction under GA, and sedation as failure to do so may result in fracture or propagation of a simple fracture into a complicated on.

The issue of shoulder immobilisation following reduction is controversial. Traditionally, sling immobilisation for 3 weeks have been advocated in order to reduce the chances of recurrent dislocation. This concept has been challenged more recently as some studies show even higher rates of recurrent dislocation following immobilisation. There also a number of studies that have demonstrated that immobilisation in external rotation rather than internal rotation is better for the healing of an associated labrum tear and results in fewer recurrent dislocations. It is, however, important to mention that recent studies on external rotation brace have not matched the outcomes of earlier studies on external rotation brace and their use remains controversial.

Regardless of whether immobilisation is used or not, isometric exercises are initiated as soon as pain subsides. This is followed by range of movement and isotonic exercises. More vigorous exercises, including rotator cuff strengthening, are initiated once full passive range of movement is achieved.

The redislocation rate is very high in young athletic population (as high as 90% in some studies). Because of these some advocate surgical intervention following first time dislocation in such athletes. Surgery is in the form of a stabilisation procedure and is thought to significantly reduce the redislocation rate (as low as 10%).

Return to sport

With both operative and nonoperative management, the athlete should only be allowed to return to sport only after achieving full strength and range of movement. With none operative management this may take 2–3 months. Following surgery, the average return to sport is between 4 and 6 months, but may be as long as 12 months.

Further reading

Atoun E, Narvani A, Even T, et al. Management of first time dislocations of the shoulder in patients over 40 years of age: the Prevalence of iatrogenic fracture. J Orthop Trauma 2013; 27(4):190-193.

Dala-Ali B, Penna M, McConnell J,et al. Management of acute shoulder dislocation. Br J Sport Med 2012; 19:1–7.

Liavaag S, Brox JI, Pripp AH, et al. Anatomical Bankart repair compared with nonoperative treatment and/or arthroscopic lavage for first-time traumatic shoulder dislocation. Arthroscopy 2012; 28:565–575.

Soldal LA, Svenningen S. Immobilization in external rotation after primary shoulder dislocation did not reduce the risk of recurrence. J Bone Joint Surg Am 2011; 93:897–904.

Related topics of interest

Shoulder – impingement syndrome/rotator cuff disease

Key points

- Primary impingement is rare in young individuals, and clinicians must exclude other pathologies that can lead to secondary impingement
- Soft tissue imaging is important to exclude rotator cuff tears
- Full thickness tears do not heal on their own and best surgical outcomes are with early repair particularly with acute traumatic tears

Overview

Recognised more than 150 years ago, this syndrome is one of the most common causes of shoulder pain in athletes. It is particularly common in activities that involve repetitive overhead movements such as swimming, tennis, volleyball, throwing sports and baseball but are seen in many other types of sports as well.

Pathology

The rotator cuff consists of four muscles that include the supraspinatus, infraspinatus, teres minor and the subscapularis. The pathology of rotator cuff disease is complex and multifactorial. Furthermore, it is a spectrum of conditions. An attempt to demonstrate the pathophysiology of the process has been made by the **Figure 34**.

As demonstrated in the **Figure 34**, mechanical impingement of the rotor cuff tendon and tendinopathy of the tendon are interlinked as impingement of the tendon can aggravate tendinopathy, and tendinopathy may lead to mechanical impingement by causing swelling of the tendon in the subacromial space. Therefore, the process can develop into a viscous cycle or a positive feedback system. The percentage contribution of impingement and tendinopathy to the pathological process and symptoms production would be different in each individual athlete. Tendinopathy is characterised by degenerative changes in the tendon.

There are conditions or circumstances that initiate this cycle/positive feedback system or increase the gain of the system. These include the following.

Primary impingement

This refers to the direct mechanical impingement of the supraspinatus tendon by structure in the coracoacromial arch [acromion, coracoacromial ligaments and the acromial clavicular joint (ACJ)]. As the humerus flexes, abducts and internally rotates, the narrowing of the subcromial space becomes significant and mechanical impingement of the tendon can occur. This position is employed frequently in sports such as swimming, tennis and those that involve overhead throwing. Other factors that contribute to primary impingement include:

- Curved or hooked acromion
- Thickening of the coracoacromial ligament
- Prominent ACJ

Secondary impingement

This is thought to be the most common of impingement in young athletes.

The following pathologies can lead to secondary impingement:

1. A weak serratus anterior may not stabilise the scapula adequately that can lead to exaggerated angulation of the acromion and therefore mechanical impingement
2. In glenohumeral stability, there can be migration of the humeral head anteriorly leading to impingement of the supraspinatus tendon by the coracoacromial arch structures
3. If the delicate balance between the rotator cuff muscles and deltoid is disturbed (i.e. weak rotator cuff muscles), deltoid contraction can cause excessive migration of the humeral head that in turn may lead to impingement

modification by the athlete. A short course of NSAIDs may be prescribed. Some athletes found other modalities such as ultrasound, massage and cryotherapy helpful in controlling the pain. Subacromial cortisone injection can also provide some pain relief and prevent it causing muscular inhibition, therefore allowing adequate physical therapy. Initially, the physical therapy programme should include stretching and range of movement exercises as contracture of the capsule in athletes can worsen the impingement. Following this, the athlete must progress to strengthening exercises concentrating on all the muscle groups utilised in the athletes sport including rotator cuff muscles, scapula stabilizers, even lower limb and trunk muscles.

It is of vital importance to detect and treat any underlying causes that could have lead to impingement/tendinopathy. Instability must be addressed and dealt with (see the topic on Shoulder - instability). Abnormal scapulohumeral rhythm must be corrected. Any imbalance between deltoid and rotator cuff contraction must be rectified as excessive elevation of humeral head can lead to or exaggerate impingement/tendinopathy process. As important is the amendment of any poor technique and training regime.

Surgery is indicated if there is complete rotator cuff tear or partial tear greater than 50% (see below) or if there is no symptomatic relief despite about 6 months of nonoperative treatment. This would in the form of either arthroscopic or open procedure. Arthroscopy combined with examination under anaesthesia, will reveal other pathologies such as labral disease, instability, tight capsule and glenohumeral degenerative changes. If it is detected that impingement/tendinopathy is secondary to occult instability, it may be more appropriate to address the instability first with a stabilization procedure. The impingement/tendinopathy itself may be addressed by careful debridement, bursectomy or acromioplasty.

Prognosis

Two thirds of patients with impingement/tendinopathy respond to nonoperative management. Surgery results in satisfactory outcome in over 80% of the patients.

Return to sport

As with other sports injuries, return to play is permitted once the athlete is pain free and has regained the majority of his muscular strength in order for he/she to perform their sport safely. The time this happens is dependent on many factors including the athlete, sport, underlying cause and type of treatment. Majority of athletes with nonoperative management return within few weeks. With operative management, the accepted time for return to sport is usually within 3 months postoperatively.

Rotator cuff tears

They frequently occur on a background of impingement/tendinopathy in a chronic setting with slow creeping process but occasionally may be as a result of a single traumatic event.

Clinical features

Common symptoms include:
- Pain (worse in with abduction above 90°)
- Night pain
- Weakness

It is of vital importance to establish whether onset of symptoms has been associated with any initiating traumatic event or not.

The following test can aid in diagnosis of rotator cuff tears:
1. **Drop arm test:** The athlete is instructed to slowly lower the arm from an abduction position. In presence of a tear, this manoeuvre loses its smoothness and is no longer smooth.
2. Test for supraspinatus (**Figure 35**). A downward force is directed to the arm as the shoulder is abducted 90° and internally rotated. This test will reveal any weaknesses in the supraspinatus by comparing both sides.
3. Test for infraspinatus (**Figure 36**). The athlete is asked to externally rotate the shoulder against resistance, with the elbow flexed to 90° at the side.
4. 'Gerber's lift-off test' for subscapularis (**Figure 37**). The athlete places arm behind his body with dorsum aspect of the hand facing the lower back. Clinician then places the palm of his hand against

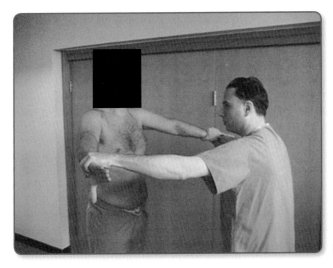

Figure 35 Test for supraspinatus.

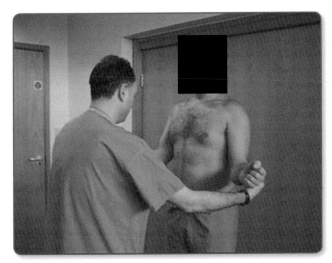

Figure 36 Testing the infraspinatus.

the palm of the athletes hand and then instructs the athlete to push his hand away from the back against resistance. Other tests for subscapularis include 'belly-press test' (**Figure 38**) and 'bear hug test'. In belly-press test, patient is asked to keep pushing the elbow forward at the same time as pushing on their abdomen with their hand flat on the belly. With subscapularis weakness, patient can only main pressure on the abdomen by flexing the wrist and moving the elbow backwards. With 'bear-hug' test patient is asked to maintain the hand of the concerned

shoulder on the opposite shoulder while the examiner applies external rotation force to the hand. Inability to maintain the hand on the opposite shoulder may suggest subscapularis pathology.

Investigations

Ultrasound and magnetic resonance imaging (MRI) (**Figure 39**) are the investigations of choice to confirm the tears (see Topics Imaging – ultrasound (US) and Imaging – magnetic resonance imaging (MRI)).

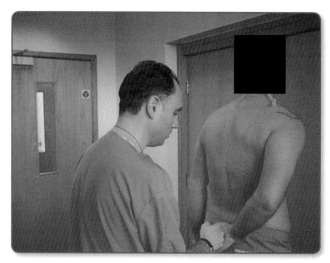

Figure 37 Gerber's lift-off test for subscapularis.

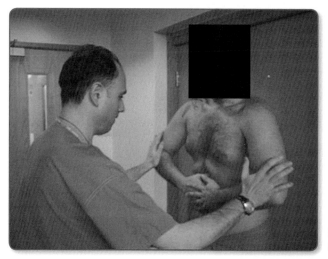

Figure 38 Belly-press test for subscapularis.

Treatment

Partial thickness tears

Treatment of partial thickness in athletes in athletes depends on a number of factors including exact sport, other associated abnormalities, athletes symptoms and degree of the partial thickness tear. Generally speaking treatment of partial-thickness tears of less than 50% is similar to that of tendinopathy/impingement.

Symptomatic partial thickness tears that involve more than 50% of the tendon thickness may require surgical repair. It is, however, important to mention that partial thickness tears in overhead/throwing athletes with internal rotation deficit may be a secondary finding. In such athletes outcome of repair may be disappointing and athlete may not return to same level of performance (see topic Shoulder - overhead and throwing athlete). Management here should focus on primary pathologies such as tight posterior inferior capsule and should mainly be nonoperative with physical therapy. Platelets rich plasma (PRP) injections may also, in

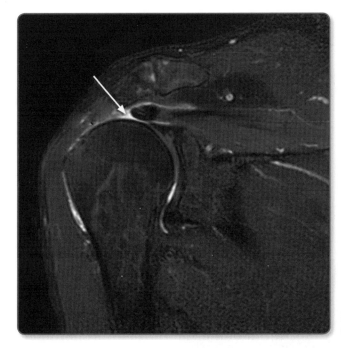

Figure 39 MRI illustrating a supraspinatus tear.

future prove to be an effective option in such patients, however, further studies are required.

Full thickness tears

Decision on how to manage full thickness tears requires an appreciation of their natural history. There is evidence that suggest:

1. Although asymptomatic rotator cuff tears are common (particularly in those above 60), a significant proportion of them do become symptomatic with time
2. When do become symptomatic, they are larger in size than when they were asymptomatic
3. Symptomatic full thickness tears do not heal and often enlarge
4. Following repairs, failure rates are greater with larger tears particularly in those older than 60
5. In presence of acute traumatic tears, the earlier repair leads to better surgical outcome

As a result of the above findings we suggest

1. Arthroscopic repair of all acute traumatic tears (**Figure 40** and **41**)
2. Arthroscopic repair in symptomatic degenerative full thickness providing patients are fit enough to have surgery, there are no contra-indications to surgery and they can comply to postoperative rehabilitation programme
3. Otherwise they may be managed none operatively with physical therapy programme consisting of:
   a. Range of motion exercises
   b. Strengthening
   c. Correction of the scapula-thoracic mechanics
   d. Correction of rotator cuff balance
   e. Anterior deltoid exercises
   f. Attention to the kinetic chain as a whole and core stability

In those that have arthroscopic repair, optimal outcome is dependent on adherence to a strict postoperative rehabilitation programme. It is also important to warn patients that they may not notice a significant improvement in their outcome for as long as 6 months postsurgery.

Return to sport following surgical repair is also dependent on many other factors including the patient and the sport. Overall

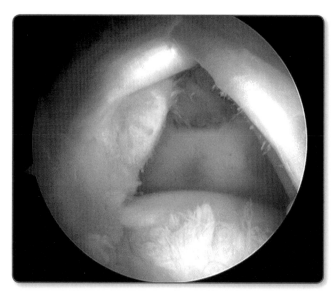

Figure 40 Arthroscopic picture if the supraspinatus tear of the same patient as figure MRI images

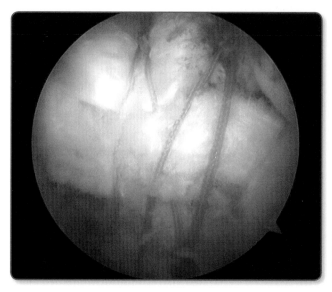

Figure 41 Picture following arthroscopic double row supraspinatus repair of the same patient as in Figures 86.6 and 86.7

athletes are expected to fully participate in sports between 8 and 12 months following surgery.

Calcific tendinopathy

The commonest site for this is the supraspinatus tendon. Calcium is deposited on the supraspinatus tendon as consequence of tendinopathy. Pain is usually intense. There is localised tenderness over the anterior upper part of the shoulder. Plain radiograph will illustrate the calcium deposits. Cortisone and local anaesthetic injection as well as 'needling barbotage' under ultrasound guidance can improve the pain. In those who do not respond to none operative management, surgical removal of the calcium deposit is successful in relieving the symptoms.

Further reading

Levy O, Narvani AA. Biomechanics of the shoulder and elbow (2010). In: Fabrizio Margheritini, Roberto Rossi (eds), Orthopedic sports medicine. Milan; Springer-Verlag, 2012:145–158.

Hughes A, Even T, Narvani AA et al. Pattern and time phase of shoulder function and power recovery after arthroscopic rotator cuff repair. J Shoulder Elbow Surg 2012; 21:1299–1303.

Mall NA, Kim HM, Keener JD, et al. Symptomatic progression of asymptomatic rotator cuff tears: a prospective study of clinical and sonographic variables. J Bone Joint Surg Am 2010; 92:2623–2633.

Related topics of interest

Shoulder – instability

Key points

- Shoulder instability may manifest in a variety of clinical features
- With 'Stanmore Classification', those with Type I instability respond well to surgery whereas those with Type III should be managed by a variety of nonoperative strategies that address muscle patterning abnormalities
- There is a shift towards treating first time Type I dislocators with arthroscopic stabilisation, particularly young athletes

Overview

Shoulder instability covers a wide range of pathological conditions that result in an abnormal motion for that joint and may manifest with a variety of clinical features including pain, subluxation or dislocation of the shoulder. It is not the same as joint laxity that refers to increased degree glenohumeral translation but still lying within the physiological range. First reported over 2000 years ago, its management still remains very controversial.

Epidemiology

Shoulder instability is a common problem in athletes. Although primary shoulder dislocation rates are comparable in younger and older patients, recurrent dislocation rate is much more common in adolescent population. Recurrent dislocation rates following primary dislocation are reported to lie between 70% to 100%, 15% to 65% and 0% to 20% in age groups 20 years and under, 20 and 40 years and 40 years or older, respectively.

Predisposing factors

Proposed risk factors include:
1. Increased joint laxity
2. Involvement in sports that are either violent or force the glenohumeral joint into extreme positions
3. Excessive retroversion of the humeral head
4. Neuromuscular conditions such as cerebral palsy
5. Young age

Pathophysiology

Both static and dynamic factors contribute to shoulder stability. Static factors include:
1. Bony articulation
2. **Labrum:** As the glenoid only covers around 25% of the humerus, the contribution of the labrum to the stability of the glenohumeral joint is very significant. As well as adding to the depth of the glenoid and increasing the contact area of the glenoid and the humeral head, the labrum also acts as a chock block resisting glenohumeral translation. The labrum also acts as a site for the insertion of the glenohumeral ligaments
3. **Capsule and its thickenings that form the various glenohumeral ligaments.** The superior glenohumeral ligaments primary function is thought to be limitation of anterior and inferior translation of adducted humerus. The middle glenohumeral ligament resists excessive anterior translation of the humerus when the arm is abducted between 60° and 90°. The inferior glenohumeral ligament (IGHL) is the strongest of the three glenohumeral ligaments, consists of three distinct parts (anterior band, axillary pouch and posterior band), and functions, like a hammock, as the primary restraints against anterior, posterior and inferior translations when the humerus is abducted further than 45°
4. Adhesion–cohesion between the intra-articular fluid and joint surfaces
5. Negative intra-articular pressure producing a vacuum effect

Dynamic stability is provided by the musculature around the shoulder. These include:
1. **Rotator cuff muscles (supraspinatus, subscapularis, infraspinatus and teres minor):** These cause compression of the humeral head into the glenoid cavity during motion

2. **Scapular rotator muscles (trapezius, rhomboids, latissimus dorsi, serratus anterior and levator scapulae):** These contribute to posterior and inferior stability of the glenohumeral stability during motion by allowing the glenoid to stay in an anteverted and superior position in order to articulate with a retroverted humeral head

3. **Long head of the biceps:** There are some reports suggesting that biceps contributes to anterior glenohumeral joint stability in external rotation and abduction by resisting the increased external rotation forces that exist in such position. However, the exact role of LHB in providing stability remains controversial

The fine balance between static and dynamic stabilisers of the shoulder joint is critical in providing the overall shoulder joint stability. This fine balance may be disturbed in a number of ways:

1. Labrum lesions:
   a. Detachment of the anterior–inferior labrum from the glenoid rim, together with its attached IGHL complex, is known as 'Bankart's lesion'. This can lead to increased anterior translation of humeral head with abduction and external rotation. In addition, there may also be excessive anterior and posterior humeral head translation with flexion, and inferior translation with extension and internal rotation of the shoulder
   b. 'Reverse Bankart's' lesion refers to detachment of the posterior-inferior part of the labrum from the glenoid rim and can lead to increased posterior and inferior humeral head translations
   c. Superior labral anterior–posterior lesions can also lead to shoulder instability

2. **Capsular lesions:** It has been argued that for a complete dislocation to occur as a consequence of capsule lesions, there must exist capsular deformation on the involved side as well as the opposite side of the joint (in order for the humerus to translate excessively, a capsular lesion in one direction must be accompanied by another lesion or capsular laxity in

the opposite direction, this is known as 'circle concept'. The capsular lesions may be in the form of tears, redundant capsular pockets or just stretched tissue. Occasionally capsule is torn from the humerus. This is known as 'HAGL' lesion (humeral avulsion glenohumeral ligament)

3. **Glenohumeral ligaments dysfunction:** These can occur either as the result of labrum or capsular lesions (see above)

4. **Muscular Dysfunction:** This may occur as a result of peripheral and central nervous system lesions, muscular and tendon pathologies

5. **Proprioception dysfunction:** It has been shown that ligaments and capsule contain neural structures and mechanoreceptors that provide proprioception feedback information that may contribute to stability by mediating muscular reflex stabilisation.

6. **Altered bony anatomy:** These rarely cause instability on their own. Examples include altered versions of the glenoid or the humerus

It is important to appreciate that for each patients, more than one of the above factors may play a part in making the shoulder unstable; therefore, when managing such athletes all the above factors must be considered.

Clinical features

History

The important features in the history include:
- Presence/absence of trauma
- Pain in the shoulder without any history of trauma may be due to shoulder subluxation
- Age
- Previous episodes
- Previous treatment (including type of physical therapy and surgery)
- Psychosocial issues

Examination

This should include:
- Specific tests for general laxity (hyperextension of the thumb, fingers elbows and the knee)

- Specific tests for shoulder laxity (anterior/posterior draw tests, Sulcus sign)
- Specific tests for shoulder instability (anterior/posterior apprehension tests)
- Detection of rotator cuff impingement and assessment of rotator cuff function.
- General shoulder girdle posture and detection of any muscular patterning disorder

Investigations

Imaging

Plain radiographs
Demonstrating acute dislocations plain films may reveal a Hill–Sachs lesion (defect in the humeral head).

CT/CT arthrography
CT (computed tomography) allows assessment bony architecture and in combination with arthrography identifies any associated labral tear.

MRI/MR arthrography (Figure 42)
As well as identifying labral/capsular pathology, these will also illustrate associated rotator cuff pathology. MR (magnetic resonance) arthrography is reported to be more sensitive and specific than MRI (magnetic resonance imaging) alone.

Electromyography
This investigation will detect any abnormalities in muscle patterning and as muscle coordination plays an important part in stability, electromyographic studies can be of great value in athletes with atraumatic multidirectional instability.

Examination under anaesthesia
Complete examination (see above) under anaesthesia may be of great value in assessment of stability; however, on its own may not be able to distinguish between laxity and instability.

Arthroscopy
Although an invasive procedure, arthroscopy is the gold standard in identifying the structural damages in the shoulder.

Classification
Based on the clinical features and investigations, in order to plan an effective

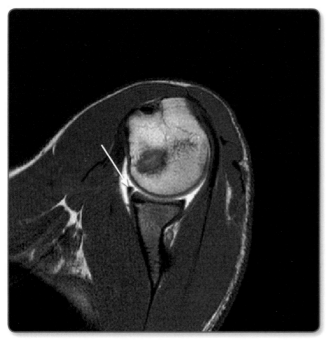

Figure 42 MR arthrogram showing anterior labrum tear.

treatment, the instability must be classified. There are many different classifications. One of the most commonly used classification system is the Thomas and Matsen classification. With this system, there are two general types of instability: TUBS and AMBRI.

TUBS stands for Traumatic Unidirectional Bankart lesion treated by Surgery.

AMBRI stands for Atraumatic Multidirectional Bilateral usually treated by rehabilitation but if surgery required, it should be by Inferior capsular shift.

Although the Thomas and Matsen classification is easy to remember, it has its limitation in that it is very rigid, and does not have a distinct category for patients who suffer from habitual instability with muscle patterning disorder and no structural damage in their glenohumeral joint.

A less rigid but more inclusive and practical system, is the Stanmore classification. With this system, the patients are divided into three main polar groups. Type I patients have a good history of trauma with some structural damage to their joint. In Type II patients, there is no history of trauma, but structural damage is present. With Type III patients there is neither a history of trauma nor any structural damage. The pathology with this type is muscle-patterning problem. In this system each type forms the angle of a triangle. Furthermore this system is a dynamic classification that allows for a shift in the pattern of instability with time.

Treatment

Management of acute dislocation is discussed in the acute shoulder dislocation Topic. Management of shoulder instability will be discussed here using Stanmore classification.

Type I (history of trauma and articular surface damage and Bankart lesion and unilateral laxity and normal muscle patterning)

Treatment of this group is by surgery.

Most Type I recurrent instabilities can be treated by arthroscopic labral repairs. However contra-indications to arthroscopic labral repairs include:

- Patients with large Hill–Sachs lesions that engage in early abduction and external rotation
- Significant glenoid bone deficiencies (>20-25%)
- Significant capsular deficiencies

In such circumstances, modified Laterjet procedure is usually procedure of choice. Although there is a lot of excitement about 'arthroscopic Laterjet', most surgeons perform the open procedure.

It is also important to mention that in recent years, particularly in young athletes (with Type I instability), arthroscopic stabilisation following first dislocation is gaining increasing popularity. This is based on the high risk of further dislocation following first dislocation in young athletes, particularly those involved in collision sports.

Type II (no clear history of trauma, but with a damaged articular surface, dysfunctional capsule and normal muscle patterning)

Those patients who do not have any underlying muscle patterning abnormality, and are pure Type II, may benefit from surgical intervention. Surgery is in the form of capsular plication and various capsular shift procedures. Laser/radio frequency capsular shrinkage procedures (capsulorrhaphy) have gone out of fashion in recent years and are utilised a lot less frequently.

Those patients who, in addition, have an associated element of muscle patterning disorder (subtype II (III)) require correction of their muscle patterning abnormality before surgery could be considered. Surgery should only be offered if underlying structural instability remains a problem despite correction of muscle patterning abnormality.

Type III (no clear history of trauma, no articular surface damage, but with abnormal muscle patterning)

Athletes in this group must be treated nonoperatively as they require correction of their inappropriate muscle recruitment. These athletes should undergo biofeedback exercises

presence of LHB instability, there may be some clicking and mechanical symptoms.

Clinical test is overall not that much accurate. There is usually tenderness over the LHB in the bicipital groove. Speed's test involves resisting forward flexion of the arm from 90° with extended elbow and supinated arm. This is positive when the manoeuvre produces pain in the bicipital groove. With Yergesson's test, resisted supination of the arm from a fully pronated position with the elbow flexed in 90° produces bicipital pain.

O'Brien's 'three-pack examination' for LHB pathology include:

1. **Tenderness in the bicipital groove:** It is a sign of pathology of LHB within the bicipital groove
2. **O'Brien test (active compression test):** With the shoulder in 90° of forward flexion and 15° of adduction, the patients is asked to resist a downward force first with the arm in pronation and internal rotation and then with the arm in external rotation and supination. This test points towards pathology at the LHB anchor (where it attaches to the superior labrum) when the first manoeuvre does produce anterior shoulder pain that is relieved be the externally rotating and supinating the arm (second manoeuvre)
3. **Throwing test:** Patient brings the arm into throwing position with external rotation and abduction. Bicipital groove pain with this motion may suggest LHB pathology, where it exists the bicipital groove

Investigations

These include:

1. **Ultrasound:** This is quite reliable for complete ruptures and dislocations. It also offers the advantage in that it is a dynamic test. It has its limitation in detecting partial thickness tears
2. **Magnetic resonance imaging (MRI):** Agreement with arthroscopic findings in detecting LHB pathologies is poor; however, MRI arthrography does improve the accuracy
3. **Arthroscopy.** Gold standard where a definite diagnosis of LHB pathology is made

Differential diagnosis

These include superior labrum anterior posterior (SLAP) lesions, anterior labrum tears, acromioclavicular joint pathologies and rotator cuff lesions.

Treatment

As LHB lesions are often associated with other shoulder pathologies such as rotator cuff tears, it is important to exclude these and treat them adequately if they coexist.

Nonoperative

These measures include:

1. Activity modification, biomechanical assessment and appropriate adjustment of technique
2. Analgesia
3. Physiotherapy
   a. Range of motion and correction of posterior-inferior capsule tightness exercises
   b. Strengthening
   c. Correction of the scapula-thoracic mechanics
   d. Correction of rotator cuff balance
   e. Attention to the kinetic chain as a whole and core stability
4. Corticosteroid injections

Operative

Options include:

1. Synovectomy
2. Debridement (when the tear involves less than 25% of the tendon)
3. Proximal insertion of the biceps (SLAP) repair
4. Tendon transfer
5. Tenotomy
6. Tenodesis (fixation of the LHB to bone or less commonly soft tissue)

Tenotomy and tenodesis are by far more the most commonly used surgical options (**Table 23**).

Tenodesis may be performed by a number of different techniques that include:

- Open V arthroscopic
- Osseous V soft tissue fixation
- Fixation above or below the bicipital groove.

Table 23 Tenotomy V tenodesis	
Advantages of tenotomy	**Advantages of tenodesis**
Technically easy to perform quick	Minimises cosmetic deformity (Popeye sign)
Avoidance of implant complications	Maintains the length tension relationship better
Little postoperative rehabilitation	Avoidance of cramping pain, however, could be associated with bicipital groove discomfort
Acceptable pain relief	

- Different fixation techniques include:
  - Anchors
  - Interference screws

Return to sport

With both operative and nonoperative management, the athlete should only be allowed to return to sport after achieving full pain free range of movement and strength as well as cardiovascular fitness. With tenodesis this may take as long as 6 months.

Further reading

Ahrens P, Boileau P. The long head of biceps and associated tendinopathy. J Bone Joint Surg (Br) 2007; 89:1001–1009.

Khazzem M, George MS, Churchill S, Kuhn JE. Disorders of the long head of biceps. J Shoulder Elbow Surg 2012; 21:136–145.

Related topics of interest

- Shoulder – impingement syndrome/rotator cuff disease (p. 259)

- Shoulder – superior labrum anterior posterior (SLAP) lesions (p. 282)

Shoulder – overhead and throwing athlete

Key points

- Shoulder complaints are common in overhead and throwing athletes
- Pathologies include posterior capsular contractures, internal rotation deficit, internal impingement, articular-sided rotator cuff tears, labral lesions, instability and scapular dysfunction
- Nonoperative treatment should always be attempted first and should focus on increasing the range of motion and improving scapular functioning, whereas operative treatment should be directed towards treating the primary pathology

Overview

The overhead throwing athlete is an extremely challenging patient in sports medicine with unique physical characteristics. A wide variety of disorders may present in the overhead thrower. The goal should be to accurately diagnose and efficiently direct treatment. The treating clinician must pay special attention to the acuity and severity of the injury with particular focus on the specific biomechanics of the sport in question. Nonoperative rehabilitation, arthroscopic and open techniques, applied judiciously, can improve shoulder biomechanics and return athletes to the sports arena as quickly and as wholly as possible.

Epidemiology

Shoulder injuries in athletes are highly prevalent in overhead and throwing sports including javelin, tennis, volleyball, baseball, water polo and swimming.

Pathology

The dominant shoulder of a thrower exhibits increased external rotation and diminished internal rotation compared with the contralateral arm. This lack of internal rotation has been referred to as glenohumeral internal rotation deficit.

Adaptations in bone and soft tissue are responsible for increased external rotation. During development, humeral retroversion decreases from about 80° to 30°. Repetitive throwing during growth is hypothesised to restrict this physiologic derotation. It has been shown that professional pitchers show 17° greater humeral retroversion in their throwing shoulder when compared with their nondominant side.

Soft tissue adaptations also occur. The anterior capsule and glenohumeral ligaments become lax, whereas the posterior capsule and glenohumeral ligaments stiffen. Repetitive microtrauma to the anterior capsule, particularly during the cocking phase of throwing, leads to anterior laxity and more external rotation.

The following leading theories have been described that explain the occurrence of the rotator cuff and labral lesions commonly encountered in the overhead throwing athlete.

Internal impingement theory

This theory describes internal impingement as occurring in the 90° abducted and 90° externally rotated (ABER) position. In this position, the posterosuperior rotator cuff contacts the posterosuperior glenoid labrum and can be pinched between the labrum and greater tuberosity. Although physiologic in a static position, forceful and repeated contact of the undersurface of the rotator cuff and the superior labrum during overhead activity can explain the development of partial-thickness rotator cuff tears and superior labrum anterior posterior (SLAP) lesions which commonly coexist in throwers.

Posterior capsular contracture theory

This proposes that the primary pathological process is posterior capsular contracture that occurs as a consequence of repetitive

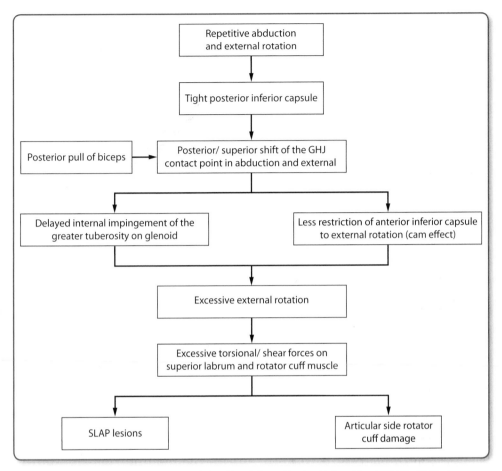

Figure 43 Glenohumeral internal rotation deficit (GIRD). From Margheritini and Rossi (2011) with kind permission of Springer Science+Business Media

throwing. The reasoning is that the posterior capsule must withstand tensile forces of up to 750 N during the deceleration and follow-through phases of throwing. These posterior tensile forces are resisted by both the eccentric contraction of the rotator cuff, primarily the infraspinatus, and the posteroinferior capsule (posterior band of the inferior glenohumeral ligament). With repetitive infraspinatus eccentric contraction, the muscle and the posteroinferior capsule become hypertrophied and stiff. The posterior contracture shifts the centre of rotation of the shoulder to a more posterosuperior location, creating posterosuperior instability with shoulder in abduction and external rotation. Additionally with this shift, there

is less obstruction to external rotation by the anterior capsule referred to as the cam effect. The humeral head can consequently externally hyper-rotate, producing increased shear in the rotator cuff tendon and more pronounced internal impingement. Furthermore, a peel-back phenomenon occurring during late cocking, consisting of a torsional force applied to the biceps anchor, contributes to SLAP lesion development.

Scapulothoracic function

The scapula plays a critical role in energy transfer from the trunk to the humerus. During cocking, when the humerus is terminally externally rotated and abducted, upward scapular rotation helps maintain glenohumeral articular congruency. Weakness, inflexibility or imbalance of the periscapular and posterior rotator cuff muscles disturb the normal anatomic static and dynamic relationships of the scapula. Abnormal scapulothoracic motion has been referred to as scapular dyskinesis. The abnormally positioned thrower's scapula has been labelled SICK (scapular malposition, inferior medial border prominence, coracoid pain and dyskinesis of scapular movement). The SICK scapula predisposes the shoulder to labral and rotator cuff tears.

Clinical features

History

Initial symptoms may be vague, such as loss of control, velocity or difficulty warming up.

Typical shoulder-related symptoms include anterosuperior or posterosuperior shoulder pain in the late cocking phase. Popping, locking and snapping may occur with unstable labral tears. Instability symptoms may be related to rotator cuff dysfunction and excessive anterior capsular laxity.

Clinical examination

A systematic examination should include the hip, knee and lower back assessment.

Muscular atrophy and scapular winging should be noted. Tenderness should be accessed at the glenohumeral joint lines, the acromioclavicular joint, the long head of the biceps tendon, and the coracoid process.

Active and passive range of motion of the glenohumeral and scapulothoracic joints is measured.

Muscle strength testing should aim to isolate the muscle being tested and compare the injured with the contralateral, uninjured side. The supraspinatus can be isolated in the 'empty can' position. The subscapularis is best assessed using the 'lift off' test, or the internal rotation lag sign, which is more sensitive. A proper examination assesses range of motion of both shoulders in both adduction and 90° of abduction.

An overhead athlete will typically have reduced internal rotation and increased external rotation. The Jobe's relocation test is also a provocative manoeuvre that reproduces the symptoms of internal impingement. In this test, the patient is supine and the arm is placed into 90° of abduction and 10° of forward flexion, and the shoulder is forced anteriorly. Pain represents a positive test. Pain subsequently subsides with a posteriorly directed force.

Many tests have been described to assist in diagnosing SLAP lesions. The O'Brien active compression test has good sensitivity and specificity for type II SLAP lesions. The arm is positioned in 15° of adduction and 90° of forward elevation. The examiner applies downward force on the forearm while the hand is both pronated and supinated, and compares the resulting pain and weakness. A positive test occurs when the patient reports pain that is worse in the pronated position.

Speed's biceps tension test is also sensitive for SLAP lesions. This test is performed through having the patient resist downward pressure with the arm in 90° of forward elevation, with the elbow extended and the forearm supinated. Although this test is more suggestive of biceps tendon damage, an unstable biceps anchor will cause the test to elicit pain.

A positive apprehension relocation sign for posterior shoulder pain may suggest a SLAP lesion in the posterior labrum as part of a spectrum of internal impingement.

Investigations

Imaging

Radiographic evaluation includes the standard three views of the shoulder (anteroposterior, axillary and outlet views) to help exclude other bony abnormalities. Magnetic resonance imaging (MRI)-enhanced arthrography outperforms plain MRI when diagnosing SLAP lesions. The diagnostic feature of the MR arthrogram is contrast between the superior labrum and the glenoid that extends around and under the biceps anchor on the coronal oblique view. The axial views visualise possible extension into the anterior and or posterior labrum. Partial thickness rotator cuff tears will also be identified (**Figure 44**).

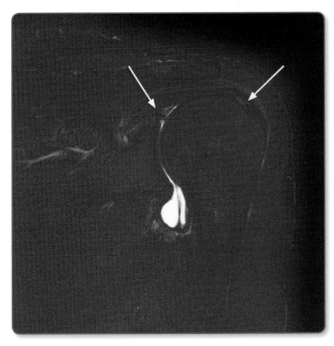

Figure 44 MR arthrogram coronal image of a volleyball player showing fraying of the superior labrum and undersurface of the supraspinatus.

Some recommend MRI with the shoulder in both the abducted and externally rotated (ABER) position. These views may further enhance visualisation of the articular side of the rotator cuff and superior glenoid and may be helpful in diagnosing delaminating tears of the rotator cuff (**Figure 45**). Up to 40% of professional pitchers have completely asymptomatic partial articular-sided supraspinatus tendon avulsion lesions.

Differential diagnosis

This would include various pathologic conditions such as:
- Articular sided rotator cuff tears
- Labral tears and/or cysts
- Long head of biceps pathology
- Anterior instability

Associated Injuries may include:
- Coracoid pain from pectoralis minor contracture and tendinopathy
- Superior medial angle scapular pain from levator scapula insertional tendinopathy
- Subacromial origin pain from acromial mal-position and decreased subacromial space from upward tilting
- Acromioclavicular joint pain caused by anterior joint incongruity
- Sternoclavicular pain
- Thoracic outlet syndrome radicular pain, and subclavian vascular problems such as arterial pseudoaneurysm or venous thrombosis

Treatment
Nonoperative
These measures include:
1. Activity modification, biomechanical assessment and appropriate adjustment of technique
2. Analgesia
3. Physiotherapy
   a. Range of motion and correction of posterior-inferior capsule tightness exercises
   b. Strengthening
   c. Correction of the scapula-thoracic mechanics
   d. Correction of rotator cuff balance
   e. Attention to the kinetic chain as a whole and core stability
   f. Image-guided corticosteroid injections

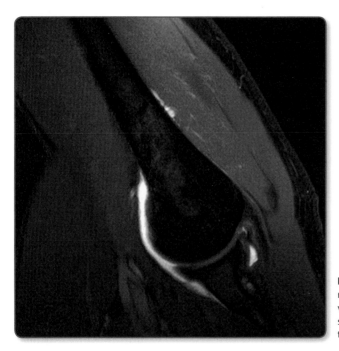

Figure 45 The abducted external rotation (ABER) view of the same volleyball player as **Figure 44** showing some increased signal of the cuff at the insertion site.

Operative

- This indicated only after nonoperative measurements have failed
- The operative approach should be pursued in a methodical fashion and focus on treating the primary abnormality
- In presence of tight posterior inferior capsule, which has to be confirmed by examination under anaesthesia, posterior inferior capsular release may be performed
- In presence of SLAP lesion, partial thickness rotator cuff tears and long head of biceps lesions, SLAP repair, rotator cuff repair and long head of bicep tenodesis may be considered, but the athlete must be counselled that following these procedures, particularly in cases of high level throwing athletes, they may not return to the pre-injury performance level

Return to sport

With both operative and nonoperative management, the athlete should only be allowed to return to sport after achieving full pain free range of movement and strength as well as cardiovascular fitness. With surgery this may take as long as 12 months.

However, as mentioned above, it must be emphasised that elite overhead athletes may not return to their prior performance level. According to some reports, return to pre-injury level of competition after SLAP lesion repairs and rotator cuff repair is the case in only 35% of elite overhead throwing athletes.

Further reading

Braun S, Kokmeyer D, Millett PJ. Shoulder injuries in the throwing athlete. J Bone Joint Surg Am 2009; 91:966–978.

Levy O, Narvani A. Biomechanics of the shoulder and elbow (2010). In: Margheritini F, Rossi R (eds.), Orthopedic sports medicine. Milan; Springer-Verlag, 2010.

Neri BR, ElAttrache NS, Owsley KC, et al. Outcome of type II superior labral anterior posterior repairs in elite overhead athletes: effect of concomitant partial-thickness rotator cuff tears. Am J Sports Med 2011; 39:114–120.

Van Kleunen JP, Tucker SA, Field LD, et al. Return to high-level throwing after combination infraspinatus repair, SLAP repair, and release of glenohumeral internal rotation deficit. Am J Sports Med 2012; 40:2536–2541.

Related topics of interest

Shoulder – superior labrum anterior posterior (SLAP) lesions

The first description of tears involving the Superior Labrum extending from Anterior to Posterior (SLAP) was described first by Snyder. This injury is now increasingly being recognised as a source of pain and disability especially in overhead athletes.

Pathology

The aetiology of SLAP lesions remains unclear, but three proposed mechanisms have been postulated to cause these injuries. These include:

- **Traumatic cause:** Fall onto an outstretched arm resulting in impaction of the humeral head against the superior labrum and the biceps anchor
- **Repetitive overhead activity:** It causes eccentric contraction of biceps muscle, creating tension on the long head of the biceps tendon especially during the arm deceleration and follow-through phases of throwing in the overhead athlete
- **'Peel-back' mechanism:** The rotation produced when the shoulder is placed in a position of abduction and maximal external rotation may cause a torsional force at the biceps anchor

In addition, concomitant pathology such as rotator cuff tears (especially partial thickness tears) and glenohumeral instability is frequently present in association with SLAP lesions.

Classification

The original classification by Snyder described four types of SLAP lesions. This has been expanded by Maffet et al. to include three further types of injuries (**Table 24**). The most common lesion is Type II that has been subclassified into three different types (**Table 24**).

Clinical features

History

- Vague shoulder pain
- Clicking, popping or snapping that is exacerbated with overhead activity most notably the late cocking phase of throwing
- May have associated symptoms of instability if the lesion extends to the anterior labrum

Examination

- No single test is sensitive or specific enough to determine the presence of a SLAP lesion accurately
- The resisted supination external rotation test and the biceps load test have been shown to be the most valuable in diagnosing a Type II lesion

Table 24 Classification of SLAP lesions	
Type	**Description**
I	Frayed or degenerative labrum with attachment of the labrum to the glenoid
II	Detachment of the superior labrum and biceps from the glenoid rim (1) anterior, (2) posterior and (3) combined anterior and posterior lesions
III	A bucket-handle tear of the labrum with an intact biceps anchor
IV	A bucket handle tear of the labrum that extends into the biceps tendon
V	Anteroinferior Bankart-type labral lesions in continuity with SLAP lesion
VI	Biceps tendon separation with an unstable flap tear of the labrum
VII	Extension of the superior-labrum biceps tendon separation to beneath the middle glenohumeral ligament

Investigations
Plain radiographs
These are normal in cases of isolated SLAP injuries but may demonstrate bony pathology (Hill Sachs or Bankart lesion) if there is concomitant glenohumeral instability.

Magnetic resonance imaging /magnetic resonance arthrography (see Figure 46).
Magnetic resonance (MR) arthrography with the arm in abduction and external rotation has been shown to be more sensitive and specific than magnetic resonance imaging (MRI) alone in diagnosing a SLAP lesion. MRI findings that suggest damage to the labrum or long head of biceps (LHB) tendon include the following: (1) increased signal at the labrum/ anchor interface or at the superior glenoid fossa, (2) displacement of the superior labrum away from the glenoid surface and (3) presence of a glenoid-labral cyst. As well as identifying labral pathology MRI will also illustrate associated rotator cuff pathology.

Arthroscopy
Arthroscopy remains the gold standard in diagnosing a SLAP lesion.

Treatment
Nonoperative
- Includes activity modification, anti-inflammatory medication and physical therapy focused on restoring normal shoulder motion followed by closed chain rotator cuff and scapula strengthening exercises
- Loss of glenohumeral internal rotation is commonly found in overhead athletes and may be a source of some of the patient's symptoms. Posterior capsule stretching to restore internal rotation may be beneficial in reducing the abnormal contact between the supraspinatus tendon and the posterosuperior labrum

Operative
- Type I and III lesions are usually debrided whilst Types II and IV are treated either

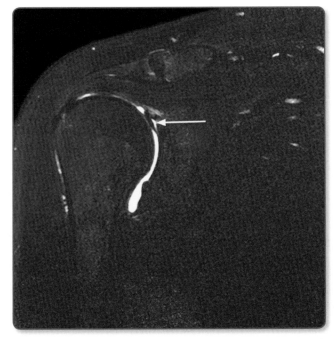

Figure 46 MR arthrogram demonstrating a SLAP lesion. MR, magnetic resonance.

with repair (suture anchor) or long of biceps tenodesis
- Concomitant partial thickness rotator cuff tears can be debrided (involving <50% of articular surface) or repaired (involving >50% of articular surface)

Return to sport

- Postoperative rehabilitation involves a period of immobilisation for 3–4 weeks followed by active-assisted and passive exercises. Resistance exercises are commenced at 8 weeks postsurgery and after 4 months a sport-directed throwing program can be commenced. Contact sports are usually resumed after 6 months
- Short to medium term follow-up of patients who have had a SLAP repair have demonstrated that in 90% of cases the results are either good or excellent. However, the results are less successful in patients involved with repetitive overhead activities

Further reading

Dessaur WA, Magarey ME. Diagnostic accuracy of clinical tests for superior labral anterior posterior lesions: a systematic review. J Orthop Sports Phy Ther 2009; 38:341–352.

Dodson CC, Altchek DW. SLAP lesions: an update on recognition and treatment. J Orthop Sports Phy Ther 2009; 39(2):71–80.

Related topics of interest

Skin infections

Key points

- Common among athletes
- May be bacterial, viral or fungal
- Many are contagious; therefore, measures should be taken to prevent spread

Overview

Skin infection amongst athletes is very common due to the nature of close contact in sport, occlusive clothing and footwear. Many of these types of infections are contagious and may result in serious consequences to the athletes themselves or the team. They include bacterial, viral and fungal infections. Rapid diagnosis and treatment of the condition is essential in minimising the disruption to the individual and the team. The prevalence of skin infection in college athletes in the United States was estimated to be 57% bacterial, 47% viral and 7% fungal.

Bacterial skin infection

The most common bacterial skin infection amongst athletes is staphylococcal infection. These bacteria live on the skin and mucous membranes (e.g. in nose) of humans. *Staphylococcus aureus* is the most important of these bacteria in human diseases. Other staphylococci, including *Staphylococcus epidermidis*, are considered commensals, or normal inhabitants of the skin surface.

Streptococcal infection is also very common and alongside *Staphylococcus* causes a variety of skin conditions including impetigo and ecthyma, which is the deeper form of impetigo, erysipelas, folliculitis or boils, cellulitis and secondary infection in wounds.

Impetigo

This is a bacterial infection of the skin that may manifest itself in two ways:

1. Vesiculopustular (nonbullous) type which is much more common resulting in golden yellow crusts
2. Bullous type

Aetiology

The micro-organisms responsible for impetigo are *Streptococcus pyogenes* and or *S. aureus* which are highly contagious.

Signs and symptoms

Symptoms are usually slight itching of the skin and some enlargement of the regional lymph nodes. The nonbullous form results in pustules that evolve in to honey coloured crusted plaques. The bullous form has fluid filled sacks that can rupture easily. They mostly occur on exposed skin of the hands, face and legs, where laceration, bites and abrasions can easily occur.

Treatment

Treatment of the lesions includes soaks of tepid water with some white vinegar several times a day and gently removing the crusts. Topical antibiotics such fucidin and mupirocin are commonly used and are affective when small areas of the skin are involved. It is essential that the athlete is aware of new lesions appearing and the importance of treating them promptly with the topical preparation. Systemic antibiotics are used if the area involved is extensive, if there is recurrent disease or if there is little response to topical treatment. The antibiotic of choice is flucloxacillin taken for 7 days.

Return to sports

Avoid close contact sports or going to the gym until crusting and blistering has stopped. Athletes can return to sports after 72 h of receiving treatment provided no new lesions have occurred in the previous 48 h. The affected area should be protected with a non permeable bandage that cannot be dislodged during sports.

Folliculitis/furunculosis and carbuncles

This encompasses a group of conditions that cause inflammation of the hair follicles. This can be as a result of infection, occlusion or irritation. Infection can be bacterial, yeast or fungal. Bacterial infection of the hair follicles results in furuncles and carbuncles. The former representing infection of one follicle and surrounding tissue and the latter involving clusters of furuncles all joining under the skin surface to form a carbuncle. The risk factor to developing this condition in athletes is occlusive tight clothing, excessive friction from clothing, externally humid environments, excessive sweating and hyperhidrosis, nasal carriage of infective strains and skin abrasions and injury.

Aetiology

The two most common bacteria responsible for this condition are S. aureus and Pseudomonas spp., these latter being responsible for outbreaks in hot tubs and swimming pools.

Signs and symptoms

It presents as a rash or red lumps of the hair covered skin. It can cause irritation and purities. Small pustules may also be present in the centre of the lesions. Deep folliculitis causes more erythema of the surrounding tissues that may result in scarring and hair loss. If this is widespread or results in formation of carbuncles there may be more systemic symptoms of fever, pain and malaise.

Treatment

Mild superficial folliculitis may resolve without treatment. Topical antiseptic agents such as chlorhexidine and povidone-iodine are frequently used. Deeper folliculitis may respond to oral antibiotics that include flucloxacillin, erythromycin and ciprofloxacin depending on the causative bacteria. In recurrent or persistent disease antibiotics will need to be continued for 4–6 weeks. Carbuncles are best treated surgically with incision and drainage.

Cellulitis

This is infection of the dermis and the subcutaneous tissue. The most common bacteria that cause cellulitis are group A beta-haemolytic streptococci (Streptococcus pyogenes) and S aureus. Athletes have increased risk of developing cellulitis due to injury or athlete's foot that can both result in breaking of the skin.

Signs and symptoms

Commonly affects the lower limbs. In most cases, there is evidence of damage to the skin through trauma or ulcers. There is erythema, warmth, swelling and pain in the affected area. The progression of the infection in to the lymphatics is represented by red lines streaking away from the infection site. Cellulitis can cause systemic symptoms such as fever and malaise and if left untreated can be potentially very serious.

Treatment

Treatment in mild to moderate cases is with 5–10 days of oral antibiotics such as penicillin, flucloxacillin, cefuroxime or erythromycin. If systemic symptoms are present or a wide area or deep structures are involved intravenous antibiotics are needed. Athletes should not return to sport until the infection has cleared.

Viral skin infection

Herpes simplex

Eighty percent of the population are asymptomatic carriers of the herpes simplex type 1(HSV1). About 30% have experienced cold sores at some time. In the United States, this has been called herpes gladiatorum or mat herpes due to the high prevalence amongst wrestlers.

Aetiology

The virus has two types: HSV1 usually causes perioral or cutaneous symptoms and HSV2 is responsible for genital herpes. The virus lays dormant in sensory nerves supplying the skin. During an attack the virus spreads down the nerve on to the surface of the skin and multiplies. Immunity develops after the initial attack but is not complete and recurrence is triggered by a variety of factors including stress, sun exposure, trauma and fatigue.

Signs and symptoms

During the primary infection there may be a prodrome of fever, malaise and lymphadenopathy. After an incubation period of 5–10 days, recurrent small grouped vesicles appear, especially around oral or genital areas, which have an erythematous base. The primary symptoms are burning and stinging. The vesicles rupture quickly and crust over within a few days. The crusted lesions may take a couple of weeks to heal completely.

Treatment

Treatment is with oral antiviral medication. Aciclovir, valaciclovir and famciclovir can all be given.

Return to sports

Vesicular lesions must be dried before the athlete can compete. The dried scabs should be covered with occlusive dressing to provide further protection.

Viral warts

Warts or verrucae are benign epithelial proliferations due to infection with various forms of human papillomavirus (HPV). More than 80 HPV subtypes are known. The presentation varies according to the site of the wart. Plantar warts appear on pressure bearing areas and are flat in appearance. In general, infectivity is low but this is increased if the wart is wet or bleeding secondary to trauma.

Warts are usually asymptomatic, but plantar warts can be painful and impede an athlete's performance.

Treatment

Warts can be treated with topical salicylic acid preparations or through cryotherapy. Multiple treatment sessions may be needed to resolve the lesions.

Molluscum contangiosum

Molluscum contagiosum is characterised by single or multiple rounded, dome-shaped waxy papules 2–5 mm in diameter that are umbilicated and contain a caseous plug, caused by a virus in the Poxviridae family. Typically, there are no symptoms, but patients can develop localised eczematous reactions and lesions can become pruritic and may suppurate.

Molluscum contagiosum most commonly develops on the face, hands and forearms, but can be seen on any other surface of skin, including genitalia. They are more common

in swimmers, gymnasts and wrestlers. Spread is through skin-to-skin contact and autoinoculation.

Even though the infection is self-limiting, it is advisable for athletes involved in contact sports to be treated.

Treatment

The treatment of molluscum contagiosum is exactly the same as for warts.

Return to sports

Contact sports can be resumed 48 h after resolution of papules.

Fungal skin infections

Dermatophytosis is a group of fungal infections that invade and grow in dead keratin. The most common species belong to the Epidermophyton, Microsporum and Trichophyton genera. Clinical classification is according to site.

Tinea pedis

Athlete's foot is a very common fungal skin infection in sports people, mostly due to *Tinea rubrum* or *Tinea mentagrophytes*. The hot moist environment in sports footwear is an ideal environment for these fungi to grow and invade the intertriginous web spaces as well as the plantar aspect of the foot.

The commonest presenting symptom is itching, which worsens after the removal of socks. There may also be burning or pain from secondary infection with complicating cellulitis and lymphangitis. Commonly there may be fungal nail infection present. Tinea pedis can present in three forms.

1. There may be scaly eruption in the intertriginous space, with or without erythema, maceration or fissuring
2. Eruption of vesicles and bullae on the mid foot
3. Hyperkeratotic scales with minimal erythema on the plantar surface of the foot

Diagnosis can be reached through clinical history and examination, and confirmed by direct microscopic visualisation of hyphae from skin scrapings.

Treatment

Treatment is with the use of topical or oral antifungal medications. Topical creams such as miconazole, terbinafine and clotrimazole are given for a duration of 1–6 weeks depending on the type and severity of the condition. Oral terbinafine, fluconazole or itraconazole are treatments of choice in particularly severe or chronic disease. Wet dressings using Burrow's solution applied three times daily can relieve symptoms if maceration or vesicles are present.

It is important that old shoes and socks be discarded to prevent recurrent infections.

Return to sports

There are no specific NCAA guidelines for return to sports with tinea pedis, but it is advisable to refrain from competition until dissolution of symptoms or to adequately cover the area with nonpermeable bandage.

Tinea capitis and tinea corporis (ringworm)

Tinea capitis is a fungal infection of the scalp and Tinea corporis of the body. Both are caused by dermatophytes of the genus *Trichophyton*.

Patients typically present with scaly, erythematous and pruritic ring-shaped plaques. The scalp may have bald patches and, on closer inspection, it can be seen that the hair shafts have been broken.

Scalp and body ringworm are especially common amongst wrestlers and athletes who wear occlusive clothing. Spread is by skin-to-skin contact and there can be tinea corporis outbreaks amongst wrestlers.

Diagnosis is usually clinical and can be confirmed by visualising hyphae from skin scrapings in 10% potassium hydroxide preparations under a microscope.

Treatment

Treatment is with topical or oral antifungals. Tinea corporis can be treated by applying terbinafine 1% or clotrimazole 1% twice daily and until 2 weeks after disappearance of the lesions, or orally with ketoconazole, itraconazole, or fluconazole. Tinea capitis should be treated with oral antifungals as above.

Return to sports

Athletes involved in contact sports with extensive tinea corporis should be disqualified until at least 72 h after topical treatment has been started, and those with tinea capitis should have had oral therapy for at least 2 weeks.

Tinea cruris

Tinea cruris is a fungal infection of the groin area and is also known as 'jock itch'" It is very common amongst athletes and is caused by *T. rubrum* or *T. mentagrophytes*. The lesions occur in the crural folds, usually sparing the scrotum, and appear as sharply demarcated, centrally clearing erythematous macular lesions, with or without vesicle formation. Pruritus is a common symptom.

Treatment

Treatment involves drying the affected area and using drying powder 2–3 times daily, and also topical antifungals, e.g. 1% clotrimazole or 1% terbinafine once or twice daily for 2 weeks. Resistant cases are treated orally.

Return to sports

There are no specific NCAA guidelines for return to sports with tinea cruris.

Measures to minimise spread of skin infections

Measures to minimise spread include:
- Clean hands often with soap and water or alcohol gels
- Do not share sports equipment or towels; shower if possible on site after training or the event
- Cover all breaks of skin with a waterproof bandage
- Wash all clothes and towels on a high temperature setting
- Wipe gym equipment with an antimicrobial wipe regularly
- Report any skin problems promptly so as to minimise spread and to initiate treatment
- Try and minimise stress, get adequate sleep, maintain good skin hygiene which helps boost immunity

Further reading

Hall JC, Hall BJ. Skin infections: diagnosis and
treatment. Chapt 18; 2009:238–245.

Related topics of interest

Sport and exercise at altitude

Key points

- Up to 2500 m altitude rapid adaptation occurs with some reduced aerobic performance
- Between 2500 m and 5500 m slower acclimatisation can occur
- Above 2500 m there is the risk of developing acute mountain sickness (AMS), high altitude cerebral oedema (HACE or HACO) or high altitude pulmonary oedema (HAPE or HAPO)
- HACE and HAPE are dangerous conditions and it is essential that immediate steps are taken to resolve them, usually descending at least 1000 m

Physiological effects of altitude

Aerobic exercise at altitude is limited by the fall in oxygen partial pressure. In mountain terrain, it will usually also be cold. This is covered in the topic on Sport and exercise in the cold (see topic Cold - hypothermia), so this section will deal entirely with the problems of exercise in a hypoxic environment. Note in passing that some of the problems discussed will also be relevant for subjects with low arterial oxygen due to lung disease.

Not a lot happens up to about 1500 m. Above this the lowered oxygen has several immediate effects, which represent an immediate adaptation. Continued exposure to low oxygen levels causes profound longer term acclimatisation. Above 6000 m, if not acclimatised you lose consciousness in minutes. With acclimatisation, it is possible to survive for some time at altitudes of 6000 m or above, but eventually illness develops (see below). No human settlements are found above 5000 m (**Table 25**).

Immediate adaptation (over a few minutes) consists of an increase in heart rate and pulmonary ventilation, with the latter causing more CO2 excretion, a lowered $PaCO_2$ and respiratory alkalosis. These adaptations are enough to allow average levels of physical activity. However, maximum aerobic exercise is limited and VO_2max is only 85% of normal. There were no world records in distance events at the Mexico City Olympics. But note that there were records in explosive events where the reduced air resistance was helpful.

After the initial adaptation the CO_2 sensitivity of the central chemoreceptor system resets to operate at lower levels suited to the hyperventilation. The resting heart rate drops back towards pre-altitude values (although the maximum heart rate is reduced). The haemoglobin content of the blood rises by around a third over 26 weeks. As discussed in the topic on blood doping and altitude training (See topic on Drugs in sport - blood doping, erythropoietin and altitude training), many athletes deliberately

Altitude (m)	Atmospheric pressure (mm Hg)	Inspired oxygen partial pressure (mmHg)	Arterial oxygen saturation (%)	Maximum exercise rate, VO₂max∗ (% sea level value)
0 (Sea level)	760	160	98	(100)
2300[+]	580	120	95	85
6500	360	75	70	50
8848[‡]	250	52	54[§]	30

Table 25 Arterial O_2 saturation and VO_2max at different altitudes

[*]After acclimatisation.

[+]Mexico City, 1968 Olympic Games.

[‡]Mount Everest summit.

[§]8400m. Grocott et al, New Eng J Med 2009; 360; 140-149.

train at altitude to get this boost in oxygen-carrying capacity. However, although it is an important adaptation for exercise at altitude, the increments in sea level performance may be small.

There is often substantial weight loss at altitudes above 4500 m. Some loss of appetite clearly occurs, and at higher altitudes there is poor absorption from the gastrointestinal tract. Maintaining an adequate energy intake, therefore, requires some attention. It is also important to have plenty of iron to support the haemoglobin synthesis during acclimatisation (**Table 26**).

Altitude illnesses

Above 4000 m AMS is common. It has been described as like a really bad hangover. With acclimatisation, symptoms usually disappear. The risk is that the condition will progress to HACE or HAPE (see below). If possible, those affected by AMS should descend, and then reascend more slowly. Certainly, they should not ascend further. Acetazolamide is helpful in treating AMS.

HACE is a medical emergency. Cerebral oedema can come on rapidly in hours and can be fatal. It is most common above 5000 m during rapid ascents. Subjects should be moved immediately to a lower altitude. If this is not possible, oxygen can be given if available. Special pressure bags are taken by some high altitude expeditions where the subject is placed in a bag pumped by foot up to a high pressure. The equivalent of 1500 m descent can be achieved and this can be enough to reduce HACE. Dexamethasone (hydrocortisone) is reported to be effective. It is crucial to pick up the early signs of HACE. These include ataxia, exercise intolerance and odd behaviour.

HAPE is more common than HACE. It is also a dangerous condition although most people survive. Actions are essentially the same as for HACE, i.e. get to lower altitude or adopt other strategies to raise PaO_2. Nifedipine is reported to help. Again, it is important to spot early signs such as exercise intolerance and a dry cough. The cause of HAPE is raised capillary pressure in the lungs, so it is different from the classical pulmonary oedema from raised pulmonary venous pressure seen in heart failure.

Golden rules

The International Society for Mountain Medicine (www.immed.org) stresses these three golden rules:
1. If you feel unwell at altitude it is altitude illness until proven otherwise
2. Never ascend with symptoms of AMS
3. If you are getting worse (or have HACE or HAPE) go down at once

Table 26 Adaptation and acclimatisation at different altitudes		
1500–2500 m	Medium altitude	Adaptation sufficient
2500–5000/5500 m	High altitude	Adaptation not sufficient – acclimatisation necessary to avoid acute mountain sickness (AMS)
5000/5500–8848 m	Extreme altitude	Acclimatisation not possible

Further reading

West JB, Schoene RB, Luks AM, et al. High altitude medicine and physiology, 5th edn. London: Hodder Arnold, 2013.

Grocott MP, Martin DS, Levett DZ et al. Arterial blood gases and oxygen content in climbers on Mount Everest. N Engl J Med, 2009; 360(2):140-149.

Related topics of interest

- Cold – hypothermia (p. 46)

- Drugs in sport – blood doping, erythropoietin and altitude training (p. 71)

Neuropsychological tests may be used to objectively assess cognitive domains such as reduced attention and the ability to process information, slowed reaction times and impaired memory and can help overcome a reliance on subjective symptoms when advising the concussed athlete on a safe return to play.

The athlete with prolonged symptoms

In a small number (5–10%) of cases, postconcussive symptoms might either be persistent or consistently reprovoked by exertion. These athletes should be referred to clinicians with specific expertise in concussion management for consideration of additional investigations that might include formal neuropsychological testing, balance assessment, and neuroimaging together with multimodality treatments.

The child and adolescent athlete

It is recognised that the recovery time frame after concussion may be longer in children and a more circumspect approach to management is recommended. An additional consideration in any assessment is the potential need to include patient and parent input as well as teacher and school input when appropriate. Child and adolescent athletes need to return safely to school before they can return to sport and a step wise approach to return to learning is recommended.

Long-term consequences

A small number of studies have suggested an association between repeated sports concussions during a career and cognitive impairment later in life and reported neuropathological evidence of chronic traumatic encephalopathy has been observed in retired football athletes. No consensus has been reached on the significance of such observations at this stage and there is no evidence currently that low exposure to contact sports places athletes at risk of these conditions. Clinicians need to be mindful of the potential for long-term problems in the management of all athletes.

Further reading

McCrory P, Meeuwisse W, Johnston K, et al. Consensus statement on concussion in sport. Br J Sports Med 2009; 43:i76–i84.

British journal of sports medicine. Sport concussion assessment tool 2. Br. J. Sports Med. 2009; 43:i85-i88.

Collie A, Maruff P, Darby D. Computerised neuropsychological testing in sport. Br J Sports Med 2001; 35:297–302.

Brukner P, Khan K. Brukner and Khan's Clinical Sports Medicine, 4th edn. New South Wales; McGraw-Hill Australia, 2012.

Stress fractures

Key points

- Magnetic resonance imaging (MRI) remains the gold standard imaging modality
- Most stress fractures can be treated conservatively 6 weeks. However, those with tenuous blood supply may require surgical intervention
- Tibial shaft stress fractures are the most common. Ninety percent affect the posteromedial aspect. Those affecting the anterior cortex (tension side) are prone to nonunion (beware the 'dreaded black line')

Overview

Briefhaupt originally described stress fractures in military recruits in 1855. Ninety-five percent occur in the lower limb, principally in the tibia and metatarsals. In the upper limb the ulna is most commonly affected followed by the scapula. Regarding incidence, no difference exists with respect to gender, race or geographical location.

Epidemiology

Stress fractures often result from participation in a new or unaccustomed activity and/or change in training regime, including intensity, duration and frequency of training. Distance running remains the most common precipitating sport.

Predisposing factors include hard unforgiving training surfaces, biomechanical causes (e.g. pronated feet, pes cavus, excessive external tibial torsion, limb length inequality, and muscle fatigue), bone density (e.g. osteoporosis, which may be related to amenorrhoea or oligomenorrhea in female athletes or increasing age), previous surgery (e.g. second metatarsal stress fracture following surgery for hallux valgus or rigidus), poor nutrition, reduced bone vascularity and genetic factors.

Pathology

A stress fracture occurs after accelerated bone remodelling in response to repetitive submaximal stresses. When bone is subjected to increased stress (load), remodelling occurs in the form of resorption from osteoclasts and bone formation by osteoblasts. If repetitive subthreshold loading continues, particularly when osteoclastic activity overwhelms the reparative capacity of bone, repetitive microtrauma's result in macrofracture of the bone.

The piezoelectric phenomenon underlying Wolff's law, which states that bone remodels itself in direct response to the applied forces, may be used to explain the pathology of certain stress fractures. Tensile stresses create electropositivity, resulting in bone resorption, while compressive forces create electronegativity initiating bone formation. Cyclical tensile forces, therefore, result in cortical thinning, osteoporosis and development of a stress fracture.

Two variants exist: normal bone that becomes fatigued through abnormal loading (i.e. fatigue fractures) and pathological bone that may fail under comparatively normal loads (i.e. insufficiency fractures). In both, fatigue failure of bone progresses through crack initiation in areas of discontinuity, propagation along cement lines and in the presence of continued stress loading, crack propagation leading to complete failure.

Clinical features

The typical history is of insidious onset of pain precipitated by a new or unaccustomed activity. Initially pain is diffuse and may only be present during the exacerbating event. If the intensity of training persists, the pain becomes localised and constant disturbing sleep and daily life. In females, a menstrual history is paramount to exclude the triad of amenorrhoea, eating disorder and osteoporosis.

On examination, look for asymmetry and swelling, signifying localised periosteal thickening or callous formation, and palpate and percuss for tenderness of the underlying fracture. Range of motion may be restricted, or symptoms reproducible upon axially loading the fractured bone. The 'hang' test used for femoral shaft fractures is highly suggestive and is used to clinically assess the adequacy of healing before resuming weight bearing.

Investigations

Plain radiographs are often unremarkable and may take 2–6 weeks to show changes. X-rays may show a periosteal reaction, a fracture line or callus formation.

A radioisotope bone scan is highly sensitive but poorly specific (focal uptake is also seen in infection and tumour). It may be difficult to localise the area of increased uptake particularly in the foot where numerous bones exist in close proximity. However, it can detect changes in bone at the phase of accelerated remodelling, thus can show stress-induced changes within the first 24 h. A negative scan, however, makes the diagnosis highly unlikely and urges consideration of alternate diagnoses. An MRI scan (**Figure 47**) is regarded as the gold standard, having the best sensitivity and specificity and capable of detecting periosteal and bone marrow oedema as well as the fracture line itself early within the evolution of stress-induced changes.

Differential diagnosis

- Strains and sprains
- Contusions
- Delayed onset muscle soreness
- Shin splints (medial tibial stress syndrome)
- Exertion-related chronic compartment syndrome
- Tumours of bone, especially osteoid osteomas
- Referred pain from the spine
- Morton's neuroma
- Plantar fasciitis
- Metatarsophalangeal joint synovitis

Treatment

Most stress fractures heal within 6 weeks of relative rest, requiring strict non or protected weight bearing with crutches. Ice, massage, compression or bracing and nonsteroidal anti-inflammatories are useful adjuncts. Healing is assessed clinically by absence of local tenderness and by the ability to undertake precipitating activity without pain. Look for and treat predisposing factors, including biomechanical factors and faulty techniques through athlete education.

Expected outcome and therefore treatment is proportional to the vascularity of bone and, whether the tension or compression aspect is fractured. The more problematic fractures shall be discussed.

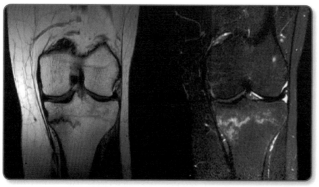

Figure 47 MRI images demonstrating tibial stress fracture. Notice bone oedema seen on fat suppressed views.

Specific fractures

Femoral neck stress fractures

There is gradual onset of poorly localized groin pain aggravated by activity. May involve the superior aspect of neck (tension side) or inferior aspect (compression side). Inferior stress fractures are more benign and can be treated with initial nonweight bearing (NWB) for 6 weeks followed by progressive loading. Displaced or tension fractures require cannulated screw fixation followed by 6 weeks of NWB.

Tibial shaft stress fractures

It is a common cause of shin pain in athletes undertaking impact running and jumping sports. Stress fractures of the anterior cortex (the tension side) are more resistant to treatment and prone to nonunion 'the dreaded black line'. Anterior cortical drilling or intramedullary nailing with or without bone grafting have been successfully employed for anterior cortex stress fractures.

Navicular stress fractures

Seen in sprinting, jumping or hurdling sports. Affects the middle third, which is relatively avascular and prone to delayed union. Treatment is strict NWB in a cast for 6–8 weeks, if tenderness remains continue for another 2 weeks. If displaced, percutaneous screw fixation is warranted. Delayed or nonunion requires internal fixation with or without bone grafting.

Metatarsal stress fractures

Most commonly affects the neck of the 2nd and seen in ballet dancers.

Following two stress fractures require special treatment.

Base of the second metatarsal

It requires athlete to be NWB on crutches for up to 12 weeks, especially with Lisfranc complex involvement. Displacement best appreciated on a computed tomography is managed by percutaneous screw fixation.

Fifth metatarsal

The Jone's fracture affects the metaphyseal–diaphyseal junction, resulting from an inversion plantarflexion injury or overuse. It is prone to be delayed or nonunion, thus percutaneous screw fixation is recommended.

Return to sport

Avoid disuse muscle atrophy and maintain cardiovascular fitness while the stress fracture heals through cross training (cycling, swimming or rowing machines). As the athlete returns to his or her primary sport, time spent on cross-training is gradually decreased.

Once the initial inflammatory stage subsides, specific exercises – such as stretching, and muscle strengthening – should be performed, supervised by the physiotherapist in conjunction with cross-training.

Further reading

Brukner P, Khan K. Brukner and Khan's Clinical Sports Medicine, 4th edn. New South Wales; McGraw-Hill Australia, 2012.
Johnson DH, Pedowitz RA. Practical orthopaedic sports medicine and arthroscopy, 1st edn. Lippincott, Williams and Wilkins, 2007.
Miller MD, Sekiya JK. Sports medicine: core knowledge in orthopaedics, 1st edn. Mosby Elsevier, 2006.

Related topics of interest

Team physician

Key points

- Preparation and planning is key
- Good mechanisms to cope with highly pressurised environments.
- Medical indemnity cover is essential

Roles and responsibilities

- The main role of a team physician is to organise, treat and coordinate the medical care for their team or athletes
- A multitude of specialist skills are required ranging from expertise with musculoskeletal problems to coping with psychological issues
- Be confident in the management of complex injuries, which will require a structured rehabilitation programme
- Know the types of acute and chronic injuries common to that sport
- Be proficient in management of medical conditions to optimise performance for the athlete
- Arrange pre-season testing for the squad
- Give nutritional advise to your athlete
- Organise and undertake presigning medicals
- Protect confidentiality of your athlete
- Have emergency protocols in place for match days
- Ensure you have all the required equipment for your team
- Know the antidoping code in detail, the procedures for drug testing and when a therapeutic use exemption is required
- Arrange training and education for medical staff, coaches and athletes
- Work within a multidisciplinary team
- Keep accurate medical records
- Ensure your indemnity covers your role

Qualifications/training required

- You need General Medical Council registration to practice in the United Kingdom (or equivalent if practicing elsewhere)
- The level of training required varies from sport to sport but a diploma (or Masters) in sports or musculoskeletal medicine is invaluable
- Medical indemnity cover is essential. The work as a team physician will be outside the remit of your normal medical practice and you must ensure it covers all aspects of athlete treatment
- Cardiopulmonary resuscitation training (i.e. Advanced Life Support courses)
- A recognised pitch side trauma course must be undertaken. Treating acute injuries and medical problems outside of hospital is very different to hospital medicine
- There are now specialist training schemes running in several countries, e.g. United Kingdom and Australia, to become a consultant in sports and exercise medicine

Ethics and doping

- The team physician needs to have an in depth understanding of confidentiality principles
- The team physician will often be under pressure to let player's return to play earlier than you feel may be recommended. It is essential for the physician to be aware of their responsibility to the athlete and the basic ethical principles (autonomy, beneficence, nonmaleficence, justice)
- Be aware of the World AntiDoping Agency code in detail
- Ensure that the athletes are aware of the antidoping code. Educating the team and management staff at least once a season is recommended
- During a season, some athletes may require treatment with drugs that are prohibited or may ask about certain drugs or supplements. See the Drugs in sport Topics for further details

Multidisciplinary team (MDT) approach

- Communication is of paramount importance. The key approach to working effectively is to use a multidisciplinary team treatment model
- Assessment, treatment and management of an individual should be discussed within the medical team (e.g. physiotherapist, sports therapist, psychologist, other physicians or surgeons) as all specialists have an important role
- Meetings with management and coaching staff are essential to ensure they have updates on player injuries and medical treatment plans. Note: occasionally this is not possible if there are confidentiality issues
- Chronic injuries will require an organised rehabilitation programme, which needs to be well structured with regular reviews to ensure progress for the athlete
- Keep accurate medical records. This needs to be documented in medical files or on a secure computer system

Preseason

- Preseason testing will depend on available resources with regards to blood tests, imaging etc. The team physician is responsible for the health of the athletes and any impact this could have on their performance or safety for them or their competitors
  - Update the athlete history regarding any current or new medical problems and medication. Investigate further as required
  - Depending on the sport, ensure cardiac screening has been undertaken and is up to date for all your athletes
  - Check on player immunisations especially if the team will be travelling abroad
  - Together with the medical team, assess for any ongoing musculoskeletal injuries, fitness tests and develop prehabilitation programmes individually for the athletes to prevent injuries where possible problems have been indentified

- Educate the team and coaches on antidoping, nutrition, injuries etc.
- Carry out a risk assessment to check that all facilities and equipment are adequate across your training/playing sites

Presigning medicals

- Medicals are often required prior to signing players. The team physician is responsible for advising management whether an athlete is 'fit' to be signed from a medical perspective
- Create a thorough medical screening pro forma. This should include cardiac screening and a detailed medical and musculoskeletal history including a thorough examination of all systems and joints
- Contact the player's previous club medical team to gather as much information prior to the presigning medical
- Following the medical, you can conclude if a player requires further tests and inform management of your findings

Match days

- Always have a briefing with the on-site medical team/healthcare professionals so you are aware of the number of other medical staff (including paramedics) at the event and their roles. If it is at your usual ground this is still important so to build relationships and check everything is in place on the day
- If you are in a different setting, ensure you know all the emergency access/egress routes, where the medical room is, and the plans in place for an emergency
- Know distances to local hospital emergency departments and have their phone numbers
- Recheck all your equipment. With all medication and equipment, ensure you have a mechanism to carry out regular checks and that they are in date
- It is imperative to regularly practice field of play scenarios with your team. Everyone should be clear on his or her roles when required
- Have agreed messages (hand signals, microphone) to communicate between

the medical team during field of play. Keep them simple
- Assessing player's pitch side and determining if they are safe to return to play is completely your responsibility. This is an important point to remember when placed under pressure from the coaching staff or team
- Be up to date with concussion guidelines as these are common in sport

Medical equipment

- Medical equipment and what you have as a carry-on bag will depend on the sport but the basics are the same, and should contain the following:
    - Airways (oropharyngeal airways, nasopharyngeal airways)
    - Breathing (oxygen, masks)
    - Circulation (intravenous lines and fluid e.g. saline)
    - Cardiac defibrillator and drugs for a cardiac arrest
    - Stethoscope, otoscope, ophthalmoscope, sphygmomanometer and sats machine
    - Entonox and injectable analgesia (i.e. opiates) for serious injuries
    - Bandages, nasal sponges, scissors, suturing equipment, dressings, scissors, wound irrigation, gloves, sharps bin, notepad and pen.
    - Medications – emergency drugs, analgesia, antibiotics, anti-inflammatories, inhalers, nebuliser and any other relevant drugs
- Pitch side equipment involves spinal boards with head blocks, basket stretchers, scoops, box splints etc., but the requirement will depend on your sport
- Ensure that the equipment required for that sport is provided. If you feel anything is unsuitable you need to inform the event organiser immediately

Travelling with a team

- Travelling with a team carries extra responsibilities, as there is often a lack of additional support. Preparation is important
- Circulate a pretravel questionnaire to all members of the travelling party, as you will be responsible for the coaching staff and players. This should include a medical history, medications, allergies, recent illnesses, and include vaccine and immunisation status. If vaccines are required then this needs to be advised well ahead of a trip
- Check the country's climate you will be staying in, contact the hotel and enquire about food, medical rooms. Also check if it is safe to drink tap water
- Find out about local hospitals, services provided and distances from your accommodation. If going on a long trip abroad, a recce trip may be advisable
- Carry simple medications on a plane-analgesia, antidiarrhoeal medications, antiemetics, antihistamines, inhaler, stethoscope and anything else depending on the illnesses within your group
- Jet lag occurs when travelling past at least three time zones, worse if travelling in an easterly direction. This can be minimised by adjusting sleeping time, adequate hydration, no caffeine, alcohol, etc. Send out an information guide to all the team prior to departure
- Decide whether extra time is required for acclimatisation
- Check the suitability of your medical room, IT availability and mobile phone reception
- You will be on-call 24 h a day but plan sports medicine clinics around training, so you can get some rest and relaxation
- Have a contingency plan in case of contagious illnesses such as traveller's diarrhoea.
- Ensure you have a code of conduct within the medical team

Further reading

Cook J, Harcourt P, Milne C. Providing team care and travelling with a team. In: Brukner P, Khan K (eds), Clinical sports medicine, 3rd edn. Australia: McGraw-Hill, 2006:954–968.

MacAuley D (ed.). The team physician. In: Oxford handbook of sports and exercise medicine, 1st edn. Oxford; Oxford University Press, 2007:789–818.

Micheli LY, Pigozzi F, Chan KM, et al. Team physician manual: international federation of sports medicine (FIMS), 1st edn. Abingdon; Routledge, 2012.

Related topics of interest

• Drugs in sport – overview (p. 74)

Tendon overuse injuries

Key points

- Injuries to the muscle–tendon complex are among the commonest injuries sustained in football players
- The management of tendon injuries can be frustrating and prolonged. The recurrence of Achilles and patellar tendon injuries in AFL players was 23% and 20%, respectively
- This high rate of recurrence results from early return to play in a competitive professional environment. It is, therefore, important to understand the exact aetiology and pathogenesis of these injuries

Achilles tendinopathy

Aetiology

Excessive loading of the tendon during vigorous physical training is considered to be the main pathological stimulus for Achilles tendinopathy. The tendon may respond to this repetitive excessive overload beyond physiological limit by either inflammation of its sheath or damage with failed healing response of its body, or by a combination of these two mechanisms. Tendon damage can also occur even if the tendon is stressed within its physiological limits, as frequent cumulative microtrauma may not leave enough time for recovery and repair.

Relative poor vascularity of the tendon, dysfunction of the gastrocnemius-soleus, age, gender, body-weight and height, pes cavus deformity and lateral instability of the ankle are common intrinsic factors that predispose to Achilles tendinopathy. Changes in training pattern, poor technique, previous injuries, footwear and environmental factors such as training on hard, slippery or slanting surfaces are extrinsic factors that predispose to Achilles tendinopathy.

In Achilles tendinopathy, pain and swelling are located in and around the tendon, 2–6 cm proximal to the Achilles tendon insertion on the calcaneus. Initially, pain occurs after exercise. As the pathology progresses, pain may occur during exercise, and, in severe cases, it may interfere with activities of daily living. The 'painful arc' sign helps to distinguish between lesions of the tendon and paratenon. In paratendinopathy, the area of maximum thickening and tenderness remains fixed in relation to the malleoli from full dorsiflexion to plantar flexion. Lesions within the tendon will move with movement of the ankle,

Investigations

Ultrasound scan and magnetic resonance imaging (MRI) will help identify the location and extent of the lesion. Magnetic resonance scanning helps to differentiate between paratendinopathy and tendinopathy of the main body of the tendon.

Management

Recovery is slow due to low oxygen consumption, slow synthesis of structural protein, and can be further slowed down by continuing excessive load. Conservative management aims to identify and correct the possible aetiological factors, at times using a symptom-related approach. It includes relative rest, analgesia, physiotherapy and orthoses. Reducing training intensity and duration or a reduction in other aggravating activities may be beneficial, as tendon loading stimulates the repair and remodels the collagen fibres. Achilles tendinopathy is not inflammatory in origin: nonsteroidal anti-inflammatory drugs should, therefore, not be used. Aprotinin (two to four injections of 62,500 IU with local anaesthetic in the paratendinous space) may offer lasting pain relief.

Physiotherapy techniques include cryotherapy, deep friction massage, soft tissue mobilisation, gentle stretching and eccentric strengthening exercises. Eccentric strengthening exercises are performed by standing on tip-toes on a step, and dropping the heel(s) down below the level of the step in a controlled manner, then raising the heels back to start position. The exercises are done with the knee straight (to eccentrically strengthen the gastrocnemius) or slightly flexed (soleus). The calf raises back to starting position are controlled with the asymptomatic leg.

Surgery is recommended if nonoperative management has proved ineffective for at least three months.

The surgical technique for Achilles tendinopathy is based on the principles of excision of fibrotic adhesions, removal of degenerated nodules, and making multiple longitudinal incisions in the tendon to identify and excise intratendinous lesions and restoring vascularity, and possibly stimulating the remaining viable cells to initiate cell matrix response and healing.

Longstanding tendinopathy may predispose to Achilles tendon rupture, as ruptured tendons show more advanced degenerative changes than tendinopathic tendons. Acute Achilles tendon ruptures are more common in racquet sport players than among footballers. Patients present with sudden onset of pain, snapping sensation in the calf, and absent calf squeeze test.

Insertional Achilles tendinopathy may present alone or as a triad, in combination with retrocalcaneal bursitis and Haglund's deformity. It presents with early morning stiffness, pain localising to insertion of Achilles tendon that worsens after exercise, climbing stairs, running on hard surfaces, or heel running. Radiographs may reveal calcification at the insertion of the Achilles tendon or a spur (fishhook osteophyte) on the superior portion of the calcaneum (**Figure 94.2**). Conservative management produces 85–95% success rate with rest, ice, modification of training, ice, heel lift/orthoses. Surgery to excise the spur, the tendinopathic tendon and bursa help alleviate symptoms if conservative management fails.

Patellar tendinopathy

In patellar tendinopathy, anterior knee pain starts insidiously, and a specific activity may make the pain worse. Pain is well localised to a small area over the anterior aspect of the knee, and early in the pathological process, it may ease completely while exercising. With time and continued activity, the pain worsens and limits sporting performance.

Eventually, anterior knee pain can develop during activities of daily living, and can even be present at rest.

Examination reveals tenderness at the junction of the patella and the patellar tendon. Palpation of the tendon attachment at the inferior pole of the patella is the classic physical examination technique for detecting patellar tendinopathy, but mild tenderness at this site is not unusual in a normal tendon in athletes.

Investigations

MRI will demonstrate an oval or round area of high signal intensity at the tendon attachment on T1, T2 and the proton-density-weighted images. It identifies the exact location and extent of tendon involvement and helps to exclude other conditions such as bursitis and chondromalacia. Ultrasonography should include both knees and shows a focal hypoechoic area combined with swelling of the surrounding tendon (**Figure 94.3**).

Management of patellar tendinopathy

Conservative management includes measures to reduce the load on the tendon, eccentric strengthening exercises, remedial massage, cryotherapy and drugs:

1. Decreasing load on the tendon can be achieved by reducing overall activity, correcting biomechanics to improve the energy-absorbing capacity of the limb. For example, pes planus and hyperpronation should be addressed if present. Shoe orthoses are helpful. Low flexibility and weakness of quadriceps, hamstrings, iliotibial band, calf muscles, gluteal, lower abdominals must be corrected
2. Eccentric strengthening is the keystone to successful management of tendinopathies including patellar tendinopathy. The key exercise is a drop squat from standing to about 100°–120° of knee flexion. Patients perform 3 sets of 10 repetitions per day. Symptoms may resolve after 6–8 weeks of exercises
3. **Cryotherapy and other physical modalities.** Cryotherapy decreases blood flow and metabolic rate, thereby limiting

tissue damage. Other modalities include ultrasound, heat, interferential therapy, magnetic fields, pulsed magnetic and electromagnetic fields, TENS and laser. The true effects of these modalities remain unknown

4. Remedial massage decreases the loads on the tendons improving muscle-stretching capabilities. Deep friction massage may activate mesenchymal stem cells to stimulate a healing response
5. **Medications.** The use of 'anti-inflammatory' medication seems paradoxical in this condition, though they are the most commonly used for controlling symptoms. Infiltration of corticosteroids by means such as iontophoresis has a dramatic effect on symptoms arising from inflamed synovial structures. Corticosteroid injections are not recommended in management of tendinopathy

Patellar tendon surgery is performed when the patient has not improved with at least 6 months of conservative management. The surgical methods for management of patellar tendinopathy include drilling of the inferior pole of the patella, resection of the tibial attachment of the patellar tendon with realignment, excision of macroscopic degenerated areas, repair of macroscopic defects, scarification (i.e. multiple longitudinal tenotomy of the tendon), percutaneous needling, percutaneous longitudinal tenotomy and arthroscopic debridement.

The mean time for return to preinjury level of sport varied from 4 months to more than 9 months. A long-term study of outcome reported that only 54% of open patellar tenotomy and 46% of arthroscopic tenotomy returned to previous levels of sport activity.

Quadriceps tendinopathy

It is much less frequent than patellar tendinopathy. Patients with quadriceps tendinopathy complain of pain at the proximal pole of the patella. The pain is typically insidious and is often associated with a recent increase in jumping, climbing, kicking or running.

Physical examination reveals tenderness over the superior pole of the patella and discomfort with resistance to extension with the knee hyperflexed. Patients should be evaluated for malalignments such as femoral anteversion, increased Q angle and tibial torsion. Quadriceps strength and hamstring flexibility should also be assessed.

Investigations

Degenerative changes such as calcification in the tendon or spur formation at the superior pole of the patella may be present on radiographs. MRI may demonstrate degenerative changes at the posterior insertion of the tendon.

Management

Conservative management consisting of activity modification, anti-inflammatory medications and physical therapy is successful in the vast majority of patients. Once the pain improves, physiotherapy for quadriceps strengthening exercises and increasing hamstring flexibility is initiated. Surgery is rarely required.

Semimembranosus tendinopathy

Semimembranosus tendinopathy, a rare cause of medial knee pain, may be primary or secondary to primary knee abnormality such as patellofemoral disorders.

Semimembranosus tendinopathy causes aching pain at the posteromedial aspect of the knee, aggravated by prolonged jogging, climbing or lifting. Clinical examination reveals tenderness at the posteromedial corner of the knee just inferior to the joint line. A thorough knee examination is mandatory to exclude intra-articular pathology.

Investigations

Bone scan demonstrates increased tracer uptake at the posteromedial aspect of the proximal tibia. MRI scanning will confirm the diagnosis and exclude a medial meniscal tear or pes anserinus bursitis.

Management

The initial management of rest, hamstring stretching exercises and analgesia is successful in vast majority of patients with semimembranosus tendinopathy. Surgical intervention is advised after failed conservative management of at least 3 months.

Popliteus tendinopathy

Popliteus tendinopathy causes knee pain along the posterolateral portion of the knee. It is insidious and occurs on weight bearing with the knee in flexion of 15° to 30° or during the early part of the swing phase. There may be a recent increase in activity levels, especially downhill running, or running on a banked surface.

Examination reveals localised tenderness over the insertion of the popliteus over the lateral femoral condyle. This tendon is best palpated with the leg in the 'figure-of-four' position. If there is no rest pain, the patient is run downhill prior to the physical examination to assist in localising the pathology. An injection of local anaesthetic into the tendon sheath may help in diagnosis.

Investigations

Plain radiographs are usually normal, but in patients with chronic involvement radiodensities in the area of the popliteus tendon may be seen. MRI helps exclude intra-articular pathology or a tendon avulsion.

Management

Most cases are acute, and respond to a 2-week course of rest and analgesics. Upon return to activity, training modifications and avoiding downhill running can help alleviate the stresses imposed on the popliteus tendon. Chronic cases usually require a longer period of restricted activities.

Tibialis posterior tendinopathy

Tibialis posterior pathology and valgus flat foot-pronation deformity are closely related. Repeated excessive pronation leads to tibialis posterior overuse. On the other hand, tibialis posterior tendinopathy causes eversion of the hindfoot and fall of the medial longitudinal plantar arch resulting in a pronated valgus flatfoot.

Examination will reveal whether there is a flatfoot, a valgus hindfoot ('too many toes sign'), and abduction of the forefoot. Subtle signs of tibialis posterior tendinopathy are detectable by the toe raise test (inability to perform a single foot tip toe raise). The position of the calcaneus is checked. In a normal foot, hindfoot is inverted. In tibialis posterior tendinopathy, the hindfoot remains neutral or valgus. Oedema and tenderness are present around the tibialis posterior tendon or at its insertion. Flexion and inversion of the hindfoot against resistance are assessed and compared to unaffected limb.

Investigations

Ultrasonography and MRI provide information about the extent of the condition and the degree of tendon pathology.

Acute and chronic paratendinopathy

The synovium surrounding the tendon can be hypertrophic and oedematous, but the main body of the tendon is not, or only minimally, involved. Symptoms onset is gradual and relatively nonspecific. Pain worsened by prolonged weight bearing and walking. Pain is also elicited by retromalleolar palpation, passive eversion and abduction, active inversion and adduction. Local swelling is often present, particularly in the posteroinferior portion of the retromalleolar sulcus. Rarely, in chronic paratendinopathy, intratendinous calcifications can be found at ultrasonography or MRI.

Partial and complete rupture

Partial tears are more frequent in younger athletes, and total ruptures are more typical of middle-aged or former athletes. The patient has a pronated forefoot and an acquired flatfoot on the affected side. Pain and swelling are generalised on the medial aspect of the ankle, the tibialis posterior is inactive on manual testing and the patient is usually unable to perform a single leg heel rise. Clinical signs of tendon failure may be absent, but local pain and swelling, pain on resisted eversion and inversion and an enlarged tibialis posterior tendon can point to the diagnosis.

Management includes rest, analgesia and orthotics with a longitudinal arch support which prevents eversion. For total rupture and avulsion of the tendon, surgery is mandatory.

Flexor hallucis longus tendinopathy

The tendon of flexor hallucis longus (FHL) inserts into the distal phalanx of the big toe. Hyperpronation strains the FHL tendon at the retinaculum predisposing it to intratendinous pathology.

Clinical features include pain and discomfort in the medial retromalleolar region elicited by flexion of the toes. Sometimes, hyperaesthesia or crepitation may be present. Fullness between the Achilles tendon and the tibia due to oedema and inflamed synovium within the tunnel are present. The hallux is stiff, with limited dorsiflexion at the metatarso-phalangeal joint when the ankle is extended. MRI is the imaging modality of choice. Early recognition of tendinopathy of FHL is important. In the acute phase, rest, analgesia and avoidance of extreme plantar flexion can be helpful. Surgical management is controversial. Conservative management is preferred, as the scar tissue produces by surgery may lead to persistent pain.

Conclusion

Tendinopathy of the lower limb in athletes is secondary to overuse, insufficient warm up or various other mechanical factors. Reducing training intensity, duration or addressing other aggravating factors is beneficial in the early stages of tendinopathy. Eccentric strengthening exercises are effective in tendinopathies. We do not recommend nonsteroidal anti-inflammatory medications and corticosteroids. Aprotinin injections in the peritendinous region are beneficial for short to medium term relief. If conservative measures fail, surgical management may relieve symptoms, but the success depends on the tendon affected, the severity and chronicity of the condition.

Further reading

Tallon C, Coleman BD, Khan KM, et al. Outcome of surgery for chronic Achilles tendinopathy. A critical review. Am J Sports Med 2001; 29:315–320.

Leadbetter WB. Tendon overuse injuries: diagnosis and treatment. In: Renstrom PAFH (ed.), Sports injuries: basic principles of prevention and care. London: Oxford, 1993:449—476.

The team physiotherapist

Key points

- Screening
- On field acute management
- Load management, rehabilitation and return to play

The team physiotherapist is a very important role that varies considerably from working in a sports clinic. Travelling and working with a team is often extremely variable but equally challenging in its role. It is often all encompassing when travelling as you are working in close proximity to the team and will often be on call from the moment you get up till late at night. The role will vary depending on the level of other medical support you have available to you full time, a sports physician and/or massage therapist. There will need to be close relationships established with the sports physician, exercise physiologist, massage therapist, head coach, surgeon and radiologist. It is important to have a very good team of trusted medical practitioners working together for the benefit of the team and player.

Screening

The role of the physiotherapist will be to treat and manage acute injuries occurring within match play or training situations and refer appropriately where necessary and to ensure longer term injuries are rehabilitating appropriately. Another important area for the physiotherapist will be trying to reduce the injury rate and quicken the return time of any athletes injured. One major area that has progressed over the recent years is screening and 'prehabilitation'. An important role is to create a screening and base-testing programme to help identify areas of concern that can be addressed with athletes before they manifest as injuries or overload. A thorough past history is necessary to identify any previous risk factors and injuries, particularly soft tissue injuries such as hamstring strains, as the biggest risk factor for a strain is to have previously has a hamstring strain. Identifying any spinal pathology

or tendon pathology that may need strict load management is another crucial area to be aware of. The screening programme will be variable dependant on the specific requirements of the sport. Components tested may include relative flexibility around the pelvis or shoulders for a throwing sport. Baseline testing of specific components of the sport like hamstring strength for field sport and various agility markers like 6 m hop test and figure eight timed run. Specific control exercises around the pelvis and baseline shoulder and hip strength to examine ratios of internal versus external rotation to identify any areas that may expose the athlete to an injury. Examining muscle patterning is another feature to look at which helps to address faulty movement patterns like in a squat pattern. Any of these findings may be used to create a specific programme to target any weaknesses or areas of improvement for the athlete and these parameters can be used as baseline markers on returning an athlete from injury.

On field

On field management and treatment is another critical component of the team physiotherapist. It is important to be prepared for all eventualities in the field of play, especially planning for any head injuries or major incidents on the pitch. Thus, it is critical to know who is the doctor on duty and where the paramedical support will be situated. The team physiotherapist's kit bag is a particularly important piece of kit. This will need to be repacked and assessed and maintained on a weekly basis to ensure supplies are at an appropriate level.

Kit bag

- Strapping, 2.5 cm, 3.8 cm, 5 cm
- Elastic bandages 2.5 cm, 5 cm
- Compressive bandages 5 cm, 7.5 cm, 10 cm
- Gauze
- Sterile solutions for wound and eye injuries
- Gloves
- Slings

- Magic spray (ice spray)
- Ice bag
- Vaseline
- Deep heat or other muscle rubs
- Salt tablets
- Painkillers
- Oxygen
- Resuscitation equipment
- Splints
- Collars

On field assessment

- Danger to athlete
- Mechanism of injury
- Is the player responsive and conscious
- Can the player remember what happened
- What did they feel, any popping, cracking or sound heard
- Can they move the injured region
- Active and passive movements
- Joint stability testing
- Can they stand if lower limb
- Can they continue? Test injury for example hop for lower limb
- Can they return to field of play safely, if not emergency intervention or manage locally

All injuries on the field of play should be attended to immediately and then follow the Rest, Ice, Compression and Elevate (RICE) principles. Reassessment will usually occur the following day with a decision taken regarding the severity and need for further investigations like X-Rays or scans etc. After a thorough assessment and diagnosis a comprehensive treatment programme can be instigated to allow prompt recovery with optimal loading of the injured segment. Recovery processes following training and competition are another area that the physiotherapist can have input with. Ice baths, recovery sessions, compression garments, monitoring sleep, massage and nutrition all have a powerful effect on an athlete's recovery and it is necessary to ensure an athlete is doing everything possible to maximise their performance.

Communication

Communication within the medical and coaching staff is critical to the success of any team. It is important to have open and direct lines of communication between the coach and exercise physiologists and be able to flag issues as they occur. Being aware of the athletes training cycle and being able to have input into the cycle can be important in monitoring athlete's wellbeing and injury status. When working within a team taking good stats to help identify what stage of training or game many of your soft tissue injuries are occurring can help to identify areas of overtraining or too higher intensity or insufficient strength work. These injury patterns may become apparent over extensive periods of time and then corrective work or rest periods can be implemented to minimise further soft tissue injuries.

Load management

Load management is another area that physiotherapists are now helping to have input in. We are constantly striving to prevent breakdown of tissues and carefully monitored training programmes particularly with the use of GPS data can give accurate information about the athlete's current level of fitness and the need for rest or a change in their training cycle. These data need to be carefully interpreted for each individual, as one athlete's breaking point will be another athlete's peak training load.

Return to play

Returning athletes following injury requires extensive sports-specific and functional training. Lower limb pathology needs to be taken through a range of exercises from hopping, pivoting, cutting, noncontact game play and then mimicking contact type situations. Upper limb pathology has to have extensive high-end functional training and to ensure at least 90% full strength glenohumeral joint with specific scapula and trunk stability. When deciding when an athlete is ready to return to sport it is critical they undergo specific strength testing and functional testing. They should hit 90% of the contralateral side in testing to ensure sufficient return of strength. The final call on when an athlete returns to sport may ultimately be guided by the medical team and this information can be relayed to the coach; however, it may often be the coach that has the final say about returning an athlete to full competition. This is where open lines of communication and a good rapport need to be established to ensure athletes are not rushed back into the fold too early.

Further reading

Brukner P, Khan K. Brukner and Khan's clinical sports medicine, 3rd edn. New South Wales; McGraw Hill, 2007.

Orchard J, Best TM, Verrall GM. Return to Play following muscle strains. Clin J Sport Med 2005; 15:436–441.

Thermoregulation and fluid balance in hot conditions

Key points

- Sweating provides good thermoregulation in hot conditions but requires fluid replacement and is relatively ineffective if humidity is high
- Replacement fluids should contain some sodium
- Heatstroke is a medical emergency and facilities for checking core temperature and for rapid cooling should be available at events
- Training or competition involving continuous high intensity activity should not be attempted if conditions are too hot and humid, as indicated by WB-GT > 28

Thermoregulation while exercising under hot conditions

The high metabolic rate during exercise is a major challenge to our thermal homeostasis. The heat generated during exercise of short duration does not increase overall body temperature much. This is because the thermal capacity of the body is large enough to absorb the heat load from short bursts of high activity. The situation for endurance events is quite different. A marathon runner, weight 70 kg, doing a 3-h time, will have a metabolic rate of around 900 kcal/h. Unless it is very cold, simply vasodilation and trusting to passive heat loss is not enough. Fortunately, we can sweat at up to 4 L/h (man is a very sweaty animal). Evaporation uses 600 kcal/L, so sweating can dissipate up to 2400 kcal/L, easily enough to keep our marathon runner cool. But the water and electrolyte lost in sweat has to be replaced. So this is why heat balance and fluid and electrolyte balance are inextricably linked.

Two conditions need to be met for sweating to be effective. Firstly, sweat must be able to evaporate easily. This does not happen if the relative humidity is high. If we take our runner and assume a relative humidity of 80% with an ambient temperature of 35°C, then maximal sweating will now dissipate barely 1000 kcal/h, only just enough to maintain a stable body temperature. This calculation is for the highest recorded sweat rates. Most people cannot sweat more than about 2–3 L/h continuously, so with high temperature and humidity, body temperature can rise dangerously when exercising hard. The second point is that to continue sweating you need to drink to replace the lost fluid, and you need to drink a lot. Over 2 L/h is a lot to drink.

In practice, body temperature does rise in a controlled manner during exercise. The rise depends mostly on how vigorously we are exercising and rather little on environmental temperature. During intense exercise the core temperature may rise to 40°C or even higher in some tolerant individuals (41.9°C has been reported with no ill effects). If core temperature reaches above 40°C, then risk of heatstroke is high. Survival limit is 44°C, so the margin between the temperatures reached normally during intense exercise and temperatures that cause illness or death is extremely narrow.

How much and what to drink?

As pointed out above, thermoregulation during endurance exercise depends on sweating. It is therefore, necessary to drink regularly or dehydration occurs. The amount of fluid needed depends on how much we sweat, something that can be assessed by weighing. In games with breaks (e.g. half time in soccer games), this could be done and fluid accurately replaced. In practice, we depend on feeling thirsty. Annoyingly, our thirst mechanism is not reliable over short time periods and most people do not drink enough during endurance sports events. An indication of hydration can be obtained from observing urine colour. If adequately hydrated then urine should not be too dark in colour, and urine should be being passed regularly. Obviously during an event it is not feasible to check urine colour and volume. The best way to find the correct balance is to train under the same conditions as the prospective event and keep careful notes of amounts drunk and whether hydration was adequate. As discussed below, training in the heat will also help with acclimatisation.

Sweat contains significant amount of sodium chloride, so over several hours it is important to replace salt as well as water. The optimal replacement fluid under these circumstances will, therefore, contain some sodium chloride. Carbohydrate drinks can help performance by delaying muscle glycogen depletion and hence fatigue. So the most popular choice for endurance athletes is a carbohydrate plus electrolyte drink, of which many are available commercially.

Treatment of heat-related problems: exhaustion, heatstroke, hyponatremia

If someone collapses during a sports event on a hot day, heatstroke due to dehydration is the most likely cause. Signs of heatstroke include mental confusion, disorientation, fatigue and nausea. However, there are other possible causes of symptoms and so a rectal temperature should be obtained. Oral temperature can be misleading, as the high respiratory volumes during exercise will keep the mouth cool. If heatstroke is confirmed by a rectal temperature of 41 °C or above then immediate steps need to be taken to cool the subject and to give fluid. The sooner this is done, the better, so facilities should ideally be available at the event itself. Cooling can be achieved by immersion in cold water or using frequently changed cold wet towels. This can get the core temperature down by around 0.2°C /min, so achieving 2°C in about 10 min. But remember that if the subject is pale and vasoconstricted, these procedures may be less effective than expected. Cold packs over major vessels (neck, groin, axilla) may be useful. If treated promptly, most cases of heatstroke resolve without complications.

Occasionally, illness can be due to a fall in blood sodium level (exertional hyponatremia) due to drinking too much water. It is important to distinguish this condition from heatstroke, particularly as a different fluid replacement strategy is required. Clearly, such subjects will not have an extreme rectal temperature, but if they have been exercising hard the rectal temperature may still be elevated. Other signs that can help with diagnosis are dilute urine and tightness of rings, watchstraps, etc. (due to tissue swelling). Serum sodium below 130 mEqu/L indicates severe hyponatremia where IV hypertonic saline is indicated. Mild hyponatremia (130–135 mEqu/) can be rectified by eating some salty food.

Acclimatisation and precooling

Heat acclimatisation is essential if planning to compete in a hot climate. It is surprisingly straightforward to achieve. Exercise sessions of 40–100 min duration in a hot room and at intensity sufficient to cause lots of sweating will be enough to trigger useful adaptations. Principal changes are sweating comes on earlier, is at a higher rate, and has slightly lower electrolyte content. So the key here is getting your sweat glands trained. But note, for this to work you need to drink plenty. Repeating exercise sessions in the heat daily for 7–14 days is enough to produce good adaptation. Heat acclimatisation is lost over weeks rather than days, and significant gains are still present at 3 weeks after the last heat training session.

Lowering the core temperature by precooling using cold suits or ingestion of cold drinks has shown some useful improvements in performance in endurance events in the heat. Such strategies do not work for sprint or other short duration, high power and sports.

Prevention of heatstroke

The key matters in prevention have already been mentioned. The first is to drink enough, and to include some electrolyte in the drinks. The second is to prepare for the event by training in the heat enough to get heat acclimatised. There may also be days when endurance events or strenuous training will not be possible outdoors. The

Clinical features

- History of direct blow
- With severe contusion, the athlete usually has to stop their activity following the blow
- Localised pain and tenderness
- Swelling
- Bruising
- Knee effusion with more severe injuries
- Reduced range of knee movement depending on the severity of the injury (see above)
- Palpable mass (with myositis ossificans this may develop up to 4 weeks after the injury)

A possible complication of muscle contusion is development of compartment syndrome. As this is mainly a clinical diagnosis, its features must be looked for by clinicians managing athletes with contusion injuries.

Investigations

Plain radiograph will also demonstrate the developing myositis ossificans as well as help to exclude other pathologies such as fractures.

Further imaging such as US, computed tomography and magnetic resonance imaging will aid to distinguish myositis ossificans from other differential diagnosis (see below). Additionally biopsy may be indicated to exclude the other conditions.

Differential diagnosis

Appearance of myositis ossificans on the plain radiograph may resemble a series of benign and malignant lesions, these include:

- Benign
  - Osteochondroma
  - Osteomyelitis
  - Juxtacortical chondroma
- Malignant
  - Periosteal osteosarcoma
  - Parosteal osteosarcoma
  - Synovial sarcoma

Treatment

Vast majority of athletes with contusion and myositis ossificans are treated none operatively.

- In the acute phase of the injury, efforts should be concentrated at limiting the haematoma and reducing pain. This usually involves using:
  - Rest
  - Ice
  - Compression
  - Elevation
  - Immobilisation of the knee in 100°–120° of flexion started within 12 h of the injury and sustained for duration of about 24 h. This is thought to have a tamponade effect, therefore, reducing the size of the haematoma
- Athlete may progress to rehabilitation phase once adequate pain control is achieved. During this phase, attention is focused on:
  - Flexibility (Over stretching however, may result in rebleeds)
  - Muscular function
    - Muscular strength
    - Isometric
    - Isotonic (concentric and eccentric)
    - Isokinetic
    - Power
    - Muscular endurance
    - Muscular coordination
  - Proprioception
  - General fitness
- Next stage of nonoperative management involves focusing on functional and sport-specific exercises and finally return to sport.
  - Walking, running, sprinting, drills
  - Sport specific skills

NSAIDs and irradiation may play a part in prevention further heterotopic bone formation, but further research is required to establish this role.

Surgery (excision) has a very limited role in management of athletes with myositis ossificans and should only be considered in those athletes with painful bony mass, persistence loss of motion and function despite adequate nonoperative management and in whom at least 6-12 months has elapsed since the original injury.

Return to sports

As with other sports injuries return to play is permitted once the athlete is pain free, able to achieve a full range of movement and has regained enough strength to perform their sport specific activities. Functional testing that includes assessment of the ability to sprint and to perform specific sporting activities without pain should also be performed before permitting the athlete to return to play and declaring him or her fit.

The actual time taken for the athlete to return to play depends on the severity of the injury and may be as much as 10 weeks in athletes with severe contusions. The majority of the athletes, however, are able to return to their sports within 4 weeks.

Further reading

Larson CM, Almekinders LC, Karas SG, et al. Evaluating and managing muscle contusions and myositis ossificans. Phys Sports Med 2002; 30(2):41-50.
Negoro K, Uchida K, Yayama T, et al. Chronic expanding hematoma of the thigh. Joint Bone Spine 2012; 79:192–194.
Tyler P, Saifuddin A. The imaging of myositis ossificans. Semin Musculoskelet Radiol 2010; 14:201–216.

Related topics of interest

Thigh pain (anterior) – quadriceps

Key points

- Athlete optimisation is important in reducing risk of quadriceps tendon injuries
- Treatment is mainly nonoperative with a targeted specialist rehabilitation programme
- As with hamstring injuries, an inadequate rehabilitation programme and early return to play can lead to recurrent injury and chronic pain

Overview

Quadriceps refer to a group of muscles on the anterior aspect of the upper leg formed by rectus femoris, vastus medialis, vastus intermedius and vastus lateralis. Commonest injuries to quadriceps muscles include strains and contusion. This Topic highlights quadriceps strains, whereas muscle contusions and quadriceps tendon injuries are covered elsewhere. Quadriceps tendon ruptures are also not discussed here.

Quadriceps strain

These injuries occur in athletes who participate in sports which involve eccentric contraction of quadriceps at high speeds such as sprinting, track and field, rugby, soccer, American football and other running sports. Most quadriceps strains involve exclusively rectus femoris as it is the only of the group that cross both the hip joint and the knee joint.

Predisposing factors

Like other muscular injuries, risk factors could be divided into:
1. Sports related:
   a. Participation in sports that involve eccentric contraction of the quadriceps at high speed (see above).
2. Athlete related:
   a. Poor posture
   b. Muscle imbalance
   c. Limb length inequality
   d. Previous injury
   e. Inadequate management and recovery from previous injury
3. Training and technique related:
   a. Poor technique
   b. Fatigue
   c. Lack of warm up
   d. Inadequate flexibility

Pathology

As mentioned above, rectus femoris is the most vulnerable muscle of the quadriceps for sustaining muscular strain injuries due to the fact that it crosses both the hip and the knee joints. Injuries commonly occur at the musculotendinous junction and more likely to be distal than proximal although proximal intramuscular rectus femoris tears have also been described. As with hamstring injuries, the primary mechanism of injury appears to be violent eccentric contraction causing stretch injury to the musculotendinous junction (due to large force generation with eccentric contractions).

This stretch injury is divided into three main grades:

Grade I: This a mild strain as only a few muscle fibres are torn with a small structural integrity disruption at the musculotendinous junction.

Grade II: This is a moderate strain with a partial tear, but some of the fibres at the musculotendinous junction do remain intact. There is some strength loss.

Grade IIIA: Complete tear/rupture of the muscle (usually at the musculotendinous junction).

Grade IIIB: Characterised by bony avulsion at the bone attachment sites.

Clinical features

Clinical features are dependent of the grade of the injury as demonstrated in **Table 29**.

Table 29 Grading of the quadriceps muscular injuries

Grade	Symptoms	Signs
I	– Pain in the anterior thigh – Presentation may be acute or chronic – There may be a history of a specific event that started the symptoms (i.e. sprinting); however, it is not uncommon for the athlete to continue his or her exercise and present after a good delay, i.e. the following day – Degree of weakness (may be secondary to pain) – Presence of any of the predisposing factors (see above)	– Small degree of haemorrhage and swelling – Localised tenderness – Pain produced by passive stretching of the quadriceps muscle – Pain produced by resisted active contraction of the quadriceps muscles – Lack of objective function loss
II	– Athletes more likely to present with an acute injury – Athlete may or may not be able to continue with his or her exercise – More pronounced weakness (actual muscle weakness not just pain related) – Athletes will usually limp but are able to fully bear weight	– Greater degree of haemorrhage and swelling – Presence of a painful palpable lesion in the muscle – Passive stretching causes greater degree by pain – Smaller degree of resistance felt by clinician before onset of pain during active knee extension against resistance – True muscle weakness
III A and B	– Similar to grade II injuries but more severe – Athlete likely to discontinue his or her exercise and present acutely	– Similar signs to grade II, but more obvious – Muscle palpable defect when the muscle contracts may be felt

Investigations

Plain radiograph may help to exclude femoral stress fracture and myositis ossificans.

Magnetic resonance imaging can be of great use by revealing the:

1. Extent of the injury
2. Grade of the injury
3. Which muscles are involved

Differential diagnosis

Differential diagnosis include:

1. Quadriceps muscle related:
   a. Quadricep muscular contusions and haematoma (see below)
   b. Myositis ossificans (see below)
2. Femur related:
   a. Stress fractures
3. Low back pathology:
   a. Referred pain from low back
   b. Lumbosacral radiculopathy

4. Tumours:
   a. Soft tissue tumours
   b. Osteosarcoma of the femur
5. Others
   a. Chronic compartment syndrome
   b. Apophysitis
   c. Nerve entrapment
   d. Sartorius and gracilis strains

Treatment

As with hamstring injuries, the vast majority of athletes with quadriceps muscular sprain injuries are treated nonoperatively.

1. In the acute phase of the injury, efforts should be concentrated at reducing the pain. This may involve using:
   a. Rest
   b. Ice
   c. Compression
   d. Elevation
   e. NSAIDs

2. Once pain control is achieved, the athlete may progress to rehabilitation phase. During this phase, attention is focused on:
   a. Flexibility
   b. Muscular function
      i. muscular strength
         isometric
         isotonic (concentric and eccentric)
         isokinetic
      ii. power
      iii. muscular endurance
      iv. muscular coordination
   c. Proprioception
   d. General fitness
3. Next stage of nonoperative management involves focusing on functional and sport specific exercises and finally return to sport.
   a. Walking, running, sprinting, drills
   b. Sport specific skills
4. Management must also include correction of any of the predisposing factors that could have contributed to the injury in the first place (see above).

Surgery may have a role in those athletes with grade III injuries who demonstrate gross retraction of the quadriceps when they contract.

Return to sports

As with other sports injuries return to play is permitted once the athlete is pain free, able to achieve a full range of movement and has regained enough strength to perform their sport specific activities. Functional testing that includes assessment of the ability to sprint and to perform specific sporting activities without pain should also be performed before permitting the athlete to return to play and declaring him or her fit.

The actual time taken for the athlete to return to play depends on the extent of the injury, and can vary from 2 days to 10 weeks; however, the majority of the athletes return to their sports within 4 weeks.

Prognosis

Most quadricep strains usually heal following an appropriate and accurate nonoperative regime; however, as with hamstring injuries, an inadequate rehabilitation programme and early return to play can lead to recurrent injury and chronic pain.

In a small number of patients, excessive scar formation may lead to impingement of the femoral nerve (dysfunction of the femoral nerve may also occur secondary to mechanical pressure caused by spasm of psoas muscle that can be associated with quadriceps injuries).

Further reading

Douis H, Gillett M, James SL. Imaging in the diagnosis, prognostication, and management of lower limb muscle injury. Semin Musculoskelet Radiol 2011; 15:27–41.

Hägglund M, Waldén M, Ekstrand J. Risk factors for lower extremity muscle injury in professional soccer: the UEFA injury study. Am J Sports Med 2013; 41:327–335.

Related topics of interest

Thigh pain (posterior) – hamstring

Key points

- Most are treated nonoperatively with appropriate physiotherapy regimes
- Inadequate rehabilitation programme and early return to play can lead to recurrent injury and chronic pain
- Surgery should be considered if there is complete detachment of the musculotendinous complex from the origin or insertion

Overview

Hamstrings refer to a group of muscles on the posterior aspect of the upper leg formed by semimembranosus, semitendinosus and bicep femoris. Their injuries are extremely common in athletes and account for a significant lost playing time. As they cross both the hip and the knee joints, they have the ability to contribute to both hip extension and knee flexion, but as a consequence can be placed under tremendous forces depending on the positions of the hip and knee joints.

Epidemiology

Commonest strain-related injuries faced by sports clinicians, these injuries are common in sports that involve eccentric contraction of the hamstring at high speeds such as sprinting, track and field, rugby, soccer and other running sports. They are reported to be more common in the 15–25 age groups.

Predisposing factors

Risk factors could be divided into:
1. Sports related:
   a. Participation in sports that involve eccentric contraction of the hamstrings at high speed (see above)
2. Athlete related:
   a. Poor posture
   b. Muscle imbalance (hamstring to quadriceps ratio of less than 50%)
   c. Limb length inequality
   d. Tight hip flexors and anterior hip tilt (may be due to rapid growth in adolescence)
   e. Previous injury
   f. Inadequate management and recovery from previous injury.
3. Training and technique related:
   a. Poor technique (poor running style; overstriding)
   b. Fatigue
   c. Lack of warm up
   d. Inadequate flexibility

Pathology

The primary pathology in hamstring strains appears to be stretch injury to the musculotendinous junction. As eccentric contractions generate a much greater forces than concentric contractions, they are more likely to induce such stretch injuries. Hamstrings span across two joints, therefore likely to undergo eccentric contractions during various sporting activities.

The initial phase of the injury (first 24 h) is accompanied with a haemorrhagic response around the injured muscle fibres. This is then followed by necrotic changes of the injured muscle fibres, oedema and increase in number of the macrophages in the area (24–48 h). After 48 h as the number of inflammatory cells in the area increase, there is also an intensification of fibroblastic activity.

This stretch injury is divided into three main grades:

Grade I: This a mild strain as only a few muscle fibres are torn with a small structural integrity disruption at the musculotendinous junction.

Grade II. This is a moderate strain with a partial tear but some of the fibres at the musculotendinous junction do remain intact. There is some strength loss.

Grade IIIA. Complete tear/rupture of the muscle (usually at the musculotendinous junction).

Grade IIIB: Characterised by bony avulsion at the bone attachment sites.

Clinical features

Clinical features are dependent of the grade of the injury as demonstrated in the **Table 30**.

Investigations

1. Plain radiograph may reveal the avulsion fractures with Type IIIB injuries. It may also demonstrate calcifications in patients with chronic hamstring pain.
2. In addition to excluding other injuries, MRI can be of great use by revealing the:
   a. Extent of the injury
   b. Grade of the injury
   c. Which muscles are involved

Differential diagnosis

Differential diagnosis include:
- Hamstring muscular contusions and haemotoma
- Referred pain from low back
- Lumbosacral radiculopathy
- Femoral stress fractures
- Chronic compartment syndrome
- Apophysitis
- Myositis ossificans
- Nerve entrapment

Treatment

In most cases treatment is nonoperatively:
1. In the acute phase of the injury, efforts should be concentrated at reducing the pain. This may involve using:
   a. Rest

Table 30 Classification of hamstring injuries		
Grade	Symptoms	Signs
I	– Pain in the posterior thigh – Presentation may be acute or chronic – History of a specific event that started the symptoms (i.e. sprinting) – Those with chronic presentation may complain of tightness/pull while participating in sports or some post exercise pain – Degree of weakness (may be secondary to pain) – Presence of any of the predisposing factors (see above)	– Small degree of haemorrhage and swelling – Localised tenderness – Pain produced by passive extension of knee with hip flexed at 90° – Pain produced with active knee flexion against resistance – Lack of objective function loss
II	– Athletes more likely to present with an acute injury – Sudden onset of pain in posterior thigh during activity (i.e. sprinting) – More pronounced weakness (actual muscle weakness not just pain related) – Athletes may recall an audible pop at time of the injury	– Greater degree of haemorrhage and swelling. – Presence of a painful palpable mass in the muscle that will not retract with active contraction of the muscle – Passive extension of the knee restricted to a greater degree by pain – Smaller degree of resistance felt by clinician before onset of pain during active knee flexion against resistance – True muscle weakness
III A and B	– Similar to Grade II injuries but more severe	– Similar signs to Grade II, but more obvious. – Painful mass that retracts with active contraction of the muscle (Grade IIIA) – Grade IIIA injuries closer close to bone attachment sites than Grade II injuries

b. Ice
c. Compression
d. Elevation
e. NSAIDs

2. Once pain control is achieved, the athlete may progress to rehabilitation phase. During this phase efforts are made to restore flexibility, muscular function, proprioception and general fitness:

   a. **Flexibility:** This is dependent on range of movement of the joint and soft tissue flexibility. Joint flexibility may be aided by active and passive exercises. Stretching will promote soft tissue flexibility as well as being beneficial in increasing muscular relaxation and preventing formation of excessive adhesions

   b. **Muscular Function:** Any muscular functioning rehabilitation programme must address muscular strength and power, muscular endurance and finally but as important muscular coordination

   Muscular strengthening involves gradual progression from isometric to isotonic to isokinetic exercises. Progression into the different forms of the muscular strengthening exercises is dependent on the pain relief achieved with each type of exercise (i.e. once the athlete regains the ability to perform isometric exercises pain free, then isotonic exercises may be started). Isotonic exercises, which involve movement of the joint against a constant resistance, may be concentric or eccentric. As eccentric exercises produce large forces in the muscle, they should only be initiated after the athlete can perform concentric exercises comfortably.

   Muscular power training usually should in most cases occur in the later stages of rehabilitation and would involve fast isotonic and isokinetic exercises, progressively faster functional exercises, and activities which are relevant to the athletes sport such as hopping and jumping.

   Muscular endurance is enhanced by low force, high repetitive exercises (load may be increased gradually).

   Enhancement of muscular coordination involves athlete and muscular education, and correction of abnormal muscular patterning.

   c. **Proprioception:** Musculoskeletal injuries can result in impairment of proprioception due to damaged nerve endings and nerve pathways. If this impairment is not addressed in the rehabilitation programme, further injuries may occur. Correction is performed through a series of progression exercises ranging from standing on one leg to zigzag running and sideway step-ups.

   d. **General fitness:** During the rehabilitation phase, attempts must be made to maintain the general fitness of the athlete. This may start with water exercises and progress to cycling and running once muscles have been conditioned adequately.

3. In the next stage of nonoperative management, following restoration of flexibility, muscular function, and proprioception, attention is focused on functional and sport-specific exercises and finally returns to sport. Functional exercises involve progression from walking to running to sprinting to drills. Athlete should also be taken through sport-specific exercises that should be followed by return to sport and practice of sport specific skills.

4. Management must also include correction of any of the predisposing factors that could have contributed to the injury in the first place (see above).

   Surgery should only be considered if there is complete detachment of the musculotendinous complex from the origin or insertion.

Return to sports

As with other sports injuries return to play is permitted once the athlete is pain free, able to achieve a full range of movement and has regained enough strength to perform their sport specific activities. The strength of the injured hamstring must reach at least 90% of the strength of the contralateral uninjured hamstring. A hamstring-quadriceps ratio of 0.55 must be achieved prior to return to play. Functional testing that includes assessment of the ability to sprint and to perform specific sporting activities without pain should also be performed before permitting the athlete to return to play and declaring him or her fit.

The actual time taken for the athlete to return to play depends on the extent of the injury, ranging from few days for Grade I injuries to 6–8 weeks for the more severe Grade III injuries.

Prognosis

Most hamstring strains usually heal following an appropriate and accurate nonoperative regime; however, an inadequate rehabilitation programme and early return to play can lead to recurrent injury and chronic pain. In a small number of patients, excessive scar formation may lead to impingement of the sciatic nerve (known as hamstring syndrome).

Further reading

Wood DG, Packham I, Trikha SP, et al. Avulsion of the proximal hamstring origin. J Bone Joint Surg Am 2008; 90:2365–2374.

Ali K, Leland JM . Hamstring strains and tears in the athlete. Clin Sports Med 2012; 31:263–272.

Reurink G, Goudswaard GJ, Tol JL, et al. Therapeutic interventions for acute hamstring injuries: a systematic review. Br J Sports Med 2012; 46 (2):103-109.

Malliaropoulos N, Mendiguchia J, Pehlivanidis H, et al. Hamstring exercises for track and field athletes: injury and exercise biomechanics, and possible implications for exercise selection and primary prevention. Br J Sports Med 2012; 46:846–851.

Related topics of interest

- Physiotherapy – acute injury management (p. 223)
- Physiotherapy – general principles (p. 229)
- Thigh – muscular contusions and myositis ossificans (p. 313)
- Thigh pain (anterior) – quadriceps (p. 316)

Training

Key points

- Important principles of training are overload, specificity, individuality and reversibility
- Resistance training can build up muscle strength and power
- Endurance training increases aerobic capacity through adaptations to muscles (e.g. more mitochondria), the heart (cardiac hypertrophy) and respiratory system
- Individuals vary markedly in their response to training, some showing big increases whilst others improve little

Introduction

Training for increased strength and power is rather different to training for endurance, so these two topics will be considered separately. However, in both cases, four principles are important: overload, specificity, individuality and reversibility. Overload indicates that to get changes we need to push the system a bit. Not necessarily to the limit, but reasonably close to it. Specificity is sometimes obvious (training for endurance versus strength, for example), sometimes surprising (isokinetic training at a fast velocity producing relatively small effects on strength at lower velocities). And of course, some effects are general (e.g. whatever muscle groups we exercise aerobically, if we do it hard enough and long enough then cardiac performance will improve). But overall the general rule is that all training programmes need to be sport-, activity- or muscle group-specific. Individuality indicates that training programmes need to take account of individual differences. You cannot adopt a 'one size fits all' approach. And it is important to understand that the response to training is itself variable from subject to subject. Everyone will get some improvement with appropriate training, but in some subjects the rewards will be greater than in others. Finally, reversibility means that if you stop carrying out an activity then strength and fitness levels will decline.

Resistance training, increasing muscle force and power

When beginning a strength-training programme, there will often be rapid increases in performance due to neural changes. One learns better technique with practice and there are also increases in motor unit recruitment. In this section, however, the focus will be on the physiological and biochemical changes in muscles when training for strength and power.

Resistance training to increase muscle strength and power can be done in several different ways. The traditional method is weight training with free weights. This is still widely used as the equipment is cheap and it is straightforward to progress. But a good technique is required and accidents can happen rather more easily than with other exercise methods. Rather similar exercises can be carried out using fixed gym equipment. A different approach is to use isometric contractions. Repeated strong isometric contractions certainly build up muscle maximum force, but the effects turn out to be quite specific for the muscle length used. So to increase strength and power over the range of movement of a muscle requires making contractions at lengths covering this range. By the time this is done for all the major muscle groups, the training session has become rather long. A relatively new method is to use an isokinetic dynamometer, a machine that sets a constant speed of movement and varies the load. This method is convenient for training at a range of speeds. The machine will also give performance readout for a range of movements. Finally, we will mention plyometrics. This system involves a series of jumps and so uses gravity to develop dynamic loads.

Resistance training programmes do not need to induce fatigue to be effective. Optimal training programmes involve sets of 3–12 repeat contractions at close to maximum force (typically 80%), not repeated too often. Using larger numbers of repeated contractions are less effective (in terms of performance improvement per training time).

The effects of all resistance exercise programmes are broadly the same. Muscle force increases, and does so along with increases in muscle cross-sectional area. Tendons and bones also strengthen. Speed of contraction generally stays the same, or may increase. If we look at the level of individual muscle fibres we find that they get larger, and for strength training the hypertrophy is restricted to fast muscle fibres. There also appears to be some switching of phenotype from FF to FR. This is not perhaps what one might expect as FF fibres are faster and more powerful than FR. However, overall, due to hypertrophy of the fast fibres, there can be an increase in speed. Slow (S) fibres do not appear to change to FR or FF, even with specific speed training. Neither do the slow fibres hypertrophy. At the level of the myosin molecule, different versions of the myosin heavy chain (MHC) are found in the three types of fibre, MHC I in S fibres, MHC IIa in FR fibres and MHC IIx in FF fibres. In resistance-trained muscles, there is rather more MHC IIa along with the increase in FR fibres.

Biology of muscle hypertrophy

The important stimulus for muscle growth is mechanical stress, particularly levels of stress (e.g. eccentric contractions) that produce a degree of microtrauma. The local paracrine factors released by muscle stress, for example IGF-1Ec (MGF, insulin-like growth factor 1, splice variant Ec) wake up the muscle satellite cells. The satellite cells proliferate and differentiate into myoblasts that fuse with existing fibres. This provides extra nuclei that can support increased protein synthesis. Mechanical stress and local growth factors activate a complex series of reactions in the muscle fibres that involves the mTOR protein kinase and transcription factors and coactivators that alter gene expression.

Aerobic training and skeletal muscle

At the muscle level, aerobic, endurance training leads to more S and FR fibres and less FF. There are also striking increases in numbers of mitochondria and in the activity of mitochondrial enzymes. Other metabolic enzymes also increase in activity. Notable here are enzymes involved in beta-oxidation of fatty acids. Thanks to this, more fatty acid can be metabolised by endurance-trained muscle. This is important as after about 1–2 h, muscle carbohydrate stores run down. Finally, there is a marked growth of capillaries. The main effect of the extra capillaries is probably not to reduce diffusion distances, but rather to ensure that blood flow is not too rapid through any given capillary when muscle blood flow is high. A long enough transit time is required to ensure that there is enough time for gas exchange.

Cardiovascular adaptations to aerobic training

Following aerobic training, ventricular volume increases. There is also an increase in contractility and the functional consequence is that resting and maximal stroke volumes are both elevated. The increase in resting stroke volume leads to a balancing reduction in heart rate. The reduced heart rate appears to be caused by increased vagal tone as evidenced by the increased heart rate variability seen in trained athletes under resting conditions. Interestingly, maximum heart rate is unchanged. There is also a useful increase in blood volume, with no change in Hb concentration.

Respiratory system adaptations to aerobic training

An important consequence of aerobic training is that the breathing muscles become trained themselves. This helps cope with the greater pulmonary ventilation needed to meet the increased oxygen consumption of trained muscles. There is no change in the pulmonary ventilation/oxygen uptake relationship. Resting tidal volume increases with training and the respiratory rate falls.

Individual variation in training responses

Responses to training, whether aerobic or resistance, are surprisingly variable from person to person. Twin and family studies show that 'trainability' is about 50% inherited. Genetic studies, most recently including genome wide association studies, have started to identify the loci that are most important for trainability. Eventually this will lead to a fuller understanding of the key cellular mechanisms underlying training responses. Already it is providing markers that will indicate an individual's trainability and we can expect such information to eventually be used to design personal training or rehabilitation programmes.

Recent studies also indicate that trainability reflects not just the pattern of gene expression, but also their post-transcriptional control. Important here are the micro-RNA molecules. These are a large group of short RNA transcripts that bind to messenger RNA and stop translation into protein of groups of genes. Given the powerful methods now available for investigating DNA polymorphisms and RNA sequences we are likely to see rapid progress in our understanding of the molecular mechanisms underlying training responses.

Further reading

Bouchard C. Genomic predictors of trainability. Exp Physiol 2012; 97:347–352.

Davidsen PK, Gallagher IJ, Hartman JW, et al. High responders to resistance exercise training demonstrate differential regulation of skeletal muscle microRNA expression. J Appl Physiol 2011; 110:309–317.

Harridge SD. Plasticity of human skeletal muscle: gene expression to in vivo function. Exp Physiol 2007; 92:783–797.

Whyte G. The physiology of training. Edinburgh: Churchill Livingstone, 2006.

Related topics of interest

- Muscle properties relevant to sports and exercise (p. 195)
- Exercise and health (p. 106)

Unexplained under performance syndrome

Key points

- Defined as underperformance of greater than 2 weeks duration with no alternative explanation
- Commonly due to increase in training and also called overtraining syndrome
- As there are no useful diagnostic tests, diagnosis is done from history and by excluding other medical and related reasons for underperformance
- Management is relative rest with gradual resumption of full training over weeks or months

Overview

Unexplained underperformance syndrome (UUPS) is defined as persistent unexplained performance deficit (agreed by coach and athlete) despite 2 weeks of relative rest. UUPS is normally associated with heavy training and this is the basis for the alternative designation of 'overtraining syndrome'. However, factors other than simply training levels are often involved, notably infective illness and nonsports stresses such as personal problems or exams. Hence, the designation 'underperformance' is to be preferred.

There is clearly a real difficulty for athletes and coaches in distinguishing between the 'healthy' exhaustion felt during periods of intense training and the enervating fatigue of UUPS. Athletes and coaches are inevitably pushing the boundaries in attempting to improve fitness and performance. Mostly, it works fine and the heavy training gives improved results. But if adequate rest and recuperation are ignored, then UUPS can develop.

Epidemiology

Periods of underperformance, accompanied by excessive fatigue, happen to as many as 20% of endurance athletes involved in heavy training programmes. UUPS is rarely seen in sprinters or other athletes in explosive events.

Pathology

Parallels have been drawn between UUPS and the General Adaptation Syndrome described first by Selye in the 1930s. Selye pointed out that many diseases were stress related and tended to run a similar course. Initially, the body adapted to the stress. However, if the stress continued over weeks and months, the character of the response altered and pathophysiological changes developed (e.g. gastric ulcers and hypertension). The solution is to remove the stressors. The unusual feature of UUPS is that the stressor – heavy training – is necessary for peak performance. Various coping strategies have been developed to reduce stress, such as relaxation. However, one aspect of the response to stress that does not appear to have been much considered in sports medicine is control. In animal models the 'executive rat' that can switch off the stressor shows less pathophysiology than a yoked animal receiving the same stress, but with no control over it. So one strategy for avoiding UUPS may be to ensure that the athlete is in control and fully involved in planning their training.

Clinical features

Reliable early signs would be helpful. Unfortunately, all suggestions so far are nonspecific. However, it is clearly worth watching out for fatigue building up, any shift towards more anxious and/or depressed moods, or a slightly elevated resting heart rate. But note, none of these, or the many other signs or symptoms suggested so far in the literature, gives a reliable indication of the onset of UUPS. Some coaches have found regularly giving the POMS (profile of mood states) questionnaire useful in heading off problems.

Repeated respiratory tract infections can be a prelude to, or accompany, UUPS. In some instances, it is felt that returning to training too soon after an infection may have triggered UUPS. There are reported falls in IgA in saliva and other immune system changes during heavy endurance training. However, not everyone with this pattern develops UUPS. Raised levels of the cytokine IL6 have been seen after heavy training and since IL6 is implicated in some illness syndromes it has been proposed that IL6 plays a part in UUPS.

Common features of UUPS are mood changes and interrupted sleep. These aspects, along with fatigue, are also seen in chronic fatigue syndrome (CFS). Alterations in brain 5HT have been associated with CFS, and so studies of 5HT have been carried out in UUPS. There are good reasons why 5HT might be altered with heavy training. Tryptophan, the precursor of 5HT, is bound to albumin in plasma. During exercise the increased fatty acids in plasma compete with tryptophan for binding sites on albumin and the result is an increase in free tryptophan, and so more available for making 5HT. In addition, branched chain amino acids (BCAA) compete with tryptophan for the carrier from plasma to brain. The concentration of BCAA in plasma falls during endurance exercise. The overall effect of these two changes should, therefore, be a rise in brain 5HT. Perhaps to compensate, trained endurance athletes have reduced sensitivity to 5HT agonists. Interestingly, athletes with UUPS show a greater response to a 5HTc agonist than athletes without UUPS in agreement with the idea that a disturbance in brain 5HT actions may play a part in UUPS.

Investigations

There are no standard investigations for UUPS. The aim is to rule out alternative explanations for underperformance. So looking for signs of infection, hormone alterations (e.g. thyroid) and metabolic measures are indicated. Note that a detailed research study found reasons, often medical, for underperformance in nearly 70% of athletes with an initial diagnosis of UUPS. In some instances, there were other problems

such as disturbed sleep due to jet lag and personal problems. Such possibilities should be clear from the history. Other athletes were in negative energy balance or on a diet low in protein, so a careful investigation of the athlete's nutrition is essential. Note that loss of appetite is often found with UUPS, so maintaining good nutrition may be difficult.

Differential diagnosis

This is the key for a certain diagnosis of UUPS. There are, unfortunately, a lot of possibilities that can explain a reduction in performance, fatigue and changes in mood. Medical explanations that need to be excluded include unresolved infections, undiagnosed asthma/bronchial hyperreactivity, thyroid disease, adrenal disease, diabetes mellitus or insipidus and iron deficiency with or without anaemia.

Treatment

The recommended management is never going to be popular. It is basically a large drop in training levels – perhaps even a period of complete rest – followed by a very gradual rebuilding of training levels. Note that when an athlete and coach first notice a decrement in performance the response is usually to increase training to try to compensate. So by the time medical help is sought, the situation has been made worse. Work should be built up gradually during recovery. At first light levels of training are set and the volume is gradually increased, then intensity is increased later. It typically takes 6–12 weeks to get back to high training loads.

Return to sport

UUPS is not a condition where a complete break from sport or exercise is appropriate. As soon as adequate levels of fitness have been reached, then return to competitive sport is possible. Continued monitoring, for example with the POMS questionnaire, may be worthwhile in avoiding reoccurrence of UUPS.

Further reading

Budgett R, Hiscock N, Arida RM, et al. The effects of the 5-HT2C agonist m-chlorophenylpiperazine on elite athletes with unexplained underperformance syndrome (overtraining). Br J Sports Med 2010; 44:280–283.

Budgett R, Newsholme E, Lehmann M, et al. Redefining the overtraining syndrome as the unexplained underperformance syndrome. Br J Sports Med 2000; 34:67–68.

Kreher JB, Schwartz JB. Overtraining syndrome: a practical guide. Sports Health 2012; 4:128–138.

Related topics of interest

- Training (p. 323)
- Female athlete – the triad (p. 124)
- Psychology – performance enhancement (p. 239)

Urological injuries

Key points

- Renal trauma can be life threatening, therefore assessment of haemodynamic stability is of critical importance
- Exact management of patients with renal trauma is dependent on haemodynamic stability, associated injuries and grade of injury
- 30% patients of patients with pelvic fracture have some degree of bladder damage

Renal trauma

Renal injury due to sport is almost always blunt in nature. Renal trauma can be acutely life threatening, but the majority can be managed conservatively.

Renal injuries are classified according to American Association for the Surgery of Trauma (AAST) classification as Grade 1–5 (**Table 31**). Abdominal computed tomography (CT) or direct renal exploration is used to classify injuries. The AAST scaling system is the most important variable predicting the need for kidney repair or removal, as well as predicting morbidity and for mortality after blunt injury.

Clinical features

In a patient with a suspected renal injury, the most important first step is to establish haemodynamic stability. History should be taken from conscious patients, witnesses and rescue team with regard to the setting of the incident.

Renal injury should be suspected on presence of haematuria, flank pain, flank abrasions and ecchymoses, fractured ribs, abdominal tenderness, distension or mass. Urine should be inspected grossly and then by dipstick analysis.

Investigations

Blunt trauma patients with macroscopic or microscopic haematuria (at least 5 rbc/hpf) and hypotension (systolic blood pressure <90 mmHg) should undergo radiographic evaluation. Radiographic evaluation is also recommended for all patients with a history of rapid deceleration injury and/or significant associated injuries.

An intravenous contrast CT scan is the best imaging study for the diagnosis and staging of renal injuries. Haemodynamically unstable patients requiring emergency surgical exploration should undergo a one-shot IVP

Grade*	Description of injury
Table 31 AAST renal injury grading scale	
1	• Contusion or non-expanding subcapsular haematoma • No laceration
2	• Non-expanding peri-renal haematoma • Cortical laceration < 1 cm deep without extravasation
3	• Cortical laceration > 1 cm without urinary extravasation
4	Laceration: through corticomedullary junction into collecting system or • Vascular: segmental renal artery or vein injury with contained haematoma, or partial vessel laceration, or vessel thrombosis
5	• Laceration: shattered kidney or • Vascular: renal pedicle or avulsion
*Advance one grade for bilateral injuries up to grade 3.	

with bolus intravenous injection of 2 mL/kg contrast.

Angiography can be used for diagnosis and simultaneous selective embolisation of bleeding vessels.

Treatment

Following Grades 1–4 blunt renal traumas, stable patients should be managed conservatively with bed-rest, prophylactic antibiotics and continuous monitoring of vital signs until haematuria resolves.

Indications for surgical management include:

- Haemodynamic instability
- Exploration for associated injuries
- Expanding or pulsatile perirenal haematoma identified during laparotomy;
- Grade 5 injury

In cases where surgical exploration is necessary, once controlling haemorrhage is achieved, renal reconstruction should be attempted if sufficient amount of renal parenchyma is viable.

Repeat imaging is recommended for all hospitalised patients within 2–4 days of significant renal trauma.

Within 3 months of major renal injury, patients' follow-up should involve urinalysis, individualised radiological investigation, serial blood pressure measurement and serum creatinine.

Long-term follow-up should be decided on a case-by-case basis but should at the very least involve monitoring for renovascular hypertension.

Bladder trauma

In the setting of blunt trauma, bladder rupture may be classified as either extraperitoneal with leakage of urine limited to the perivesical space, or intraperitoneal.

A fully distended bladder can be ruptured by a light blow; however, an empty bladder is seldom injured, except by crushing or penetrating wounds. Seventy to ninety percent of patients with bladder injuries caused by blunt trauma have associated pelvic fractures and up to 30% of patients with pelvic fractures will have some degree of bladder injury. Bladder injury is classified by AAST into five grades (**Table 32**).

Clinical features

The most common signs and symptoms in a patient with major bladder injury are gross haematuria (82%) and abdominal tenderness (62%).

Investigations

Retrograde cystography is the standard diagnostic procedure in the evaluation of bladder trauma. CT cystography can be used with equal efficacy if the patient is undergoing CT scanning for associated injuries.

Treatment

In the absence of bladder neck involvement and/or associated injuries that require surgical intervention, extraperitoneal bladder ruptures caused by blunt trauma are managed by catheter drainage alone.

Table 32 Bladder injury grading	
Grade	Description
I	Haematoma: Contusion, intramural hematoma
	Laceration: Partial thickness
II	Laceration Extraperitoneal bladder wall laceration < 2 cm
III	Laceration Extraperitoneal (> 2 cm) or intraperitoneal (< 2 cm) bladder wall laceration
IV	Laceration Intraperitoneal bladder wall laceration > 2 cm
V	Laceration Intraperitoneal or extraperitoneal bladder wall laceration extending into the bladder neck or ureteral orifice (trigone)

Intraperitoneal bladder ruptures by blunt trauma, and any type of bladder injury by penetrating trauma, must be managed by emergency surgical exploration and repair. Safe method of repairing the bladder wall is a two-layer closure with absorbable sutures.

Urethral trauma

The male urethra is divided into the anterior and posterior sections by the urogenital diaphragm. The posterior urethra consists of the prostatic and the membranous urethra. The anterior urethra consists of the bulbar and penile urethra. Only the posterior urethra exists in the female. Sports injuries, such as falls, and crush injuries can cause pelvic fractures, which result in injuries to the posterior urethra. Anterior urethral injuries usually result from blunt trauma such as fall astride (straddle) and kicks/blows in the perineum.

Blunt anterior and posterior urethral injury is classified to 6 grades (**Table 33**).

Clinical features

Blood at the meatus is present in 37–93% of patients with posterior urethral injury, and in at least 75% of patients with anterior urethral trauma.

Investigations

Retrograde urethrography is the gold standard for evaluating urethral injury. In the absence of blood at the meatus or genital haematoma, a urological injury is very unlikely and is excluded by catheterisation. When blood is present at the urethral meatus, do not attempt urethral instrumentation until the entire urethra is imaged. In an unstable patient, attempt to pass a urethral catheter, but if there is any difficulty, place a suprapubic catheter and perform a retrograde urethrogram when appropriate.

Treatment

Classification helps with clinical management:

- Grade I requires no treatment
- Grades II and III can be managed conservatively with suprapubic cystostomy or urethral catheterisation
- Grades IV and V will require open or endoscopic treatment, primary or delayed
- Grade VI requires primary open repair

Genital trauma

Any kind of full contact sports may be associated with genital trauma, but there is increased risk with off-road bicycling and

Table 33 Urethral injury grading		
Grade	Description	Appearance
I	Stretch injury	Elongation of the urethra without extravasation on urethrography
II	Contusion	Blood at the urethral meatus No extravasation on urethrography
III	Partial disruption of anterior or posterior urethra	Extravasation of contrast at injury site with contrast visualised in the proximal urethra or bladder
IV	Complete disruption of anterior urethra	Extravasation of contrast at injury site without visualisation of proximal urethral or bladder
V	Complete disruption of posterior urethra	Extravasation of contrast at injury site without visualisation of bladder
VI	Complete or partial disruption of posterior urethra with associated tear of the bladder neck or vagina	

motorbike riding, in-line hockey skating and rugby football. Genital trauma from sport can happen in both sexes; however, it is much commoner in men.

Blunt trauma to the flaccid penis is usually associated with only subcutaneous haematoma and usually not a tear of the tunica albuginea. These injuries are best managed conservatively.

Blunt trauma to the scrotum can cause testicular rupture and/or subcutaneous scrotal haematoma; testicular dislocation occurs rarely.

In patients with genital trauma, urinalysis should be performed. The presence of macro- and or microhaematuria requires a retrograde urethrogram in males. In females, flexible or rigid cystoscopy has been recommended to exclude urethral and bladder injury.

Blunt trauma to the scrotum can cause significant haematocele even without testicular rupture. Testicular rupture is found in approximately 50% of cases of direct blunt scrotal trauma.

High-resolution, real-time ultrasonography should be performed to determine intra- and/or extratesticular haematoma, testicular contusion or rupture. Conservative management is recommended in haematoceles smaller than three times the size of the contralateral testis. Large haematoceles should be treated surgically, irrespective of testicle contusion or rupture.

In testicular rupture, surgical exploration with excision of necrotic testicular tubules and closure of the tunica albuginea is indicated. Traumatic dislocation of the testis is treated by manual replacement and secondary orchidopexy. If primary manual reposition cannot be performed, immediate orchidopexy is indicated

Blunt trauma to the vulva is rare and commonly present as a large haematoma. Vulvar haematomas usually do not require surgical intervention. It is important to emphasise that vulvar haematoma and/ or blood at the vaginal introitus are an indication for vaginal exploration under sedation or general anaesthesia in order to identify possible associated vaginal and/or rectal injuries.

Further reading

Kristjánsson A, Pedersen J. Management of blunt renal trauma. Br J Urol 1993; 72:692–696.

McAninch JW, Santucci RA. Genitourinary trauma. In: Walsh PC, Retik AB, Darracott Vaughan E, Jr., Wein AJ (eds), Campbell's urology, 8th edn, Philadelphia: W.B. Saunders, 2002: 3707–3744.

Peterson NE. Genitourinary trauma. In: Mattox KL, Feliciano DV, Moore EE (eds), Trauma, 4th edn. New York: McGraw-Hill, 2000: 839–879.

Related topics of interest

Index

Note: Page numbers in **bold** or *italic* refer to tables or figures, respectively.